PRACTICAL NEUROPSYCHOLOGICAL REHABILITATION IN ACQUIRED BRAIN INJURY

Brain Injuries Series
Published and distributed by Karnac Books

Other titles in the series:

Anxiety and Mood Disorders following Traumatic Brain Injury: Clinical Assessment and Psychotherapy
    Rudi Coetzer
A Relational Approach to Rehabilitation: Thinking About Relationships after Brain Injury
    Ceri Bowen, Giles Yeates, & Siobhan Palmer

Orders:
Tel: +44 (0)20 7431 1075; Fax: +44 (0)20 7435 9076

E-mail: shop@karnacbooks.com

www.karnac books.com

PRACTICAL NEUROPSYCHOLOGICAL REHABILITATION IN ACQUIRED BRAIN INJURY

A Guide for Working Clinicians

Edited by

*Gavin Newby, Rudi Coetzer,
Audrey Daisley, and Stephen Weatherhead*

KARNAC

First published in 2013 by
Karnac Books Ltd
118 Finchley Road, London NW3 5HT

Copyright © 2013 to Gavin Newby, Rudi Coetzer, Audrey Daisley, and Stephen Weatherhead for the edited collection, and to the individual authors for their contributions.

The rights of the contributors to be identified as the authors of this work have been asserted in accordance with §§ 77 and 78 of the Copyright Design and Patents Act 1988.

All rights reserved. No part of this publication may be reproduced, stored in a retrieval system, or transmitted, in any form or by any means, electronic, mechanical, photocopying, recording, or otherwise, without the prior written permission of the publisher.

British Library Cataloguing in Publication Data

A C.I.P. for this book is available from the British Library

ISBN 978 1 85575 722 6

Edited, designed and produced by The Studio Publishing Services Ltd
www.publishingservicesuk.co.uk
e-mail: studio@publishingservicesuk.co.uk

Printed in Great Britain

www.karnacbooks.com

CONTENTS

ACKNOWLEDGEMENTS	ix
ABOUT THE EDITORS AND CONTRIBUTORS	xi
SERIES EDITORS' FOREWORD	xv
FOREWORD by Andy Tyerman	xvii
PREFACE by Gavin Newby	xxiii
INTRODUCTION by Gavin Newby	xxvii

PART I: GETTING STARTED: THE ESSENTIAL KNOWLEDGE AND BASIC SKILLS FOR SUCCESSFUL WORKING IN ACQUIRED BRAIN INJURY

Prelude: The very basic basics: definitions, prevalence, and consequences 3
  Hayley Entwistle and Gavin Newby

CHAPTER ONE
Behavioural neuroanatomy 13
  Rudi Coetzer

CHAPTER TWO
Neuropsychological assessment: the not-so-basic basics   27
*Aidan Jones, Simon J. Prangnell, Crawford Thomas,
and Gavin Newby*

CHAPTER THREE
Therapy and engagement   67
*Stephen Weatherhead, Rudi Coetzer, Audrey Daisley,
Gavin Newby, Giles Yeates, and Phillippa Calvert*

CHAPTER FOUR
Social consequences and social solutions: community   115
neuro-rehabilitation in real social environments
Howard F. Jackson and Gemma Hague

PART II: BEING IN PRACTICE: WORKING WITH THE
ISSUES FACED BY REAL CLIENTS WITH ACQUIRED
BRAIN INJURIES LIVING IN THE REAL WORLD.
ASSESSMENT IN SPECIFIC CONTEXTS

CHAPTER FIVE
Low awareness conditions: their assessment and treatment   159
Crawford Thomas

CHAPTER SIX
Assessment of mental capacity   179
Helen Newby and Tracey Ryan-Morgan

CHAPTER SEVEN
Driving after acquired brain injury: rehabilitation   209
and therapy
Gavin Newby

CHAPTER EIGHT
Vocational rehabilitation after acquired brain injury   225
Bernie Walsh

CHAPTER NINE
Opportunistic group work: service-based and community   245
support group examples
*Stephen Weatherhead, Bernie Walsh, Phillippa Calvert,
and Gavin Newby*

CHAPTER TEN
The use of emails and texts in psychological therapy after acquired brain injury 255
Gavin Newby and Rudi Coetzer

CHAPTER ELEVEN
Working with relationships in standard neuro-rehabilitation practice 271
Giles Yeates and Audrey Daisley

CHAPTER TWELVE
Supporting families and parenting after parental brain injury 295
Rachel Skippon

PART III: WORKING WITH PROFESSIONAL AND ORGANISATIONAL SYSTEMS

CHAPTER THIRTEEN
Leading a community acquired brain injury team: the South Cheshire experience 323
Beth Fisher

CHAPTER FOURTEEN
Thinking creatively about continuing professional development 347
Gavin Newby and Stephen Weatherhead

PART IV: MAKING SENSE OF IT ALL: REFLECTIONS AND INSIGHTS

CHAPTER FIFTEEN
Epilogue: putting it into practice in the real world 365
Gavin Newby

INDEX 375

ACKNOWLEDGEMENTS

Although one of the last tasks to be completed in writing any book, mentioning everyone who has had a hand in the creation of this book is not only crucial, but also a tall order if it aspires to be fully comprehensive. This is not only because any book has a large cast of contributors, administrative and publishing staff who have directly contributed to the writing of the book, but also because there is an even larger cast of brain injured clients, their families, clinicians, and workers from all sorts of backgrounds who have indirectly shaped and informed this book.

First, I would like to extend my heartfelt thanks to Oliver Rathbone, the Managing Director of Karnac Books, Oliver's staff, and Drs Ceri Bowen and Giles Yeates, the Series Editors of the Brain Injuries Series. I am particularly grateful for their faith that we could pull this book together, but also their patience, encouragement, and advice throughout the whole process from start to finish.

Second, the writing of this book has very much been an interactive collaboration between very knowledgeable and very busy clinicians. It is a real testament to all of the contributors that each of the chapters is both of high quality and also extremely readable. Of course, my particular thanks go to my co-editors, Rudi, Audrey, and Stephen, for their sheer hard work, determination, and good humour in pulling all of the contributions together.

Third, I would very much like to thank my employers, Cheshire & Wirral Partnership NHS Foundation Trust, not only for their support, but also their encouragement. In particular, I would like to express gratitude to my Service Manager, Beth Fisher, for her willingness to give me the time to produce this book, and our long-suffering administrator, Anne Mansfield. Anne persevered with a very unfamiliar academic format and somehow turned my dictaphone ramblings into my contributions.

Fourth, I would also like to take this opportunity to acknowledge the undoubted influence of those clinicians who have influenced my thinking and practice. The list is long, but includes: Ken Mackay, Rudi Coetzer, Andy Tyerman, John Pimm, Chris Allen, Lillian Hickey, and Arlene Vetere, to name but a few. Rudi Coetzer, in particular, gave me the courage and belief that my initial ideas could be turned into something that other people would read.

Fifth, I could not let these acknowledgements pass without showing my appreciation to my family, Helen, Cara, Ally, and Jamie, for being so understanding about why Daddy disappeared to type on the computer and seemed so distracted at times.

Finally, I wanted to make special mention of all of the brain injured clients and their families that I have had the pleasure of working with over the years. It is very much your stories, your victories, and your solutions that have shaped who I am as a clinical neuropsychologist. I will continue to do my best to continue to listen and learn from both new and existing clients in the years to come.

ABOUT THE EDITORS AND CONTRIBUTORS

Phillippa Calvert is a clinical neuropsychologist with the Acquired Brain Injury Service, Cheshire and Wirral Partnership NHS Foundation Trust. She also works as a clinical psychologist with the Hyndburn, Ribble Valley and Rossendale Complex Care and Treatment Team, Lancashire Care NHS Foundation Trust.

Rudi Coetzer is a consultant clinical neuropsychologist and Head of Service with the North Wales Brain Injury Service, Betsi Cadwaladr University Health Board NHS Wales, and Honorary Senior Lecturer, Bangor University.

Audrey Daisley is a consultant clinical neuropsychologist at the Oxford Centre for Enablement, Oxford University Hospitals NHS Trust.

Hayley Entwistle is a clinical psychologist with the Acquired Brain Injury Service, Cheshire and Wirral Partnership NHS Foundation Trust.

Beth Fisher is the Acquired Brain Injury Service Manager with Cheshire and Wirral Partnership NHS Foundation Trust.

Gemma Hague is a clinical psychologist specialising in neuropsychology and Deputy Clinical Director of the Transitional Rehabilitation Units, Haydock, St Helen's.

Howard F. Jackson is a consultant clinical neuropsychologist and Clinical Director of the Transitional Rehabilitation Units, Haydock, St Helen's.

Aidan Jones is a consultant clinical neuropsychologist and Head of Clinical Neuropsychology at the Oxford Centre for Enablement, Oxford University Hospitals NHS Trust.

Gavin Newby is a consultant clinical neuropsychologist with the Acquired Brain Injury Service, Cheshire and Wirral Partnership NHS Foundation Trust.

Helen Newby is a clinical neuropsychologist and Managing Director of Newby Psychological Services Ltd., Northwich, Cheshire.

Simon J. Prangnell is a clinical psychologist at the Oxford Centre for Enablement, Oxford University Hospitals NHS Trust.

Tracey Ryan-Morgan is a consultant clinical neuropsychologist and Clinical Director of Talis Consulting Limited & Harley Memory Clinic Limited.

Rachel Skippon is a clinical psychologist with Merseycare NHS Trust, Liverpool.

Crawford Thomas is a consultant clinical neuropsychologist with Cheshire & Wirral Partnership NHS Foundation Trust.

Andy Tyerman is Consultant Clinical Neuropsychologist & Head of Service, Community Head Injury Service, Buckinghamshire Healthcare NHS Trust.

Bernie Walsh is a specialist vocational occupational therapist with Cheshire & Wirral Partnership NHS Foundation Trust.

Stephen Weatherhead is a clinical tutor and lecturer in health research with Lancaster University's Clinical Psychology Department. His independent clinical practice specialises in family-based interventions and assessments of mental capacity post-brain injury (www.neurofamilymatters.co.uk).

Giles Yeates is a principal clinical neuropsychologist and couples therapist with Buckinghamshire Healthcare NHS Trust.

SERIES EDITORS' FOREWORD

It is with great pleasure that we introduce the latest book in the Karnac Brain Injuries Series, the first book to focus on the topic of service development. As a key figure in the UK neuropsychology field and senior member of Cheshire & Wirral Partnership's Acquired Brain Injury Service, Gavin Newby is ideally placed to edit a book that sets out to describe the context and the essential ingredients required to establish a "successful" community service. By addressing head-on some of the more substantive issues and big questions, including how to judge "success" and how to prioritise among competing demands, Dr Newby and colleagues quite possibly have produced the most reader-friendly and accessible book about brain injury and neuro-rehabilitation ever. While the answers are not always short and clear-cut, Dr Newby never fails to leave the reader wiser and, importantly, more able to navigate the terrain ahead, to short-cut and avoid the many pitfalls that await any novice to this area of work.

Key to his task, Dr Newby has assembled an impressive team to help him articulate his real world neuropsychological rehabilitation approach, many from the Cheshire & Wirral team and others who have guided and supported him in this venture, namely, Rudi Coetzer, Audrey Daisley, and Stephen Weatherhead. Dr Coetzer is locally based, from another key UK team, the North Wales Brain Injury team (also Karnac Series author of *Anxiety and Mood Disorders following Traumatic Brain Injury: Clinical Assessment and Psychotherapy*, 2010). Dr Daisley has pioneered work with child relatives and whole families within the UK, and, from her base at Oxford Centre for Enablement, offers consultancy to many rehabilitation professionals in their efforts to meet the needs of the family around the patient. Dr Weatherhead is a tutor on the Lancaster Doctoral Clinical Psychology Programme, previously with the Cheshire & Wirral team, and is also a future Karnac Series author (*Narrative Approaches to Brain Injury*, forthcoming). Together, they have managed to articulate an approach that is highly practical and relevant to both patient and family in its approach to assessment. Excitingly, the approach taken describes ways to offer accessible, creative, and opportunisitic therapy at different stages of the long post-acute care journey. However, the various authors are also careful to be mindful of the constraints posed by working within NHS budgets. In keeping with the relational rehabilitation book, Dr Newby takes a systemic frame when necessary to understand the role of the neuropsychologist within the broader spectrum of overlapping systems, be they family, friends, or health professionals.

This third volume in the Series is a welcome addition. Being a distillation of broad swaths of theory and evidence in the area, it achieves its aim to be comprehensive, yet easy to read at the same time—a succinct analysis if ever there was one! For the Series, this book marks a new venture that is to showcase the approach adopted by key teams within the UK, and the Chester team has certainly achieved that status, alongside one or two others.

We are grateful to Dr Andy Tyerman, from Aylesbury Community Head Injury Service, for writing the Foreword to this unique book.

Ceri Bowen and Giles Yeates, Series Editors

FOREWORD

I welcome this book not just for its specific content and particularly its personal and family focus, but also for what it indicates about the development of neuropsychological rehabilitation in the UK. The book's reflective approach to neuropsychological practice, which complements other UK guidance, is likely to be of particular interest to the less experienced and/or lone practitioner. Its reflective nature and style makes for an easy read. Before highlighting some of its specific contributions, I would like first, if I may, to add some personal reflections.

Back in 1979, when I started out in neuro-rehabilitation, clinical neuropsychology in the UK was grossly underdeveloped. While we had a presence in many regional inpatient neurological rehabilitation units, our contribution was often confined to formal testing, patchy input into the management of cognitive difficulties, and some limited involvement in the management of severe behavioural difficulties, most notably in the independent sector. Rehabilitation follow-up studies in the UK highlighted the importance of emotional and behavioural effects of traumatic brain injury (TBI) and related long-term personal, vocational, and family impact. Witnessing the distress of people with TBI and their relatives, very poor vocational outcome, limited leisure life and social isolation, and the wide-ranging impact on families was a powerful and sobering experience (Tyerman, 1987). This highlighted the need for a more psychotherapeutic approach to promote long-term personal, vocational, and family adjustment (Tyerman & Humphrey, 1988). Based on that experience, the priority for me was for UK clinical neuropsychologists to contribute and, when appropriate, take the lead in developing brain injury rehabilitation services that address these unmet needs—psychological, family, vocational, and social.

In the past, rehabilitation after brain injury in the UK was largely confined to the first six months, with little assistance in returning to an independent and productive role in the community (Greenwood & McMillan, 1993; McMillan & Ledder, 2001; Murphy et al., 1990). Limited access to neuropsychology was among the specific concerns raised by Headway as part of the development of the *National Service Framework for Long-term Conditions* (Department of Health, 2005). My personal take on the development of neuropsychological rehabilitation in the UK is that unmet psychological need was highlighted in the 1980s, specific community, cognitive, vocational, and family orientated services were developed in the 1990s, and then implemented (to a limited extent) and refined (where already present) in the 2000s. The role of neuropsychology was recognised in the *National Clinical Guidelines on Rehabilitation Following Brain Injury* (British Society of Rehabilitation & Royal College of Physicians, 2003). The markers of good practice of the quality requirement on "Community rehabilitation and support" of the *National Service Framework for Long-term Conditions* (Department of Health, 2005) stress the need to focus on goals that promote "participation in a full range of life roles", "a sense of wellbeing", and "long-term psychological adjustments to altered personal, family and social circumstances". This includes explicit reference to the need for access to neuropsychology.

Neuropsychological services in the UK have come on a long way over the years, both in addressing cognitive, behavioural, and emotional needs and in promoting personal and family adjustment to the effects of brain injury. However, the task is far from complete, with services remaining very patchy, especially those promoting longer-term adjustment. We have not had the resources to develop consistent and comprehensive services. Many neuropsychologists operate as sole practitioners, often in a part-time capacity, within underdeveloped and overstretched services. Under these circumstances, addressing the wide range of psychological needs of people with brain injury and their families remains a challenge.

The nature of this book reinforces the view that we have moved beyond the provision of time-limited, narrow neuropsychological provision in a limited number of specialist services. However, given the financial squeeze in the current economic climate, we might now face a struggle over the coming years to maintain the progress made to date, let alone develop further our services. We need to continue to work with people with brain injury, their families, and support groups to highlight unrecognised needs (and resultant costs) to those who commission health, employment, and social services. There is a risk that we could be forced back to a limited short-term role that neglects our major potential contribution in promoting longer-term personal and family adjustment. In the current context, this book is most welcome. The editors' intention is to produce a "realistic, straightforward and useable guide for ordinary clinicians", both in guiding those with minimal previous contact with brain injury and also in assisting experienced practitioners to enhance their clinical practice.

The Introduction is the lead editor Gavin Newby's reflective account of the complexity of clinical need and the challenges of the multiple roles required of the neuropsychologist—this is likely to be particularly helpful to the less experienced practitioner. Part I then begins with a section providing basic background information about the nature and effects of brain injury, and Chapter One gives a notably clear verbal account of neuroanatomy. (The latter I particularly enjoyed, in part because I have always found retention of such information to be something of a challenge and, as such, clear explanation and consolidation is always welcome!)

The next three chapters in Part I address central issues: neuropsychological assessment, therapy and engagement, and social issues/ community neuro-rehabilitation. In the first of these, the multiple factors, sources, and methods in neuropsychological assessment within the individual/family context is relevant to all practitioners. This is supported by practical suggestions, including those around specific assessment challenges (e.g., "profoundly impaired", challenging behaviour, dual/multiple diagnoses). The chapter on therapy and engagement focuses on psychotherapy with people with brain injury, with the innovative approach of different practitioners viewing the one case from the perspective of five psychotherapeutic models (cognitive–behavioural therapy, neuropsychoanalysis, narrative therapy, systemic therapy, and cognitive analytic therapy). This will, we hope, stimulate further development and provision of psychotherapy after brain injury. In the chapter on social issues/community rehabilitation, the account of the nature and implications of executive difficulties and associated practical management strategies are likely to be particularly helpful to the practitioner.

The chapters within Part II focus on specific assessment and rehabilitation issues. The three assessment chapters are likely to be of particular benefit to the practitioner early in their careers, but also offer valuable opportunity for reflection for more experienced practitioners. For me, the strengths of these chapters includes the following: the clarity of explanation (especially the quick reference guide) and practical suggestions in assessing low awareness conditions; the clear explanation of the principles of mental capacity and the illustrative examples across four core areas of capacity (i.e., living circumstances, managing finances, testamentary capacity, and capacity to undertake litigation); and both the legal context and practical suggestions on driving assessment. The specific rehabilitation chapters include an occupational therapist's perspective on vocational rehabilitation within a brain injury service context, examples of "opportunistic groups" (supporting mothers and community support), and a timely account of the therapeutic benefits of embracing the use of emails and texts.

While the family impact of brain injury has long been recognised, service development has been frustratingly slow, not helped in my view by a focus in national policy on pan-disability carer support rather than investment in family work within specialist services. However, the markers of good practice of the quality requirement on "Supporting family and carers" in the *National Service Framework for Long-term Conditions* (Department of Health, 2005) recognised the need to assist adjustment to cognitive or behavioural changes, including a "whole-family approach". The authors of the first of the book's two family-focused chapters argue the case for practitioners to adopt a "relational" approach to brain injury rehabilitation, together with practical suggestions about how this could be integrated into practice. The second chapter discusses the importance of the parenting role after brain injury and the need to build flexible support for parenting within the rehabilitation process, again with suggestions about how this can be achieved in working with parents and their children.

The focus in Part III switches to "Working with professional and organisational systems". In the first chapter, the author shares her experience of managing a community brain injury team and suggests twenty practical "tips" for those leading such teams. While the relevance of some tips will vary according to local service management arrangements, others will have more universal relevance, especially those relating to team leadership, networking, and maintaining the service profile. The second chapter advocates "thinking creatively" about continuing professional development, with useful practical tips about how this might be integrated with a challenging clinical role. In line with its reflective approach, the book ends with the lead editor's personal reflections, focusing on the complex needs of a recent referral, both the immediate response and anticipated interventions in the short, medium, and long term.

In summary, as illustrated above, I view this book as making a valuable contribution to the support available to the neuropsychological practitioner. Its particular strength lies in the authors' shared reflections on their practice, supported by practical suggestions and illustrations. If you are seeking systematic reviews of the evidence base for brain injury rehabilitation programmes or the wide range of specific neuropsychological interventions, then you need to look elsewhere. However, if you are relatively new to neuropsychological rehabilitation, or a lone practitioner confronted by the wide range of clinical demands, then you are likely to find this book of assistance in developing your practice. If you are a more experienced practitioner, then the chapters on specific areas of assessment (e.g., capacity, driving, low awareness), intervention (e.g., psychotherapy, therapeutic use of email and texts, family services), and professional development are likely to assist you in reflecting on your own practice and in considering developments and refinements within your own particular service context.

I would like to thank editors Gavin, Rudi, Audrey, and Stephen and all the contributors for sharing their experiences, reflections, and practical suggestions to the benefit of other practitioners.

Andy Tyerman
Consultant Clinical Neuropsychologist/Head of Service
Community Head Injury Service, Buckinghamshire Healthcare NHS Trust

References

British Society of Rehabilitation Medicine & Royal College of Physicians (2003). *Rehabilitation Following Acquired Brain Injury: National Clinical Guidelines*, L. Turner-Stokes (Ed.). London: Royal College of Physicians, Lavenham Press.

Department of Health (2005). *The National Service Framework for Long-term Conditions*. London: Stationery Office.

Greenwood, R. J., & McMillan, T. M. (1993). Models of rehabilitation programmes for the brain-injured adult. 1. Current provision, efficacy and good practice. *Clinical Rehabilitation*, 7: 248–255.

McMillan, T. M., & Ledder, H. (2001). A survey of services provided by community neurorehabilitation teams in South East England. *Clinical Rehabilitation*, 15: 582–588.

Murphy, L. D., McMillan T. M., Greenwood, R. J., Brooks, D. N., Morris, J. R., & Dunn, G. (1990). Services for severely head injured patients in North London and environs. *Brain Injury*, 4: 95–100.

Tyerman, A. D. (1987). Self-concept and psychological change in the rehabilitation of the severely head injured person. Unpublished Doctoral thesis. London: University of London.

Tyerman, A., & Humphrey, M. (1988). Personal and social rehabilitation after severe head injury. In: F. N. Watts (Ed.), *New Developments in Clinical Psychology*, Vol. 2 (pp. 189–207). Chichester: John Wiley.

PREFACE

Gavin Newby

Like many textbooks, *Practical Neuropsychological Rehabilitation in Acquired Brain Injury: A Guide for Working Clinicians* has had a long gestation—over fifteen years! Like other textbooks, this volume tries to distil the wisdom of a number of experienced practitioners into a digestible format for interested readers. However, unlike other textbooks, *Practical Neuropsychological Rehabilitation* aims to provide a realistic, straightforward and useable guide for ordinary clinicians. All of the contributors work in the UK's National Health Service or private settings and understand the challenges and complexities of working with brain injury on the one hand, and appreciate the financial and resource restrictions placed on a shrinking health economy on the other. Throughout the writing and editorial process, we have been guided by the simple wish to provide a readable and meaningful guide for practitioners working with acquired brain injury (ABI). All of the contributors have been asked to keep jargon down to an absolute minimum, to fully explain any jargon that is used, and to illustrate concepts as much as possible with real case material. At the end of each chapter, the contributors have provided a bibliography of both academic and practical resources. Where possible, they have provided internet-based resources that can be easily accessed.

We strongly believe that this textbook can pass a number of practical tests. First, we believe that any interested practitioner who might have had only minimal contact with brain injury should be able to pick up this book and understand the concepts discussed, be able to access additional resources to support their learning and get a flavour of how to apply a range of therapeutic assessment, therapeutic, service development, and practical case management techniques. Second, we believe that experienced practitioners will also be able to read this book and enhance their working with brain injury. This book is suitable for all of the practitioners who come into contact with brain injury and is not exclusively a book for experienced clinical neuropsychologists.

In Part I, the contributors have provided an introduction to the kinds of difficulties faced by clients who have suffered an ABI, their families, and the care and professional networks that work with them. Successful engagement and working with ABI clients and their families is dependent on the professional having a good, thorough, and holistic understanding of what ABI is, and how to assess it and work with its emotional consequences. In this vein, Part I contains chapters on behavioural neuroanatomy, meaningful neuropsychological assessment, community rehabilitation, and how to engage clients in therapy. The latter chapter takes the novel approach of using different perspectives on one case to look at how different models can be helpful.

In Part II, we very much focus on the actual situations that clinicians face. The particular issues addressed here include chapters on assessment in specific contexts (such as low awareness states, driving, and capacity), rehabilitation (such as vocational rehabilitation, opportunistic group work, and the therapeutic use of emails and texts), and working with the complex maze of relationship and parenting issues.

In Part III, there are chapters on working with professional organisations, with contributions on managing an ABI service and proactively ensuring ongoing continuing professional development and supervision.

Finally, in Part IV, we hope that we successfully tie together all of the insights provided in the preceding chapters to demonstrate how even one case might demand knowledge from many of the domains discussed.

Above all, we hope you will find *Practical Neuropsychological Rehabilitation in Acquired Brain Injury: A Guide for Working Clinicians* a good and informative read that helps you be enthusiastic about your work, gives you some new ideas, and helps you gain confidence in working with people who have a brain injury

Introduction

Understanding how to work with acquired brain injury, or how to be or not to be: that is the crucial question in brain injury

Gavin Newby

For a new professional, starting out in a typical acquired brain injury (ABI) team can be a daunting experience. I am sure all readers of this chapter will recognise the glassy-eyed stare of a new team member or student as they try to make sense of the tidal wave of information and the twists and turns of lives during that Monday morning referral meeting. Maybe, if you are really honest, and you delve deep into your own memory if you are an experienced practitioner, you will remember what it was like when you first started to work with people who have had a brain injury. Putting it simply, brain injury is a complex collection of lasting signs, symptoms, and deficits, superimposed on often complex webs of family, childcare, work and leisure relationships, and friendships. When you start working in brain injury (maybe if you are "long in the tooth", too), it can sometimes seem an impossible task to work out what your role is, how to do it, and where the boundaries are. This introductory chapter suggests a number of pivotal roles that you might play in working with people who have an acquired brain injury and their families. They are meant to reflect the range of roles you might be asked to play, but the reader should think of them as fluid and interchangeable.

Working with acquired brain injury: what is the problem?

Early on in my career, I distinctly remember a client telling me how their brain injury had fundamentally changed their life. He said something along the lines of:

> Imagine one minute you are normal, with normal feelings, normal thoughts, a normal range of skills, a normal family—good points and bad points and that you are the boss and in control. Suddenly it all changes—you wake up one morning and your body doesn't feel entirely your own. You don't speak as well as you used to, you don't sound good and can't get the words out. One side of your body isn't as strong as it used to be. You keep bumping into things. You have headaches. Oh God, you've got headaches. Your memory is crap and you can't be sure whether you have understood or remembered anything correctly. Everything is confusing. It is like driving along a familiar road in a familiar car and then suddenly being plonked in the middle of Paris Peripherique not knowing what the hell is going on. But the worst of it is that you don't trust yourself and nobody trusts you.

While this represents my probably half-remembered musings of an extremely severely brain-injured person at one of their lowest points, I am sure you get the point. Acquired brain injury is devastating, life changing, and, above all, confusing. In this context, I firmly believe that it is our role as professionals to bring simplicity and direction wherever we can. I have detailed below some of the labels and roles that have helped me over the years.

The pathfinder or (one hopes non-annoying) Sat Nav

Many years ago, a colleague, Andy Tyerman, likened the role of the professional in brain injury as being like a mountain guide or pathfinder. The terrain of brain injury is metaphorically rocky with twists and turns, ups and downs and uncertain end points. Many brain-injured people need guidance through the terrain from someone they trust and feel is credible. However, the guidance must be judged correctly or you will quickly be rejected.[1] The process of becoming trusted is also enhanced by taking on the subsequent roles, as appropriate, in a flexible manner.

The expert

Clients and their families need credible information. They need you to be working towards a high level of knowledge of the causes of the things that trouble them. In my experience, clients and their families often want you to be able to give them a coherent story or narrative about what happened, how and where in the brain the damage occurred, and how these difficulties have led to the difficulties they now have as they sit across the room from you. Rudi Coetzer's chapter "Behavioural neuroanatomy", and Aidan Jones and colleagues' chapter, "Neuropsychological assessment" (Chapters One and Two, respectively) stand as excellent primers in this area. How this information is delivered—most commonly through psycho-educational information or during feedback after a session—is dealt with in further detail in Jones and colleagues' chapter. After a person has experienced a brain injury, they often particularly value professionals trying to tailor complex information about neurological mechanics or cognitive dysfunction to their level of understanding. The power of having a story cannot be underestimated, and is dealt with in more detail in the narrative therapy examples discussed in Chapter Three. More often than not, clients and their families will understandably pressure you for information about prognosis—the dreaded "future". As many of you will know, when completing self-report measures such as the Semantic Differential (Tyerman, 1992, cited in Tyerman, 1999), clients will often idealise their pre-injury lives and how they hope their future will be. It is at this point that you will need to be strong and clear about what you can and cannot predict. Attaining and maintaining such credible expertise is an important function of good continuing professional development (CPD) and training. Suggestions and a rationale for continuing professional development and further training are discussed further in Chapter Fourteen.

The therapist

This might seem an obvious role. However, in my experience, some services can become overly concerned with assessment and getting a clear picture of problems. They can sometimes forget to do something with those problems. Clients and their families are often looking to you to help them not only understand their problems, but also contain and do something with them. Chapter Three looks at particular types of therapy and how they help to contain the emotional consequences of acquired brain injury. It is not the job of this introduction to prescribe a therapy and there is no clear evidence that one therapy is much more effective than others in acquired brain injury. However, it is important that brain-injured people have access to someone taking on the therapist role.

The formulator and information processor

These are essentially two roles combined into one. The formulator synthesises and brings together often a huge amount of information from disparate sources—usually collated at interview and during assessment and maybe throughout their contact with a client—into one coherent, or set of coherent, stories. In the professional literature, formulation is often framed from the point of view of the professional and their attempt to gain credibility by developing clever and often jargon-laden models. In my experience, the most important role is to bring the information together in an understandable format for clients and their families so that they can make sense of it.

This then leads into the second linked role: the information processor. Remember the Paris Peripherique analogy? In that situation, you want a sensible satellite navigation-type character not only to guide you, but also give you clear direction and make sense of the information around you. This is a crucial and valuable role. If you consider that brain injury is fundamentally a disorder of making sense of information, clients often need you to be that filter. This can be a filter for all sorts of information, not just the narrow confines of your therapy, and can include making sense of benefits information, bills, and exactly what a GP has said or meant when they last went to see him or her.

The case manager

Those of you who have been working in brain injury for even a short time will have come across case managers, especially within the medico–legal sphere. A good case manager in that context rightly takes a lead in making sense of a client's situation, helping to organise a web of professionals, services, and support staff around the client as he or she needs them. Some of you might have been lucky enough, as I have, to work in a National Health Service setting that is led by a case manager (Beth Fisher—see Chapter Thirteen for further discussion of her managerial role). In this particular context, I would suggest that all of us will need to take on aspects of the case manager role—particularly "the gopher role", as Beth calls it. The gopher role might include very practically seeking out information about the results of scans, medication changes, etc., following a client's visit to see a consultant at a hospital where the communication has not been clear. The best place to start is often the client's GP and a quick call to his or her secretary can bear fruit.

More fundamentally, the case manager role implies a professional openness to flexibly deal, where appropriate and in limited fashion, with some of the issues that spontaneously arise in sessions. Quite simply, if you do not do this, your engagement might well be scuppered at the very beginning. I remember an instructive story told by a head-injury advocate who always tells people new to brain injury a story that goes along the lines of:

> You might have a plan to work on anxiety management. You might have worked up an agenda, got your relaxation tape. But when you get to the guy's house, he is not concentrating and looks really worried. If you don't stop and ask him what's on his mind and what's troubling him you won't gain his trust. For example, he might tell you that the reason he is worried is that his passport application has come in and he doesn't know what to do with it. If you have the time and ability to help him complete that passport application, not only will you have taken a weight off his mind and helped him complete something that is really important to him, you will have engaged him and gained his trust.

Suggestions for gaining trust and engaging people with a brain injury

As you have been reading through the above roles, there are a number of common themes that come through, and I have drawn these out below.

Flexibility: You need to be flexible. Yes, you need to have an idea of what you are going to do in any particular situation or session so that it is not complete chaos, but you also need to be prepared to sometimes, and where appropriate, go with the flow, as with the example of completing the passport application.

Structure: While this might look like the antitheses of the above, there is a place for structure. This might be within the structure of your service, so that it has reasonably predictable and replicable processes, such as having a clear lead worker, clear initial assessment, feedback, and review processes, easy contact details; do not promise something you cannot deliver and answer those texts, telephone calls, or emails. The work of Andy Tyerman and the Community Head Injury Service in Aylesbury is instructive (see Tyerman & Booth, 2001 for further details).

Getting Real: In order to fully engage with head-injured people and provide therapy and intervention that has a chance of leading to a fundamental change, you have to work with the contexts that people actually live in. Everyone has a history and background, but not all of them are either nurturing or familiar to the mainly white, middle-class therapist. One of the first tasks of meaningful engagement must be to get to know the person's context and adopt the GRACES model (i.e., understand G = Gender, R = Race, A = Age, C = Culture, E = Ethnicity, S = Sexuality). As a concrete example from my own work, while alcohol and violence abstinence might be preferable, it might not be realistic if the person lives in an economically deprived area and/or their friendship culture is dominated by alcohol use and fighting. Howard Jackson and Gemma Hague's Chapter Four looks in depth at the question of constructing realistic programmes of risk management and cognitive rehabilitation.

Holding fire when appropriate: the value of therapeutic holding

Therapeutic holding is an extremely valuable and maybe currently misunderstood topic. It is multi-faceted. It contains aspects of a nurturing, containing role that would be familiar to those espoused to the theories of Melanie Klein and Wilfred Bion (Waddell, 1998). Indeed, Bion's idea of *reverie* has a great relevance here. By reverie, Klein means the point in a therapeutic relationship at which the therapist and client trust each other and the therapist can often predict and understand what the client might be feeling, much like the baby and mother interactions from which Klein's writings originally derived. Just like the infant, the brain-injured client derives a great deal of succour and comfort from the feeling and experience of another understanding them. In some ways, this kind of relationship can only take root and occur over time and when a therapy space is not filled with strict and structured agendas, is flexible and allows space for the client, their worries and troubles. This particularly militates against mental health models of restricted, highly structured, and time-limited sessions. This idea is also further developed by Rudi Coetzer and myself in Chapter Ten on using emails and texts in therapy.

This state of being can also only develop if you and your team carefully consider the timing and nature of your intervention. Some clients arrive at your team thirsty for knowledge and desperate for intervention. It is important to act sensibly, quickly, and gain trust through progress in rehabilitation. Others might be suspicious or reticent about engagement for a whole host of reasons. These reasons could include bad experiences with professionals or authority figures, pre-dating their brain injury. Indeed, they might have—from the *elephant in the room*—difficulties with insight. This might mean that they do not fully "get" why they need to see you in the first place. For these types of clients, and even those clients with whom you have a good relationship but might have finished a period of care, therapeutic holding could mean a number of spaced reviews that are led by the problems or, indeed, successes that the clients themselves bring to the session. If you are able to listen and acknowledge them, clients will have the experience of you as somebody they can trust, and will come to you when they need you, not when you think they need intervention.

> Sarah was a forty-two-year-old senior car manufacturer executive who suffered fronto-temporal contusions following a head-on car accident. When she first came to the rehabilitation service she was extremely nervous, agitated, and worried that I would say she could not go back to work. She fiercely defended her ability and demanded the right to return to work. Sensing her defensiveness and not being sure whether this was denial or a problem of insight, rather than challenging her at first, I offered her information and advice. I suggested that she might want to wait at least two to three months so that she could gain extra stamina before beginning a graded return to work programme. She appeared to accept this advice and duly returned to work after three months. At subsequent

three-monthly reviews, Sarah portrayed a very positive image—all was going well. It was only after two and a half years of struggling at work with a number of negative work reviews and suggestions of downgrading that she finally began to admit at a review that she needed help. She created a doorway with the door slightly ajar, allowing me to gently push it open.

Conclusions

From the above, the reader will undoubtedly get a sense of my wonderment at the complexity of working with acquired brain injury. There are no "cookbook" solutions, and one solution that might work for a while can be thrown out of the window with the twists, turns, and difficulties that brain-injured people and their families face. However, I hope that the reader will also get the sense that there are some "conceptual hooks" to hang your work on. Sometimes, you will come out of a session thinking "What on earth did we do there, what school of psychology/occupational therapy/speech and language therapy did that come from?" But, if you take account of some of the issues, roles, and suggestions contained in this introduction, it is more than likely that you will have massively helped your client. Something that might only take a minute to complete could have a huge effect, not only for the client, in that they achieve something, but also you have become deeply engaged in a positive therapeutic process with them. I hope that these suggestions make you feel positive and ready to take on board the challenges of acquired brain injury.

Note

1. Some strategies are suggested in Chapter Three: "Therapy and engagement".

Useful resources

Headway (2012). www.headway.org.uk/home.aspx. Accessed 29 May 2012.

Calderwood, L. (2002). *Cracked: Recovering After Traumatic Brain Injury.* London: Jessica Kingsley.

Newnes, C. (2006). Reflecting on recovery from head injury. *Clinical Psychology Forum, 159*: 34–40.

References

Tyerman, A. (1999). Outcome measurement in a community head injury service. *Neuropsychological Rehabilitation, 9*(3–4): 481–491.

Tyerman, A., & Booth, J. (2001). Family interventions after traumatic brain injury: a service example. *NeuroRehabilitation, 16*(1): 59–66.

Waddell, M. (1998). *Inside Lives: Psychoanalysis and the Growth of the Personality.* London: Duckworth.

PART I

GETTING STARTED: THE ESSENTIAL KNOWLEDGE AND BASIC SKILLS FOR SUCCESSFUL WORKING IN ACQUIRED BRAIN INJURY

PRELUDE

The very basic basics: definitions, prevalence, and consequences

Hayley Entwistle and Gavin Newby

In this book we have assumed that most of the readers will at least have some idea of what an acquired brain injury (ABI) is and will have met a number of clients with an ABI and their families. It is not, therefore, the primary purpose of this book to provide a comprehensive basic primer of what an ABI is and its effects. We would wholeheartedly recommend that the interested reader consult seminal texts such as Gurd, Kishka, and Marshall (2010) or Powell (1994) for a more comprehensive discussion.

However, if you are new to ABI or would like a short refresher, we have provided an overview of how people come to have a brain injury and the kind of problems that are likely to be seen among people accessing an ABI service.

Types of ABI

Traumatic ABI

The most frequent acquired traumatic brain injuries are usually classified as "closed", where there is no cut or break through the skull.

This is typical of road traffic accidents or assaults where there has been a blow to the head. The rapid deceleration of the brain within the skull damages the brain cells, with twists and tears causing "diffuse" damage. "Open" head injuries are those where the skull is damaged and the brain is exposed, or a foreign object enters the brain tissue. These are less common than closed head injuries, and could be caused by bullet wounds, building implements, or, in the unfortunate case of Phineas Gage, an iron bar (O'Driscoll & Leach, 1998, or see Costandi, 2010, for a recent media article). When the head is trapped between two objects a "crushing" injury can occur. Typically, this affects the brain stem and the base of the skull.

Complications might follow the initial injury and could exacerbate the initial extent of the brain damage occurring from the head injury. A reduction of oxygen to the brain is one major cause of complications and this can occur either if the injured person has trouble breathing or through general blood loss.

Non-traumatic brain injury

Damage to the brain can also occur through infections such as herpes encephalitis, tumours, metabolic conditions including liver and kidney disease or diabetic complications, toxins, and cerebral–vascular incidents such as subarachnoid haemorrhages, aneurysms, clots, and other strokes. Brain injuries might also be associated with progressive neurological conditions, such as multiple sclerosis or dementia.

Prevalence

The most easily accessible prevalence data is found for traumatic acquired brain injuries. According to figures collected by the Health and Social Care Information Centre (2011), 336,396 people who attended A&E departments in England between April 2009 and March 2010 had suffered a traumatic brain injury. This accounts for about 3–4% of UK emergency department attendees per year (Yates, Williams, Harris, Round, & Jenkins, 2006). However, these numbers do not capture those suffering head trauma that do not attend hospital. What is clear is that the number of people sustaining a head injury has been increasing since the 1970s, and reasons cited include the increased use of motor vehicles and the growing number of assaults (House of Commons Health Committee, 2001).

Severity

Traumatic brain injury severity is usually described as mild, moderate, or severe. Estimates suggest that around 5% of those admitted to A&E with a head injury are severely injured (Jennett & McMillan, 1981). The Glasgow Coma Scale (Teasdale & Jennett, 1974) is the most commonly used classification system, in which a fifteen-point scale is applied to the patient's level of consciousness; scores of less than eight are considered severe, 9–12 as moderate, and 13–15 as mild. Other estimates of severity are used based on the length of post traumatic amnesia or the duration of unconsciousness. Please see Crawford Thomas's chapter, "Low awareness states" in this volume for further details.

Classifications of ABI severity do not reliably predict the extent of the brain injury that might follow and, of course, not all head injuries will result in a brain injury. Therefore, it is difficult to estimate of the number of people sustaining a brain injury using head injury data alone. Likewise, it is difficult to forecast the day-to-day difficulties that a person with a particular classification of head injury will experience. Someone with a mild head injury could face life-long difficulties. Improvements in medical science have meant that more people suffering from severe head injury survive and, therefore, have to live with the consequences of an ABI (House of Commons Health Committee, 2001).

Typical ABI service criteria

Although there will be local variations, a typical UK ABI service will usually see those who have sustained their brain injury through head trauma and non-traumatic means, as described above. However, those whose brain injury is associated with a progressive neurological condition, such as multiple sclerosis or dementia, or tumours that are not yet medically stable, are usually supported through other services. Likewise, there will be local arrangements made as to whether stroke survivors access the ABI service or are seen elsewhere.

Problems seen after ABI

So, what are the kinds of problems seen after brain injury? Below, we provide a brief overview of some of the problems reported by people accessing our service. A more comprehensive account can be found in Gurd, Kishka, & Marshall (2010).

Brain injury has been referred to as a "hidden disability" (Department of Health. Social Service Inspectorate, 1996). Many of those who have sustained a severe ABI have no obvious physical impairments but continue to experience a range of difficulties in day-to-day life (Powell, 1994). We have heard service users comment that if they were in a wheelchair or had a visible scar it would be easier for others to appreciate their difficulties.

Physical effects

Motor impairments are common and follow damage to the brain in the motor and pre-motor areas, the basal ganglia and the cerebellum. Of course, nerve, muscle, and bone damage will also play a part. Muscle tone and power might be affected, making movement and movement control difficult. Cerebellum damage typically results in difficulties with movement co-ordination and jerky movements or tremors. Smooth and accurate movements also rely on sensory feedback and, therefore, can be impacted by damage to the sensory pathways or areas of the brain involved in sensation, such as the thalamus and the sensory areas of the parietal lobes. Any of these difficulties might mean that walking, balance, writing, speech production, and activities such as dressing and eating are challenging and extremely exhausting.

Commonly reported sensory changes include an increased sensitivity to light, changes to smell and taste, an altered sensitivity to temperature, and a reduction in limb pain sensations. Visual impairments, including some loss of visual field, are not unusual and can be hugely debilitating. These impairments could result from problems with the eyes or optic nerve as well as from damage to the visual cortex and pathways within the brain.

Hearing loss is common when the auditory cortex in the temporal lobe has been damaged. Brainstem damage has also been implicated in hearing loss, as well as in tinnitus, balance problems, and feelings of dizziness or motion sickness. Damage to the ear and cranial nerves might also play a part. Rudi Coetzer's chapter on functional neuroanatomy (Chapter Two) discusses more relationships between areas of damage, and functional consequences.

The ABI client might report some ongoing pain, particularly headaches, which can be very disabling and could impact upon thinking skills, vision, and frustration tolerance.

In addition to the seizures commonly seen around the time of injury, or early seizures occurring less than a week after the injury, clients with a traumatic ABI generally have a risk of developing epilepsy that is twenty-nine times higher than that in the general population (Herman, 2002). This is even higher for those suffering a subarachnoid haemorrhage (Herman, 2002). The prospect of a seizure can be very daunting and a person might limit his activities to avoid danger or embarrassment. Experiencing seizures will also delay a person's return to driving. There is a strong literature that suggests a continued risk of post trauma epilepsy compared to the general population for more than ten years after the index injury. An important indicative study is that of Christensen and colleagues (2009). In this Danish study, the collaborators found that the increased risk was dependent on the severity of the injury as well as whether or not there was a skull fracture. Although the risks reduced somewhat over time, the Danish study found that they continued to be present more than ten years after injury (for mild brain injury, this was an increased risk of seizures of 1.5 times that of the general population and over four times the risk for severely injured ABI clients).

Cognitive effects

Cognitive changes or some degree of difficulty in "thinking skills" usually follow a brain injury. Sometimes this may be subtle, only noticeable by close family members. Commonly reported areas of difficulty include attention and concentration, memory, processing information, planning, and problem solving. Howard Jackson and Gemma Hague discuss the social implications of some of the cognitive changes following brain injury in Chapter Five.

Many people tell us that they have problems with their attention. They might report distractibility, the neglect of environmental cues, difficulties with multi-tasking and being unable to concentrate for a sustained period of time. Attentional problems can make day-to-day cognitive activity exceptionally tiring. They can also lead to what service users describe as memory failings, given that to remember something you need to have registered the information in the first place.

Reported memory problems include not being able to remember to do things such as attend appointments, being unable to remember names or recent conversations, and forgetting where items are kept. Learning could be slower and require extra time or more presentations of the information than would have previously been necessary. These difficulties can make people very anxious and unsure of themselves.

Information processing is often slowed after brain injury, manifested in trouble following conversations or plot lines on television programmes, for example. Planning and problem solving might also be difficult. There might be a reduced flexibility to think around different issues, to generate new ideas or solutions, and to weigh up the pros and cons of alternative courses of action. This can mean that people become very troubled if routines are interrupted or problems arise, and/or they might display very rigid and concrete thinking.

Social understanding and the awareness of appropriate social behaviour can be affected and clients with an ABI can find themselves making inappropriate comments. This can cause a great deal of embarrassment and stress, more so to family members than the brain injured client herself when coupled with limited insight. Some people also report an increased tendency to cry or to laugh at inappropriate times, as if their "emotional display control switch" is broken.

Language and general communication problems might follow a brain injury. Specific difficulties with speech production or understanding what people say could occur. Reading and writing might also be affected.

Emotional effects

Given all the changes and challenges that might follow a brain injury, it is no wonder that there can be a high incidence of low mood and anxiety. Depending upon how the injury was sustained, there may be post-trauma experiences. Many of our clients struggle with the challenges to their identity, some worry about their future occupation, finances, relationships, and health, others become socially anxious and isolated. Nevertheless, as with other serious health incidents, there can also be positive emotional changes following a brain injury, such as a re-evaluation of life's priorities, the ending of unhelpful behaviours, and so on. Please see the chapters on dual diagnostic assessment issues (Chapter Two), and therapeutic work in ABI (Chapter Three) for more detailed information.

Family relationship effects

Brain injury presents challenges for families. There can be added strain on romantic relationships. Partners might have to take on new responsibilities within the household, such as managing the bills or taking on a greater share of childcare. They might have to make changes to their own working hours to provide care for the ABI client, or to balance a new shortfall in household income. Personality changes can make the person with whom they share their home feel very different to the person they married. Those closest to the brain injured person often tell us they are the ones who bear the brunt of their increased irritability and frustration. Changes in sexual interest can also be a great source of disharmony. Such things are a challenge to deal with in relationships that were supportive and fulfilling before the injury, but even more so where the relationship was not so harmonious.

On the other hand, a brain injury might cause positive changes, such as a workaholic father feeling able to spend more time with his children, or the impact of a life-threatening experience can lead to new perspectives. Relationship dynamics also change for parents of adults who sustain a brain injury, and for the children of brain injured individuals, whether young or adult themselves. Please see Chapters Twelve and Thirteen, on relationships after ABI and on parenting dependents, respectively, for a thorough discussion.

Employment effects

Given the above difficulties, it is unsurprising that around two-thirds of those with a severe traumatic brain injury are unable to return to work (Sander, Kreutzer, Rosenthal, Delmonico, & Young, 1996). The effects of loss of employment and the complexities of managing vocational rehabilitation are discussed more fully by Bernie Walsh in the chapter on Vocational Rehabilitation, later in this book.

Conclusions

While we make no claim to have provided a fully comprehensive account of the basic definitions, prevalence, and consequences of ABI, we hope that there is enough information for the reader in this chapter to have a grasp of the basics of ABI if it is new to you or feel refreshed in your knowledge if it has been some time since you have worked with such clients. The references suggested below, as well as the chapters that follow, should help to put some "meat on the bones".

References

Christensen, J., Pedersen, M. G., Peterson, C. B., Sidenius, P., Olsen, J., & Vestergaard, M. (2009). Long term risk of epilepsy after traumatic brain injury in children and young adults: a population-based cohort study. *Lancet, 373*(9669): 1105–1110.

Costandi, M. (2010). Phineas Gage and the effect of an iron bar through the head on personality. Electronic version: www.guardian.co.uk/science/blog/2010/nov/05/phineas-gage-head-personality on 3 February 2012. Accessed 29 May 2012]

Department of Health. Social Services Inspectorate (1996). *A Hidden Disability: Report of the SSI Traumatic Brain Injury Rehabilitation Project*. London: The Stationery Office.

Gurd, J., Kishka, U., & Marshall, J. C. (Eds.) (2010). *Handbook of Clinical Neuropsychology*. 2nd edn. Oxford: Oxford University Press.

Health and Social Care Information Centre (2011). Hospital Episode *Statistics: Accident and Emergency Attendances in England (Experimental Statistics) 2009–10*. Electronic version: www.hesonline.nhs.uk/Ease/servlet/ContentServer?siteID=1937&categoryID=1502. Accessed 21 January 2012.

Herman, S. (2002). Epilepsy after brain insult: targeting epileptogenesis. *Neurology, 56*: S21–S26.

House of Commons Health Committee (2001). *Head Injury: Rehabilitation. Third Report*. London: Stationery Office.

Jennett, B., & McMillan, R. (1981). The epidemiology of head injury. *British Medical Journal, 282*: 101–104.

O'Driscoll, K. & Leach, J.P. (1998). "No longer Gage": an iron bar through the head. Early observations of personality change after injury to the prefrontal cortex. *British Medical Journal, 317*(7174): 1673–1674.

Powell, T. (1994). *Head Injury: A Practical Guide*. Nottingham: Headway National Head Injuries Association.

Sander, A. M., Kreutzer, J. S., Rosenthal, M., Delmonico, R., & Young, M. E. (1996). A multi-center longitudinal investigation of return to work and community integration following traumatic brain injury. *Journal of Head Trauma Rehabilitation*, 11: 70–84.

Teasdale G., & Jennett, B. (1974). Assessment of coma and impaired consciousness. A practical scale. *Lancet*, 2: 81–84.

Yates, P. J., Williams, W. H., Harris, A., Round, A., & Jenkins, R. (2006). An epidemiological study of head injuries in a UK population attending an emergency department. *Journal of Neurology Neurosurgery and Psychiatry*, 77: 699–701.

CHAPTER ONE

Behavioural neuroanatomy

Rudi Coetzer

Introduction

Neuroanatomy is one of the core subjects of the neurosciences. While most experience some trepidation when confronted with studying neuroanatomy, there are very solid reasons for developing a robust understanding of basic functional neuroanatomy. Of particular importance to those practitioners working in brain injury rehabilitation, including neuropsychologists, is to link anatomical structure with function. To integrate diagnosis, formulation, and rehabilitation, the clinician should have a sound knowledge of which areas of the brain, when damaged, are likely to affect what functions (e.g., language, memory). In clinical neuropsychology, there is a focus on cognitive functions, but, clearly, emotional and behavioural functions have the potential to affect functional outcome after brain injury to a similar degree, or more. Where possible, structure is linked to function within this chapter. The excellent textbook written by Crossman and Neary (2000) is used as the main reference source for this chapter. As the reader will discover, I have primarily provided a narrative tour through the important neuroanatomical structures. I would again recommend Crossman and Neary as a good source of pictorial representations of the structures discussed.

Gross anatomy and bony structures

The obvious place to start with developing knowledge about neuroanatomy is the immediately visible, the bony structures that encase the brain. Fortunately, there are very few skull bones we need to know a lot about. The brain weighs approximately 1.5 kilograms and is encased by the skull. The skull is made up of several different bones. These bones fuse during a baby's early development. As regards gross anatomical features, the brain is divided into two hemispheres, left and right. In the vast majority of right-handed people, the left hemisphere is more involved in language and the right hemisphere in non-verbal and related processes. In all, there are four lobes on each side of the brain. Listing these from the front (anterior) through to the back (posterior) are the frontal lobes, the temporal lobes, the parietal lobes and finally the occipital lobes. There is one of each of these lobes in the left and right hemisphere respectively.

Let us now return to the bony structures. The ones that mostly come to the attention of neuropsychologists are the following. First, the skull base, the part the brain rests on. The skull base has a prominent opening to allow the brain stem to link up with the spinal cord. This hole is called the foramen magnum. During some types of acquired brain injury, most notably traumatic brain injury, the skull base can sometimes be damaged through transmission of mechanical force. Some of the clinical signs associated with a skull base fracture include bleeding from the ear or subsequent hearing loss. The latter happens because the cranial nerve (item 8 in the list on p. 23) involved in hearing is vulnerable to damage when the skull base is fractured. A fracture of the skull base does not necessarily always equate to a more severe traumatic brain injury. However, it is important to determine the presence of skull base fractures as it can, among other information, also give some indication of the amount of mechanical force involved in the injury a patient sustained.

The temporal, occipital, parietal, and frontal bones are important to consider as well, as these can also be fractured during a severe traumatic brain injury. Again, these types of fractures can give some indication to the clinician of the force in involved in the injury. A fracture of these bones would imply that a significant amount of mechanical energy might have been transmitted to the brain areas below and around the fracture area. Besides the location of these skull bones, there are other factors to be aware of. For example, the temporal bone is a bit thinner in places and can sometimes relatively easily sustain a depressed fracture. An example here would be when a person is hit to the side of the head by an object, such as a baseball bat.

Generally, fractures to the surface of the skull are more common where force has been applied very locally. For example, a blow with a hammer can result in a more circumscribed, depressed fracture, whereas a blunter object might cause a linear or wider fracture area on the skull. Localised or circumscribed skull fractures can result in post-trauma epilepsy or relatively specific impairment associated with underlying brain regions' functions. For example, if on the left, disturbances of language might occur. There are different types of fractures, for example hairline fractures or depressed fractures. The latter, in some cases, is much more ominous. Depressed skull fractures, for example, can often present a higher risk of the person subsequently developing post-trauma seizures or epilepsy. There are also other risks associated with depressed skull fractures, for example risk of infection where bone splinters pierce the protective coverings of the brain and enter the brain tissue, among others.

Returning to internal structures, the sharp bony protrusions (most notably the sphenoid ridge) upon which parts of the temporal and frontal lobes lie pose an obvious risk. When the brain is violently moved around during the deceleration or acceleration associated with severe traumatic brain injury, these bony protrusions can cause abrasions and contusions to the frontal and temporal lobes, most notably the anterior poles. This can result in a predictable pattern of cognitive impairment and behavioural changes: for example, executive dysfunction and memory or language impairment. Other skull bones also occasionally come to our attention. For example, fractures to the orbital bones (bones around the eye), are often mentioned in medical notes or during case presentations.

While with the developments in maxillo-facial surgery, very obvious facial scars or disfigurement is nowadays less likely, the person might well, on testing, present with cognitive difficulties common to head trauma, such as poor information processing and executive functioning. This occurs because these bones can (similar to, for example, the nose) be fractured during an assault where a person might be kicked or punched in the head, with the associated transfer of force to brain tissue. Clearly some knowledge about the bony structures surrounding the brain is important for our understanding of the forces involved in traumatic brain injury.

Cellular structure

Like all organs or structures in the human body, the brain is made up of billions of cells. The main cells in the brain are called neurons. Neurons are responsible for transmitting neuronal impulses, generally via chemical changes and electrical conduction. Neurons consist of a cell body and a disproportionately long tail, known as the axon. Groups of axons make up the white matter tracts in the brain. The cell body of the neuron has several short arms (not dissimilar to the branches of a tree), the dendrites. These play an important role in the conduction of nerve impulses. The axons of the neurons are vulnerable to acquired injury: for example, shearing and tearing occurring during traumatic brain injury, or demyelination in multiple sclerosis. This can have significant clinical implications, disrupting neuronal communication between separate anatomical regions in the brain.

Bundles of axons make up white matter tracts, as already mentioned above. Impulses are transmitted via the neurones by means of neurotransmitters: for example, dopamine, serotonin, noradrenaline, and acetylcholine. However, the neurons do not actually make contact with each other. There is a gap between neurons—the synapse. The transmission of impulses results from the release of neurotransmitters on the one side of the synapse, effecting receptors on the other side of the synapse. In this way, the gap is bridged, chemically and electrically. The release of neurotransmitters changes the electrical properties or potential, and in this way conducts nerve impulses. But what holds the neurones together, or, rather, what comprises the supporting cells? This is the function of the neuroglia. These cells are not involved in the conduction of nerve impulses. Rather, they have a "supporting role". Some of the neuroglia would include oligodendroglia, microglia, and astrocytes. Many brain tumours result from the undifferentiated growth of neuroglia. Sometimes, when brain damage occurs, there can be an increase in the microglia in the area where the damage occurred.

Topography and internal structures

Perhaps the most striking feature of the brain is the unique nature of its actual surface (cortex). The surface of the brain consists of convolutions, or, put differently, valleys and hills, covering the four lobes. These are known as sulci (valleys) and gyri (hills). These serve to maximise the surface of the cortex. Once the brain is cut open, two features tend to stand out. First, there is a change in colour. Second, the presence of rather large fluid-filled spaces in the brain. With regard to the change in colour, while grey on the surface (constituting the cell bodies of the cortex), the tissue below changes to white. These white parts are made up of nerve fibres (tails of the cell bodies) that project throughout the brain. In essence, these projections serve as connective pathways between different brain regions. For example, concentrated bundles of white matter fibres form the internal capsule almost in the middle of each hemisphere. These are important to be aware of, since certain types of stroke can involve the internal capsule. But it is not only the cortex that contains grey matter. There are also islands of grey matter deep inside the brain, some of which are called collectively the basal ganglia. The most prominent of these is the corpus striatum. The corpus striatum contains the caudate nucleus, globus pallidus, and putamen. Certain types of strokes in the basal ganglia can result in quite specific impairments of cognitive functions, as outlined below in the context of damage to the limbic system.

Perhaps the most important, from a neuropsychological perspective, of the internal brain structures is the limbic system. The limbic system consists of the cingulate gyrus, hippocampal formation, amygdala, septum, formix, and hypothalamus. Papez's circuit describes the pathways involved in the functions of the limbic system. The limbic system is closely involved in the functions of memory, motivation, and emotion. The hippocampus is specifically involved in memory. Furthermore, there is a lateralisation effect where (in the vast majority of right-handed people) the left hippocampus is closely involved in verbal and the right in more non-verbal type of memory. Where both the left and right hippocampi are destroyed, very severe memory impairment usually results. Some of the neuropathological conditions that involve structures of the limbic system include Korsakoff's amnesia, Klüver–Bucy syndrome, herpes simplex encephalitis, and temporal lobe seizures, among others. The hippocampus, because of its proximity to the sphenoid ridge, is also one of the brain areas vulnerable to injury during severe head trauma. Not surprising then, in view of the functions the limbic system is closely involved in, that neuropathological conditions affecting the limbic system almost always have profound impairment of new learning (memory) as one of its defining symptoms.

Let us now return to the spaces, or large "holes", inside the brain. These comprise the ventricular system, made up of several interconnected, fluid-filled spaces. The ventricular system communicates or is in contact with the fluid between the brain and the skull. This is how it provides much-needed cushioning and protection for the brain. The most prominent of the ventricles are the two horseshoe-shaped lateral ventricles found in each hemisphere. These connect to the midline third ventricle by means of the interventricular foramen. The "walls" on the sides of the third ventricle are the thalamus and hypothalamus. The third ventricle is connected to the fourth ventricle via the cerebral aqueduct. Between the brain stem and cerebellum lies the fourth ventricle. The fourth ventricle is connected to the subarachnoid space around the brain by three apertures: in the midline, the foramen of Magendie, and laterally, the two foramina of Luscha. The cerebospinal fluid of the ventricular system is produced by the lateral, third, and fourth ventricles. Some understanding of the ventricular system is important for the clinical neuropsychologist because sometimes the system might become blocked by, for example, tumours, or too much cerebro-spinal fluid is produced. Under both of these conditions there is an increase in pressure on the surrounding brain tissue, a condition known as hydrocephalus. Hydrocephalus tends to present with a triad of symptoms: a broad-based gait, incontinence, and cognitive impairment. Profound slowness is also not uncommon.

The brain appears to rest on a "pedestal", the brainstem. The brainstem is involved in maintaining vital, life-preserving functions: for example, breathing. It consists (from the top down) of the midbrain, pons, and medulla oblongata. The brainstem contains the reticular formation, which is directly involved in a person's level of consciousness, among other critical functions. Ten of the cranial nerves attach to the brainstem, numbers 3 to 12 in the list on page 23, connecting to some of the brain stem nuclei. The rear of the brainstem has four bumps, the superior and inferior colliculi, involved in vision and hearing pathways. Behind the brainstem, we find the cerebellum.

The cerebellum has its own convolutions, similar to the sulci and gyri of the cortex, but these are called folia. The cerebellum is involved in the integration of movement, among other things. Motor integrity contributes to many functions and can affect performance on neuropsychological tests. But the cerebellum is also thought to be involved in other functions: for example, memory and learning. Motor impairment can, of course, have a profound effect on a person's psychological wellbeing also. In the past, the brainstem and cerebellum were considered to be less important structures for many clinicians to be aware of, but this is probably not the case any more.

Finally, how is the brain "wrapped up" inside the skull? We know that cushioning is provided by the cerebro-spinal fluid, but there is further protection between the brain and the skull. Three layers of membranes cover the brain. These are found between the skull and the brain itself. Directly under the skull the lies the dura mater, then the arachnoid mater, and, attached to the brain surface, closely following its convolutions, the pia mater. The dura mater is the tough outer layer (closest to the skull) and has a protective function. In the midline, the dura mater reaches down between the hemispheres via the falx cerebri into the longitudinal fissure. From the rear of the brain, the dura mater reaches in horizontally via the tentorium cerebelli. The subarachnoid space lies between the arachnoid mater and pia mater. The subarachnoid space contains cerebro-spinal fluid and blood vessels. Knowing the structure of these three layers covering the brain is very important for understanding where some types of stroke (for example, sub-arachnoid haemorrhage), infections (meningitis), and also some of the secondary problems that might result from severe traumatic brain injury (for example, subdural haemorrhage) occur.

Lobes and their functions

One of the important points to orientate oneself is to know where the lobes of the brain start and end. Some of the major prominent sulci function, almost like borders between countries, to indicate where the different lobes of the brain start and end. The frontal lobes start from the front of the brain and extend posteriorly to the central sulcus. It does not extend below the lateral fissure, though, which is where we find the temporal lobe on each side of the brain. The frontal lobes are involved in initiation, planning, problem solving, and the direction of our behaviour, among many other things. Sometimes, these functions are collectively referred to as executive control function. However, the frontal lobes are thought to be involved in much more than cognitive functioning, including, for example, personality or patterns of behaviour unique to an individual. Furthermore, the frontal lobes and their connections have also been implicated in some of the psychiatric diagnoses.

The temporal lobes are primarily involved in language and memory. We find that the temporal lobes are delineated by the lateral fissure. Extending the lateral fissure as an imaginary line towards roughly the middle of the area posterior to the central sulcus, this signals upwards the boundary between the parietal and occipital lobes. At the top of the temporal lobe is Heschl's gyrus, which is directly involved in auditory function. Inside the lateral fissure is located the insula, a somewhat "hidden" cortical area. Unfortunately, there are no obvious boundaries or anatomical "landmarks" here. The occipital and parietal lobes are at the rear of the brain, separated by the parieto–occipital sulcus. The parietal lobes contain the primary somatosensory cortex and are involved in processing incoming perceptual stimuli. It is also primarily involved with visuo-spatial functions. The occipital lobes are fairly extensively involved in vision. Lesions in this area can lead to an interesting syndrome, Anton's Syndrome (cortical blindness), where a patient can be unaware of his or her blindness. Below follows a simplified overview of some of the main neuropsychological functions each of the lobes are thought to be involved in.

1. *Frontal lobes*: planning, problem solving, initiation of behaviours, aspects of personality and behaviour, emotional regulation, insight, and specific components of language (e.g., word production via Broca's area).
2. *Temporal lobes*: most of the language functions (including comprehension via Wernicke's area), memory, learning, and emotion.
3. *Parietal lobes*: processing of incoming perceptual stimuli, spatial relationships, body awareness, mathematical ability, some language functions, including reading and naming objects.
4. *Occipital lobes*: extensive involvement in the visual functions.

It should, of course, be remembered that the individual lobes of the brain serve many more functions than those listed above. In addition, the different lobes do not function in isolation from each other, or from other structures in the brain such as the brainstem and cerebellum. The brain mostly functions as an integrated whole.

Blood supply

While it can be a struggle to understand the blood supply or "tubing" of the brain, it is important to know about it—vascular pathology gives rise to fairly specific (compared to, say, traumatic brain injury) patterns of cognitive impairment and behavioural changes. But, for some reason, it tends to be a particularly difficult area of neuroanatomy to memorise. Perhaps, to aid visualisation, it might be helpful to change perspective. It is a lot easier looking from underneath the brain inwards from the two pairs of vessels supplying blood to the brain and imagining following the pathways from there. First, the internal carotids make a few bends and go through the cavernous sinus before reaching the brain to the side of the optic chiasm (where cranial nerve II partially crosses). Here, branches create a circular flow (or "roundabout"), known as the Circle of Willis. The Circle of Willis comprises the posterior and anterior communicating arteries. From the Circle of Willis the internal carotid divides into the two anterior cerebral arteries and the two middle cerebral arteries. The anterior cerebral arteries follow the longitudinal fissure and irrigate the medial part of the brain, whereas the middle cerebral arteries follow the lateral fissure and, accordingly, supply blood to the lateral parts of the hemispheres.

The second sources of blood supply to the brain are the vertebral arteries. These arteries enter the brain through the formamen magnum and join between the pons and medulla in the brainstem, to form the basilar artery. Between the pons and midbrain, the basilar artery divides into the superior cerebellar arteries and the posterior cerebral arteries. The posterior cerebral arteries are connected to the Circle of Willis (and, hence, the internal carotids also) via the posterior communicating arteries. The posterior cerebral arteries provide a blood supply to the occipital lobes and a small part of the lower temporal lobes. Various small arteries leave the Circle of Willis and enter the surrounding brain tissue. These are known as perforating arteries and provide a blood supply to neuropsychologically very important structures such as the basal ganglia, hypothalamus, and internal capsule, among others. Aneurysms in the Circle of Willis (for example anterior communicating artery aneurysms) have great potential to disrupt the blood supply to some of these crucial structures. Among other things, this can result in impairments of memory and executive control function. Finally, the superficial veins, deep veins, and dural venous sinuses are involved in draining blood from the brain.

The cranial nerves

Although not necessarily of primary concern from a cognitive, behavioural, or emotional perspective, the cranial nerves, nevertheless, have very important functions. The cranial nerves are involved in functions such as eye movements, sense of smell, and vision. There are twelve cranial nerves, of which ten originate from the brain stem. The twelve cranial nerves, with some of their corresponding main functions are listed below.

1. *Olfactory nerve*: involvement in sense of smell.
2. *Optic nerve*: essential to vision and seeing.
3. *Oculomotor nerve*: controls eye movement; pupil reaction.
4. *Trochlear nerve*: controls eye movement.
5. *Trigeminal nerve*: responsible for sensation.
6. *Abducens nerve*: involved in eye movement.
7. *Facial nerve*: involvement in facial movement, taste.
8. *Auditory nerve*: responsible for hearing; sensation of head position.
9. *Glossopharyngeal nerve*: involved in sensation and taste; swallowing.
10. *Vagus nerve*: involvement in sensation; swallowing and speech.
11. *Accessory nerve*: controls head and shoulder movement.
12. *Hypoglossal nerve*: responsible for tongue movement.

Which of these cranial nerves are more likely to be of relevance to the clinician working in assessment and rehabilitation within hospital settings? In all probability 1, 2, and 8 when it comes to traumatic brain injury. In fact, loss of sense of smell (anosmia) is a fairly good clinical marker of potential frontal lobe injury after head trauma. The olfactory nerves lie underneath (the base) and to the middle of the frontal lobes and are vulnerable to shearing when subjected to rotational forces. Visual problems can follow traumatic brain injury, but not all are as a result of cranial nerve 2 involvement. A skull base fracture can sever or bruise parts of cranial nerve 8, resulting in loss of hearing. Some types of stroke can affect the functioning of cranial nerve 7, resulting in facial asymmetry. Acoustic neuromas (a type of tumour) can affect cranial nerve 8. Cranial nerve 3 can be compressed by aneurysms or tumours. The general neurological examination covers the assessment of the functioning of the cranial nerves. Neuropsychological assessment examines the cognitive, emotional, and behavioural functions that constitute neuropsychological functioning, in the context of actual or suspected acquired brain injury.

Neuropsychological functions

So far in this chapter, an overview of basic, introductory level neuroanatomy has been provided. Reference was made to some of the most salient neuropsychological factors associated with certain anatomical areas. For example, in right-handed persons, language is usually represented in left temporal and frontal lobes. More specifically, word production is associated with Broca's area in the left frontal lobe, comprehension with Wernicke's area in the left posterior temporal lobe. However, it should be remembered that not only cognitive functions are mediated by brain structures. Emotion and behaviour are, of course, also outputs of the human brain. For example, the limbic system is not only involved in memory, but emotion also. Similarly, the frontal lobes are not solely responsible for executive control function. They are also involved in behaviours, personality, and so forth. Examples here include initiation and drive, or social insight. It is not always possible to make a definite and specific distinction between, for example, cognition and behaviour, and certainly there is sometimes an overlap in these and other domains of the outputs of the human brain. Furthermore, while some functions (for example, language) are much more localised with regard to anatomy, others (for example general intellectual ability) are much more widely distributed throughout the brain. Below follows an overview of some of the cognitive, behavioural, and emotional areas important to assess in most persons with various forms of acquired brain injury.

With regard to cognitive functions, these broadly include attention, language, memory, constructional ability, visuo-spatial functions, calculus, and executive control functions. For the purposes of assessment, cognitive functions should perhaps best be viewed as organised in a hierarchical fashion (Strub & Black, 2003). What this means is that more complex cognitive functions rely on more fundamental functions. For example, for all cognitive functions to "work", a prerequisite would be reasonably intact attention. Another example might be that intact language is, to some extent, a basic requirement for memory (of language). Executive control function, of course, relies fairly heavily on the integrity of most other cognitive functions. This has important implications for neuropsychological assessment, as outlined by Strub and Black (2003). The practitioner ideally would start the cognitive assessment with the most fundamental or basic functions, for example, attention, before proceeding to more complex cognitive functions, say executive control function. Building up a picture of cognitive strengths and weaknesses in this fashion prevents "contamination" (artificial lowering of performances) on higher order cognitive functions, due to problems lower down the hierarchy of cognition. All results from cognitive assessment should be gauged against the individual's own general abilities. For this reason, it is of fundamental importance to assess the person's overall level of general intellectual ability, as well as their pre-morbid ability.

Areas of behavioural functioning, while sometimes difficult to completely disentangle from cognition, include the following. Initiation (or starting off) of activities, impulsivity, apathy, and speed of activity are some of the more commonly encountered behavioural outputs to consider in the context of acquired brain injury. Initiation can be thought of as the "spark" required to start an activity. Apathy is a closely related concept, but perhaps relates more to the actual desire to start an activity. Apathy can be difficult to distinguish from depression in some cases. Nevertheless, there is a potentially useful qualitative distinction to be made in that apathy is devoid of strong emotion, whereas depression has a strong component of feelings of sadness. Impulsivity, while also a behaviour, is, of course, closely related to executive control function: it is, essentially, doing without thinking. Speed of performance usually relates to motor speed, but, of course, is difficult to fully separate from attention and obsessive behaviours, for example. Behaviours are usually objectively observable, but might, over time, start to represent more stable, predictable patterns. Relatives of the client with acquired brain injury report these as "a change in his (or her) personality since the injury". However, the person with an ABI might not recognise this. If not recognised or seen in this way by the person with acquired brain injury, levels of insight or self-awareness might be important to consider. Overall, it is important for the practitioner to assess if a person's behaviours are goal directed and how aware they might be of their own impairments or disability.

Emotion after acquired brain injury is a complex area to conceptualise. Changes in emotional expression could well be representative of biological, psychological, or social factors. In most cases, it is actually more likely to represent a combination of these factors. Examples include the following. After acquired brain injury, the areas in the brain responsible for mediating emotion (for example, the limbic system during some types of encephalitis) might be affected. This can be on a both a structural and neuro-transmitter level. The person might then present with increased anxiety, or depression, for example. But areas involved in emotional regulation may also be affected by acquired brain injury, for example, damage to the amygdala during severe traumatic brain injury. Under these circumstances, the person might present with dramatic fluctuations in emotion. However, emotion can, of course, also vary significantly for psychological reasons. The most obvious example here is a person's direct emotional reaction to the brain injury itself. Cognition also contributes to emotional experience. For example, impaired memory might make some people anxious, while others become depressed. Or perceptual difficulties might make a person anxious, as could the perceptual overstimulation associated with impaired information processing. Finally, social factors associated with acquired brain injury, for example, unemployment, can, of course, also have dramatic effects on emotional experience. While practitioners should always keep fundamental neuroanatomical concepts in mind, the expression of impairment and associated disability should always be seen in a bio-psychosocial framework.

Conclusion

It is an important skill for the rehabilitation professional to develop very early on an ability to visualise brain structures when no pictures are available. This, for example, includes being able to explain neuroanatomical concepts to students or trainees, or being able to visualise what is being discussed during a case presentation or ward round. Perhaps this is an "ecologically valid" environment for practising one's skills in this area? The point here is that at work, in the clinic, neuroanatomy is talked about (ward rounds) or written about (medical notes), rather than displayed in neat line sketches or colour photographs. The second point is to learn to associate structure with neuropsychological function, but not in a rigid way. Brain lesions hardly ever perfectly match a patient's clinical presentation. Why is this? Of course, we do not fully understand the complex reasons for this. And there might anyway be limitations to the technologies we use to determine lesions (for example, magnetic resonance imaging (MRI) scans), as well as clinical presentation (for example, neuropsychological tests). Nevertheless, in this regard, there are probably three points we should keep in mind. First, when it comes to lesions, disconnections are important to consider. Second, psychological aspects of brain injury can significantly colour presentation. Third, environmental factors can have a potent effect. Clearly, making sense of neuroanatomical data and individual presentation after acquired brain injury requires considerable skill, including that of assessing clients. The next chapter addresses the neuropsychological assessment of persons with acquired brain injury.

References

Crossman, A. R., & Neary, D. (2000). Neuronanatomy. An Illustrated Colour Text (2nd edn). Edinburgh: Churchill Livingstone.

Strub, R. C., & Black, F. W. (2003). The Mental Status Examination in Neurology (4th edn). Philadelphia, PA: F. A. Davis.

CHAPTER TWO

Neuropsychological assessment: the not-so-basic basics

Aidan Jones, Simon J. Prangnell, Crawford Thomas, and Gavin Newby

Introduction

In this chapter, we hope to give the reader a "Cook's tour" through some of the basic orientating issues relating to neuropsychological assessment that face clinical neuropsychologists in modern practice. In the "Putting into practice" chapters later in the book, we look at assessment in some specific contexts including: assessment of patients in low awareness states (Crawford Thomas), mental capacity assessments (Helen Newby and Tracey Ryan-Morgan), and driving (Gavin Newby). However, there are almost an indefinite number of contexts and confounds (ranging from pain to mood to epilepsy, to name a few) that affect the results of an assessment, and it is dealing with, and working within, these "real world" issues that forms the focus for this chapter.

With this in mind, neither this chapter nor the practice chapters that follow could possibly hope to be fully comprehensive. However, we hope that this chapter will illustrate a reasonably broad range of the patients that clinical neuropsychologists might be asked to see, from the apparently straightforward screening assessment to the complex, difficult-to-assess client. The chapter then goes on to provide an overview of the types of issues we might be asked to address, consider the questions that might be posed, and explore the contexts and practicalities of assessment. In particular, we will discuss the issues these assessments raise for clients with an acquired brain injury (ABI) and for those conducting them. We will do this from an applied practical perspective, drawing on case examples to illustrate points. In keeping with the spirit and aims of this book, we approach assessment from a practical, hands-on, feet on the ground perspective, acknowledging both the possibilities and limitations in assessing people with ABI.

For many practitioners, Lezak, Loring, Hannay, and Fischer (2004) (or earlier editions) would have been their first introduction to psychometrics in applied clinical neuropsychology settings. This is certainly still an excellent and very comprehensive primer in this area. However, for readers who wish to read more about the statistical and theoretical bases of assessment, we would also recommend Strauss, Sherman, and Spreen's (2006) excellent discussion of tests and their psychometric properties, and Gurd, Kischka, and Marshall's (2010) superb general introduction to neuropsychological assessment.

We want to start out by emphasising that neuropsychological assessment in everyday clinical practice is not simply about scores derived from standardised psychometric tests. It incorporates a broader clinical approach including interviews, discussions with family members, liaison with the clinical team and/or other agencies involved, and behavioural observations, careful formulation, and the sensitive feedback and sharing of results. Critical to any assessment is an account of the person's social, personal, and family circumstances, together with a detailed clinical history. In order for the results of psychometric testing to be validly interpreted, the clinician must have a detailed profile of the person's individual social and clinical context. This can easily be neglected if one focuses exclusively on psychometrics in isolation from other data. In essence, one of the main challenges for practitioners is to ascertain and explain why a person achieved a given profile, rather than merely report scores and confirm a diagnosis or aetiology that, in the vast majority of cases, would already be known from the history.

However, it is important to recognise that not everybody can be tested using standardised assessment. To begin with, the clinician needs to be open and creative and be prepared to consider using assessments beyond the standard battery of tests. For example, brain injured clients who present as being in vegetative or low awareness states cannot be reliably assessed using traditional paper and pencil tests. Instead, a valid picture of their responses may be gained by formalised structured behavioural observations, such as the Sensory Modality and Rehabilitation Technique (SMART; Gill-Thwaites & Munday, 1999), the Wessex Head Injury Matrix (WHIM; Shiel, Wilson, McLellan, Horn, & Watson, 2000) and the Sensory Stimulation Assessment Measure (SSAM). This area is fully discussed in Chapter Five, by Crawford Thomas, in this volume.

Before you get testing, get testing into perspective

From the authors' experiences, many of us develop our assessment practices from a loosely apprenticeship-type model. That is, maybe as assistant psychologists or trainees, we learn by doing and observing from the practices of the senior clinicians that supervise us within the environments they work in. This "getting-your-hands-dirty" approach is an entirely practical and valid way of learning some of the tools of the trade. However, it is extremely important to take a step back from the minutiae of the mechanics of testing to consider the nature and validity of testing, and the contexts within which you work. Put simply, it is important to recognise both the value and limitations of testing and that it is only one of several ways of getting your client's story in order to help them.

Pen and paper to everyday life: the validity of neuropsychological tests

Other clinicians are often cynical about neuropsychological assessment and the findings from such assessments. They might question the extent to which neuro-psychometry has face validity, given the strong environmental bias presented by the quiet testing room. Clinicians might find themselves faced with being required to make predictions about performance on everyday tasks based on the results of neuropsychological assessment. Chaytor, Temkin, Machamer, and Dikmen (2007) assert that while neuropsychological test data may predict some variance in everyday performance, several other factors, such as mood, are likely to be influential. Odhuba, van den Broek, and Johns (2005) highlight that neuropsychological tests are designed to identify patterns of cognitive impairment, not to predict functioning on everyday tasks. In other words, neuropsychological tests do what neuropsychological tests say they do. Odhuba, van den Broek, and Johns (2005) highlight the multiple factors that have an impact on everyday performance, with cognitive impairment being only one of these factors. Survey findings suggest that having to consider the confounds and limitations of test findings can lead clinical neuropsychologists to doubt the validity of psychometrics before settling on a balanced view that recognises testing guides but does not determine a view on a client's functioning (Christie, Savill, Buttress, Newby, & Tyerman, 2001).

What needs to be taken account of when reporting and interpreting test scores?

You will need to have considered a range of factors when making the decision to begin assessing someone and then evaluating information generated from that assessment. It is important to consider the person's emotional state, whether they are fatigued, their ability to sustain attention on tasks, their ability to sustain mental effort, their understanding of why the assessment is taking place or has been requested, and their motivation to engage in the assessment process. Some of these factors can be addressed in planning assessment sessions. For example, with fatigue, it might be necessary to schedule more frequent and shorter sessions over several days rather than the standard "timetabled" session. Identifying and addressing a person's concerns about the assessment process might address test related anxiety, as would paying close attention to developing and maintaining good rapport with the client. Additional time spent in engaging the person in the assessment process and developing a therapeutic relationship is a sound investment. The interested reader would do well to refer to the excellent guidance on relationship building during the testing process offered by Gorske and Smith (2008) in *Collaborative Therapeutic Neuropsychological Assessment*.

In modern clinical neuropsychological practice, there is currently a heavy emphasis on effort testing of clients with cognitive complaints (e.g., see the excellent paper "Assessment of effort in clinical testing of cognitive functioning for adults" (British Psychological Society, 2009) for UK-based guidance). In medico–legal practice, effort testing is now regarded as an imperative, with non-testing of this area being seen as poor. Whereas effort testing is no doubt useful whatever the environment, there is a danger that poor performance could be universally viewed as synonymous with malingering. The British Psychological Society's report argues that clients might fail effort tests for a variety of reasons, and that to suggest that poor performance is always wilful would be to neglect the opportunity to better understand and unpack the patient's symptoms. Furthermore, at times, an obvious and well-documented history of, for example, a severe traumatic brain injury might negate the need for routine effort testing, and perhaps also reduce its relevance.

There are times, however, when, due to the extent of a person's cognitive, physical, or communication impairment, their emotional state or medical condition, that neuropsychological testing is not the most appropriate or helpful mode of assessment. For example, during the very early recovery stages after ABI, where test results are likely to become outdated owing to the rapidly changing clinical picture, or where emerging self-awareness might cause a client to become depressed if tested at that specific time, rather than a few months later, when improvements might be more evident. In these cases, close interdisciplinary working and use of alternative modes of assessment, such as observation, become crucial. When questioning whether to assess a patient or not, it is important to consider what the clinical priorities are; it is often more important to delay assessment in order to safeguard a patient's self-esteem.

Observation: but what to look for?

Observing a patient's performance in other therapy sessions is often an excellent way of gathering meaningful information about the nature of their difficulties and a way of gauging their performance in "real life" scenarios. However, the question remains: what to look for? Observing an occupational therapy or physiotherapy session might be a useful indicator of a client's performance on specific tasks, and will yield information about their ability to plan, problem solve, concentrate, and sustain effort on tasks. Observing other aspects of the session is also important. For example, you can assess social cognition and behaviour through the manner in which the client engages with the therapist or other people present. Alternatively, you can note whether the client attends the session independently, or the level of support they require in order to be present for the start of the session (e.g., verbal reminders, assistance to get to the right location). Given that many therapy sessions occur within open-plan therapy rooms with other client sessions running alongside, it can be helpful to note how well your client can engage in the task in hand while dealing with those background distractions. It can also be helpful to gauge the nature and intensity of support required to complete a task, from a written checklist detailing components of a task through to verbal prompts and physical assistance. Often, observing a patient during an everyday functional task such as cooking a meal can provide a far quicker assessment of skills such as problem solving, planning, judgement, self-monitoring, concentration, vision, and movement. It is also more likely to encourage a patient to embark on other forms of assessment with you at a later stage if you have been present during activities that have held more meaning for them. Links between test performance and everyday functioning are easier to draw when you have witnessed, for yourself, the patient in action.

The clinical interview

The clinical interview with the client is at the heart of the assessment process. There really is no substitute for meeting the patient and some significant others in order to gain an overview of the *individual* in front of you. Over time, numerous clinical interviews become the bedrock for making sound clinical judgements and problem formulations. These judgements can not only be used to understand the client better, to guide which tests are appropriate and drive your recommendations, but also, undoubtedly, to hone the clinician's skills. One of the most important parts of the clinical interview is in assessing the extent to which a client's autobiographical memory appears intact, the extent to which they can place life events into chronological order, and, indeed, the extent to which they can highlight events of emotional currency.

The nature of a client's cognitive, physical, and communication difficulties is likely to influence how this interview takes place. For example, conducting a joint session with a speech and language therapist can facilitate communication. There might be situations where it is not possible or appropriate to conduct a direct clinical interview with the client (e.g., when a patient is in a low level of responsiveness), but it could still be possible to meet and observe them during therapy sessions. In essence, the clinical interview provides the opportunity to establish the patient's perspective on their current problems, and to establish their personal context. The perspective they offer and their personal context are crucial to later interpretations of results from neuropsychological testing. Indeed, two supposedly identical ABIs, for these reasons, can manifest very differently in two persons with similar demographics. The need for the clinician to understand each individual client cannot be overemphasised. It is frequently said by clinical neuropsychologists that when you have seen one brain injury—you have seen one brain injury.

The components of a clinical interview tend to be similar across settings, but typically include the client's view of changes in their cognitive functioning, their mood, and relevant personal information such as their occupational and developmental experiences, family situation, and their social networks. In addition to these areas, it can be helpful to explore other areas that have been shown to be related to the client's adjustment to brain injury and longer-term outcomes. For example, establishing the client's appraisals, and personal meanings, of the brain injury can be useful in identifying whether they are at risk of increased emotional distress. Appraisals characterised by themes of loss are predictive of greater emotional distress (Coetzer, 2010; Prangnell & Dean, in preparation). Furthermore, it is important to assess both a person's resources to manage the outcome of the injury and their perception of their available resources. Limited resources and perceptions of limited resources are also linked to emotional distress and difficulties in adjustment and coping.

In addition to these factors, assessing personal resilience could be a useful way of bolstering the patient's sense of their ability to cope, based on how they have managed previous adverse situations.

Filling in the picture: family assessment

Families play a crucial role in adjustment to, and recovery from, acquired brain injury. Families offer the opportunity for clinicians to corroborate the information gained from clients and to more fully understand the pre-morbid personality and characteristics of the individual who has sustained the brain injury or neurological illness. An area of neuropsychology that is somewhat underdeveloped is in assessing individual clients' social reasoning. Interviews and discussion with family frequently give clinicians insight into the extent to which their client might be recovering from a range of cognitive, emotional and social–behavioural perspectives. The clinician needs to establish who is in the immediate family and any other people that are important to family life (e.g., close neighbours). Indeed, in the third author's (GN) service, we routinely construct genograms to record the important family, friends, pets, professionals, work members of their worlds (Bowen, 1980; McGoldrick, Gerson, & Shellenberger, 1999). Having established who is in the family, it is important to get a picture of who fulfils which roles within the family, the nature of relationships between family members, lines of power and authority, and family resources for support. In addition to these issues, establishing family beliefs about illness and injury, and how the family has coped with stress and adversity in the past might provide an indicator as to the family response to the patient's injury, and if further specialist support could be required.

An ethical approach to neuropsychological assessment

An ethical approach to assessment means embracing two core principles. First, there is the need to avoid causing harm, and second, try to do some good (Collicutt-McGrath, 2007). This has a number of implications for everyday practice.

First, you must work within your professional competencies, seek supervision, and engage in additional training wherever appropriate (see Weatherhead and Newby in this volume for a more detailed discussion of continuing professional development). At a basic level, this might simply involve being well acquainted with the tests that one is using and having a clear rationale for their use. Related to this is the important task of always reviewing the relevant medical records before setting out to test a client, as interpretation of test results in isolation from the history would be limited in its meaning and usefulness.

Second, you must acknowledge the limitations of the assessment process and the limits to the validity of assessment when feeding back to others and be open about this with your clients, their families, and the referrer. For example, it is important to be aware that many tests are biased in favour of those sharing a similar cultural background to the area where the test was developed.

Third, these principles mean only doing the minimum number of tests necessary for the assessment in hand. Being selective about which tests are used with which patients can ensure they are not subjected to unnecessary testing.

Fourth, it means being open about how information from the assessment is likely to be used; that is, that it might be shared with the team, and other healthcare professionals who could be involved in supporting the person. Difficulties might arise in situations where families wish to receive feedback on assessment results when the client may not have specifically sanctioned this. While, in some settings, it would not be appropriate to share information with others, in the rehabilitation context, families might be in a position to provide the client with significant levels of practical and emotional support providing they have adequate information to do so. This issue should be addressed before undertaking an assessment. During initial meetings, it can be helpful to provide a rationale for why it can be helpful to share assessment results. This may be done collaboratively, supporting the patient to feed back to their family about the nature of their difficulties, or by arranging joint feedback sessions with the patient and family present. This can be facilitated by the provision of clear, well-written assessment reports.

Fifth, you should seek to obtain informed consent to undertake assessment, especially if mental capacity is the issue. In practice, this means explaining and providing information about the nature of the assessment and the commitment/effort required from the patient. You could also consider developing an information leaflet on neuropsychological assessment for your service. Where there is doubt about a person's capacity to make this decision (see later chapter on the assessment of mental capacity), then a decision must be taken in the patient's best interests. In this case, it is generally held that it is in the best interest of the patient for the rehabilitation team to have a greater awareness of the patient's strengths and areas for support, although it is more problematic when a capacity assessment is required and a person declines to take part. There is no easy resolution to this situation, apart from going back to the principles of not doing harm and trying to do good.

Sixth, it is important that clinicians undertaking assessments reflect on the impact that doing certain assessments can have on our relationships with patients. That is, if we already have good therapeutic relationship with a patient and then are asked to do capacity assessment close to discharge, what will the findings mean for your relationship with them and your ability to carry on working with them in the future, especially if you deem them to not have capacity and this causes them and the family a number of difficulties. In order to manage these situations, it might be useful for departments to have a protocol for these potentially difficult late assessments that sets out circumstances in which a colleague could complete the assessment instead of you, leaving you available to continue to support the person with decisions. However, lone clinicians do not have this option and need to manage this issue (this is later touched upon in the final chapter, by Gavin Newby).

Applied neuropsychological assessment in practice: actually getting down to it

Conducting neuropsychological assessments in real-world clinical settings are often subject to a number of significant limitations. These range from: the availability of suitable assessment resources, the time pressures to complete and report on an assessment, referrers' potential misunderstandings of the role of neuropsychological assessment (e.g., that it offers pin-point accuracy) data of cognitive functions, and the difficulties of assessing clients with severe physical and communication impairments. In addition, neuropsychological tests have tended to be developed in highly controlled conditions, sometimes with a relatively selected normative group of patients and control subjects.

The context of assessment

This book has emphasised the application of neuropsychological approaches in everyday settings. These "everyday" settings could include:

- acute medical settings, for example, stroke medicine, neurosurgery, cardiology;

- specialist neurological rehabilitation services;
- specific neurology clinics: for example, memory, epilepsy, Huntington's chorea;
- residential services;
- community head injury services;
- forensic and learning disability services;
- older adults' services;
- patients' own homes.

Clinical roles might vary considerably across these settings, as do resources such as time, available materials, and attitudes to, and expectations of, neuropsychological assessment. Furthermore, the demands of neuropsychological assessment are likely to vary accordingly. The general guidance provided in this chapter is intended to be relevant across all settings.

The actual content of a neuropsychological assessment will vary according to context. Depending upon the nature of the clinical problem/the questions being asked, more weight may be placed on different aspects of assessment areas. For example, someone experiencing the early stages of dementia might present with subtle changes in behaviour, yet functional brain imaging does not always, in these early stages, show any gross pathology. Neuropsychological assessment might not show any significant impairment, but behavioural responses to novel situations and evidence of behaviour change could indicate an underlying problem. This might often occur in the context of somebody with little, if any, significant previous clinical, family, or other medical history.

On the other hand, there are situations where an individual's ability to engage in social situations on a day-to-day basis and to pick up on social cues is essentially normal, yet cognitive test performance reveals specific areas of impairment. It is not particularly unusual to assess someone in the aftermath of a stroke or head injury to find them, superficially at least, to be functioning very well, but to be surprised when a brief assessment reveals very significant deficits.

The domains of neuropsychological assessment

Broadly speaking, practising neuropsychologists have to deal with four main domains, as suggested by Vanderploeg (1999):

- observed and reported data (as collated from medical records and clinical histories);
- neuropsychometric and standard questionnaire data;
- aetiological formulations: neurological, medical, psychiatric/ psychological disorders;
- functional neuroanatomical knowledge.

A useful model for considering these domains is presented in Figure 2.1. Essentially, the interpretation process is to examine each data area for internal consistency and consider the implications each data domain has on the other three.

What is the question that is being asked? And who is asking it?

Surveying the referrals to a neuropsychology service gives some indication of the range of assessments that are undertaken and the nature of questions asked by referrers. For example:

- Mr X is a fifty-eight-year-old financial manager who had a stroke two months ago and was discharged home after a brief admission to an acute stroke unit. His family have expressed concerns about

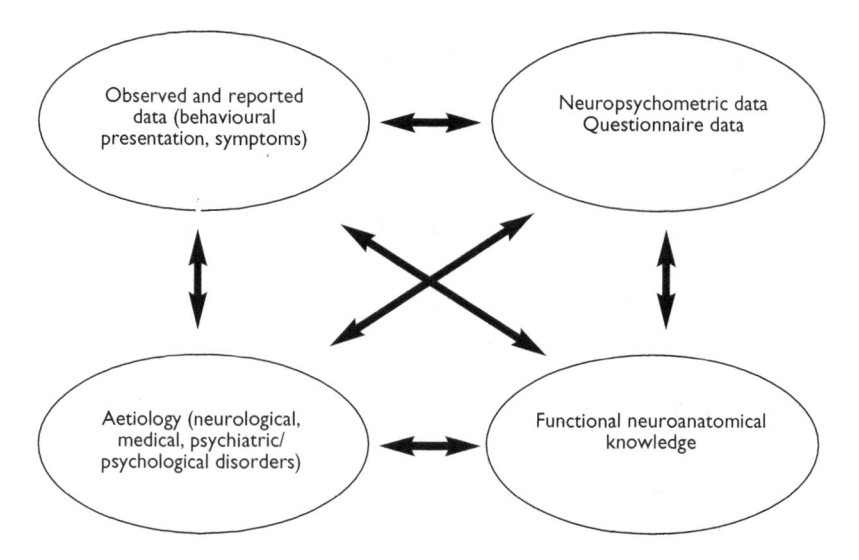

Figure 2.1. Data domains for neuropsychological assessment.

residual cognitive problems and have asked whether he has the mental capacity to manage his financial affairs after making a number of risky investment decisions.
- Mrs Z is a thirty-year-old solicitor who had cardiac arrest six months ago, sustaining a severe hypoxic brain injury. It is thought that she might be in a low awareness state and you have been asked to establish her current level of cognitive functioning.
- Mr A sustained a mild traumatic brain injury six months ago and is reporting ongoing difficulties with headaches and concentration. His GP has requested an assessment of his readiness to return to work.
- Miss H is a twenty-year-old university student who sustained a moderate brain injury twelve months ago and apparently made a good recovery. Her family have raised concerns with her GP about her mood and her tutors had noted that she is becoming increasingly withdrawn at university. They are concerned about her ability to continue and keep up with her coursework.

Essential to a valid and reliable neuropsychological assessment is a clear sense of why the assessment is being undertaken, and to ensure that the assessment itself has face validity. Educating our referrers about the nature of neuropsychological examination is essential, as this might help them to formulate more specifically which issues need to be addressed. In clinical practice, assessments might be undertaken to address some of the following questions (among others):

- Is there any evidence of brain damage?
- What is the extent of cognitive impairment?
- What is the probable functional impact of any observed cognitive impairment?
- Is there rehabilitation potential?

Furthermore, assessments might be undertaken to address specific issues:

- to establish a baseline for current cognitive functioning and to measure changes over time;
- to assess readiness for return to driving (see Chapter Seven, by Newby);

- to assess readiness for return to work (see Chapter Eight, by Walsh);
- to assess the potential effect of medication on cognitive status;
- to assess cognitive function pre-and post-neurosurgery.

It is possible that an assessment could be conducted as part of establishing an opinion on an individual's mental capacity (for further details, see Chapter Six, by Newby and Ryan-Morgan, in this volume). Alternatively, an assessment could be undertaken to consider the effects of medication on a single subject design.

In summary, a clinical neuropsychological assessment is a specialist assessment that involves the use of clinical interviewing, observation, reviewing clinical records, and psychometric and psychological testing. The assessment should integrate sources of information pertaining to the cognitive, behavioural, and emotional consequences of brain damage. This includes integrating evidence of pathology obtained from diagnostic testing or imaging, with data from the sources outlined above.

Which tests for which clients?

As already stated, a neuropsychological examination will often address a range of questions. The questions themselves will guide the extent of the assessment, the number of markers used, and the depth to which different domains of cognitive functioning are assessed. For example, a screening assessment administered to all patients admitted to a neuro-rehabilitation unit is likely to be a broader but briefer evaluation than an assessment addressing a question concerning differential diagnosis. A wide range of assessment tools are available, including those that seek quickly to assess a range of cognitive functions, through to domain specific tests that will assess certain areas of cognitive function in greater depth. For example, the Addenbrooke's Cognitive Examination (ACE), viewed by some as an extended mini mental state examination, will quickly tap into orientation, memory, verbal fluency, aspects of executive function, and visual–spatial processing. By contrast, more in-depth assessment of, for example, executive function would be addressed through the use of a battery test such as the Dellis–Kaplan Executive Function System (DKEFS). Often, in clinical practice, tests will be chosen to briefly assess specific areas or test hypotheses, and these initial results will guide the clinician as to whether or not more in-depth assessment of a given area is needed. In essence, while the purpose of the assessment will guide the selection of which tests are to be used, so, too, might the patient's cognitive, physical, and communication impairments. Different assessment protocols might, indeed, be suitable for different patients.

Extensive testing using test batteries for different areas of cognitive function are rarely used in the cut and thrust of an active rehabilitation environment where the focus is on functional rehabilitation and where patients are rapidly changing across their inpatient stay (i.e., particularly in acute illness or injury, the client can be recovering or deteriorating rapidly, making an extended assessment out of date before you have the chance to score the tests, feed back the results, and write up the report). It can be helpful to develop your own range of "packages", that is, assessments covering different cognitive functions that can be used as part of a screening assessment. An example of such a package is included in Table 2.1. These tests have been selected on the basis that they are widely available and have reasonable psychometric properties when used in a neuro-rehabilitation setting. The information derived from these assessments is combined with relevant information on personal history, results from previous assessments, use of medication, and any use of controlled substances. These packages can be used as a preliminary assessment, and acknowledge the changing nature of patients' functioning in early recovery, and the role of neuropsychologist in giving a "here and now" opinion (like our medical colleagues). Often, the most useful approach is not necessarily a long, detailed report. A section later in this chapter presents an example of a very brief report that is used to communicate the essential results from a preliminary screening in a clear and straightforward manner. Once an initial assessment is completed, it is important to remain open to the idea of assessment as an evolving process, and to remain curious about a person's strengths and weaknesses. In essence, different aspects of functioning might require testing at different times following an initial assessment, while the initial assessment itself might highlight areas requiring further assessment.

In addition to standard screening assessments that can be used off the shelf for a quick but fairly detailed profile, having a range of other assessments can also be helpful when these standard measures cannot be used: for example, when assessing patients with receptive and expressive communication difficulties.

Table 2.1. Example of assessment package used in routine practice for screening new admission to neuro-rehabilitation unit.

Domain	Test
Pre-morbid ability	Test of Premorbid Function (TOPF-UK) (Wechsler, 2011)
Immediate and delayed verbal and visual memory	BIRT Memory and Information Processing Battery (BMIPB) (Coughlan, Oddy, & Crawford, 2007)—list recall, story recall, figure recall
Working memory	Wechsler Adult Intelligence Scale Version Four (WAIS-IV) (Wechsler, 2010)—digit span
Vision	Visual Object and Space Perception Battery (VOSP) (Warrington & James, 1991)—screening, object decision, position discrimination.
Attention	Trailmaking (Delis–Kaplan Executive Function System (DKEFS) (Delis, Kaplan, & Kramer, 2001)
Speed of thinking	BMIPB—speed of processing
Language	Graded Naming Test (McKenna & Warrington, 1983)
Verbal fluency: lexical and semantic access	FAS; category fluency (DKEFS)
Planning, organisation problem solving	Behavioural Assessment of the Dysexecutive Syndrome (BADS) (Wilson, Alderman, Emslie, & Evans, 1996); Zoo Map Test, Key Search, six elements

Adopting a flexible position, thinking laterally, and a willingness to work in conjunction with other team members is important when assessing patients with, for example, significant communication difficulties. Given the reliance of neuropsychological tests on verbal comprehension and responses, such a package is likely to be more limited and tests might need to be administered in a non-standard way. While this might reduce the reliability of an assessment, it could yield ecologically valid observations that can inform the rehabilitation process. Rather than focusing solely on standard scores or percentiles, qualitative analysis of a patient's performance can provide useful information: for example, the block design task of the WAIS-IV sets certain time limits in which the designs must be replicated. Taking a more flexible approach, allowing a person to continue beyond the time limit imposed by the test might indicate whether the person is, in fact, able to do the task, but just requires more time to complete it. This information can be fed back to the rehabilitation team, who can adapt their approach accordingly.

In order to support assessment of people with communication problems, it is important to have a range of supported communication tools (communication "ramps") available. This could include pictures, alphabet charts, number and time grids, and prompts for common difficulties and concerns following ABI. All these materials can be laminated and stored so that they can be accessed easily without having to reproduce large amounts of material every time. Speech and language therapists might be available to provide support with the assessment process, and could also help with the development of these additional materials. These situations provide excellent opportunities for close interdisciplinary working. There are, of course, also many other areas where adaptation of standard testing procedures and close collaboration with other colleagues might be required, including when working with clients with severe motor impairments or perceptual constraints such as visual or auditory impairment.

The challenges of assessing specific groups

Working with two extremes: the "walking wounded" and the "profoundly impaired"

Working in neuro-rehabilitation exposes the clinical neuropsychologist to patients with a plethora of different problems and presentations. However, we can crudely divide patients into two groups: those amenable to standard forms of assessment and those where such measures cannot be usefully deployed.

On the one hand, there are ABI clients with residual cognitive impairments but who are able to communicate and have some sense of having experienced this trauma (i.e., they have a reasonable level of awareness of the injury and its effects). Lezak, Loring, Hannay, and Fischer (2004) provide invaluable guidance in assessing patients who have this kind of presentation. Indeed, these authors have suggested a general methodology of testing known as the *deficit-testing paradigm*. Clients are often referred because family members and/or work colleagues have noticed cognitive or personality changes in the client some months after the injury. Once you have made a thorough clinical assessment, involving interviews of the client and at least one person close to the client (to get an alternative view of how a brain injured client is actually functioning—essential if insight is poor), formal testing can begin. Standard tests can then be wheeled out, in order to clarify further the cognitive and other problems that are presented.

On the other hand, there are those clients who present as so severely impaired (e.g., gaining labels such as low awareness state, including, but not limited to, persistent vegetative state, minimally conscious state, "locked in" syndrome, and other similar low awareness states that have not necessarily been formally diagnosed). This is more fully discussed by Crawford Thomas in Chapter Five of this volume. However, in the context of this chapter, the following suggestions are presented. The clinician should make an initial screening of the client's cognitive status, behaviour, and emotional processing. It is important that the person being assessed is reasonably medically stable. At the very least, this means that the person's other injuries (for there are usually many) are at least stable, and that no infections or viruses are present. Also, you must consider the potential medication effects on their neuropsychological presentation. Primarily, this screening begins with clinical interviews. Of necessity, these should include as minimum the patient, significant others, and clinicians who have had direct contact with the patient. As at this end of the continuum, micro-observation and reporting become essential ingredients for a successful assessment. It is during this process that sounds/utterances or groans, eye opening (and tracking), motoric displays, and other seemingly trivial, or at least infrequent and often indistinct, behavioural patterning becomes crucial. Once again, it is the *individual* in front of you that you are seeking to understand better.

In some cases, it might well be that, based on these early observations, a particular standardised measure may be employed, such as the Wessex Head Injury Matrix (WHIM) (Shiel, Wilson, McLellan, Horn, & Watson, 2000). This formally assesses the emergence from severe head injury and, while it cannot specify exact cognitive difficulties, its natural recovery curve and associated behavioural repertoires can provide clues to what to do next as a clinician: more of that later. At this point, it might be that the clinician seeks/carries out a formal assessment of the client's ability to respond to sensory stimuli using the Sensory Modality and Assessment Technique (SMART) (Gill-Thwaites & Munday, 1999). Again, please see Chapter Five, by Crawford Thomas, in this volume for a more detailed account. One of the cornerstones of the assessment should be the recommendation for the level of stimulation allowable in the environment (including the "dosage" of family and therapeutic input).

Clients who do not easily fit into either extreme: the people in the middle

Most experienced practitioners would be struck by how many of their clients do not fit neatly into "textbook" categories or descriptions. Ironically, potentially the most satisfying patients to assess and work with are those that, by their very complex needs, cannot be easily categorised and, therefore, cannot be assessed by means of a "standard" or "routine" test battery. For the purposes of illustration, a case will be presented that encapsulates a number of the difficulties that have been outlined above and which clinicians who work in neuro-rehabilitation meet on a fairly routine basis. The case is an amalgam of a number of cases recently seen by one of the contributors.

> Patient WG was referred to the unit to assess his potential for rehabilitation. He was a forty-two-year-old man who had sustained a severe TBI (GCS 3, Coma >4 weeks) and cardiac arrest as a result of car accident some six months previously. Subsequently, he developed a very severe (Grade V) post-trauma sub-arachnoid haemorrhage. He was thought to remain in post-trauma amnesia (PTA). In any ABI assessment, severity of injury is useful to get a sense of the associated neuro-anatomical damage; however, it is essential to get more than one indicator to provide a more refined overall estimate of severity. At referral, we wondered how much hypoxic damage had occurred due to the subsequent cardiac arrest—estimates varied between a few minutes and fifteen minutes without oxygen. As a clinician, hypoxic injuries often (although not always, owing to differences in age, patency of blood vessels, etc.) can lead you to suspect problems with attention and memory.
>
> The CT head scans report stated evidence of "diffuse cerebral oedema in keeping with hypoxic brain injury, some abnormal hypo-density within

the white matter of the frontal lobes near the midline, right frontal craniotomy, subarachnoid haemorrhage in the peri-callosal region, two lacunar infarcts within the right caudate nucleus . . ." Apart from the difficulties in understanding the technical language,[1] there are a number of obvious things that are shown by these results. First, it confirmed more significant hypoxia than the original notes suggested. Second, the white matter (or architectural wiring of the brain) damage suggested ordinary communication between the frontal lobes and the rest of the brain might be affected in addition to the damage that might have occurred more directly due to the craniotomy. Remember, even blood in the wrong place in the brain acts as an irritant to brain tissue. Third, peri-callosal damage (depending on the extent) can produce further disruptions in the ability to communicate within the brain. Classically, this damage can present as various forms of callosalapraxias. Finally, the sites of the infarcts suggest (due to the implications of being at the head of the caudate nucleus) possible further unusual motoric problems. While all of the foregoing is not supposed to be definitive or seen in isolation, it is part of the picture that needs to be built up of the individual that you are assessing, as all these data facilitate the generation of ongoing hypothesis testing.

Prior to the injury the above client was described as a happy, outgoing person who worked as a security consultant undertaking work for multinational companies. He was educated to post-graduate Masters-degree level. He was a devoted family man with an apparently happy relationship with his wife and four children. He had no other reported health problems. This recent health issue was viewed as a catastrophe for his family and himself. The weight of the emotional impact was felt by all those who had worked with him and his family prior to admission. Mr WG was on a range of medication, some of which could potentially have had some cognitive or other neuropsychological side-effects. These included Tizanidine, used for treating muscle spasm and spasticity, Citalopram, an antidepressant, Phenytoin, Carbamazepine, and Clonazepam, anticonvulsant drugs.

He was said to experience considerable fatigue. Confederate reports suggested further difficulties with initiation, mobilising safely, hypersensitivity, double incontinence, poor sleeping, unusual left arm movements, and visual problems (that could have been left-sided visual inattention, field deficits, or frank blindness). He was also reported to be preservative, disorientated to time, place, or context. He appeared to have adequate short-term memory but had poor delayed memory for new material, and limited but improving insight. He was said to confabulate and appeared to have better expressive than receptive conversation skills. He challenged staff at the referring hospital a great deal, particularly during personal care, when he would swear, shout, and attempt to hit out on frequent occasions. Staff did not appear to know whether he was depressed, anxious, or both. He could not feed himself and staff considered him to have "given up", with the staff resorting to feeding him themselves.

The above suggests so many different possible hypotheses and potential avenues for investigation that you must try to filter through the possibilities and refine your ideas.

With this in mind, it is important to work as a team. Within the first few weeks after admission, the team decided to focus on medication issues and to consider the impact these might be having on his presentation. A phased withdrawal of Citalopram was initiated, alongside a reduction in the anti-seizure medication; the muscle relaxant was changed to an alternative with potentially slightly less impact on cognitive functions. During the period of medication changes, and then for another sustained period after these had been stabilised, behavioural observations, recordings, and interviews (with staff and significant others) were undertaken in order to understand his "natural" fatigue profile and sleep–wake cycle. At this point, apart from basic care, no other therapeutic intervention was allowed to ensure (as best as was practicable) that a clear baseline of these fundamental processes was obtained to facilitate the team's understanding of Mr WG's continually evolving clinical presentation.

Diagnostic and presenting complexities

As if the motivations and understandings of the referrers, the contexts of the referral, and the severity of the brain injury is not enough, we also need to consider the effect of the myriad different diagnoses and problems that clients bring with them. These can be problems such as pre-existing long-standing mental health issues, as well as the likes of pain and marital instability that have arisen since the brain injury. As stated earlier in this chapter, it would be impossible to cover every possible angle. We hope the following sub-sections will stand as a good orientation to these complexities.

Considering the role of challenging behaviour

Challenging behaviour has been defined as those behaviours

> of such an intensity, frequency or duration that the physical safety of the person or others is likely to be placed in serious jeopardy, or behaviour which is likely to seriously limit use of, or result in the person being denied access to, ordinary community facilitates. (Emerson, 2001, p. 3)

This might include behaviour such as self-harm, verbal and physical aggression, or self-stimulation. Current thinking often emphasises such behaviours come from a poor fit between the person's needs and the environment. Furthermore, consideration is given to the underlying function of the behaviour: that is, what purpose is this behaviour serving? Typically, the behaviour might represent a way of communicating some form of unmet need, be it boredom, hunger, pain, or difficulty regulating mood/arousal. It is helpful to remember that when a patient causes a problem for you, they are usually trying to solve a problem for themselves.

In practice, the use of decision-making pathways can help those working with the team to clarify the role of the neuropsychologist in the assessment and management of challenging behaviour. An example of such a pathway is included in Figure 2.2.

Typically, incidents of challenging behaviour have been assessed using observation and 'ABC' recording charts. In practice, ABC recording charts provide the opportunity to gather essential information towards understanding challenging behaviour, yet are rarely completed, and the information included on these charts is either irrelevant or incomplete. In order to address these issues, the use of "tick chart" recording sheets (see boxed text on p. 52 for example) can be useful. These charts are quicker to complete, making them more appealing to a busy team, can be tailored to the individual person, and provide more focused information. The use of the tick chart provides prompts for the team member as to the sort of information is required.

Which is the greater problem? Being asked about differential diagnosis

One of the most common questions in a neuropsychology outpatient clinic will be the extent to which the patient's presentation reflects

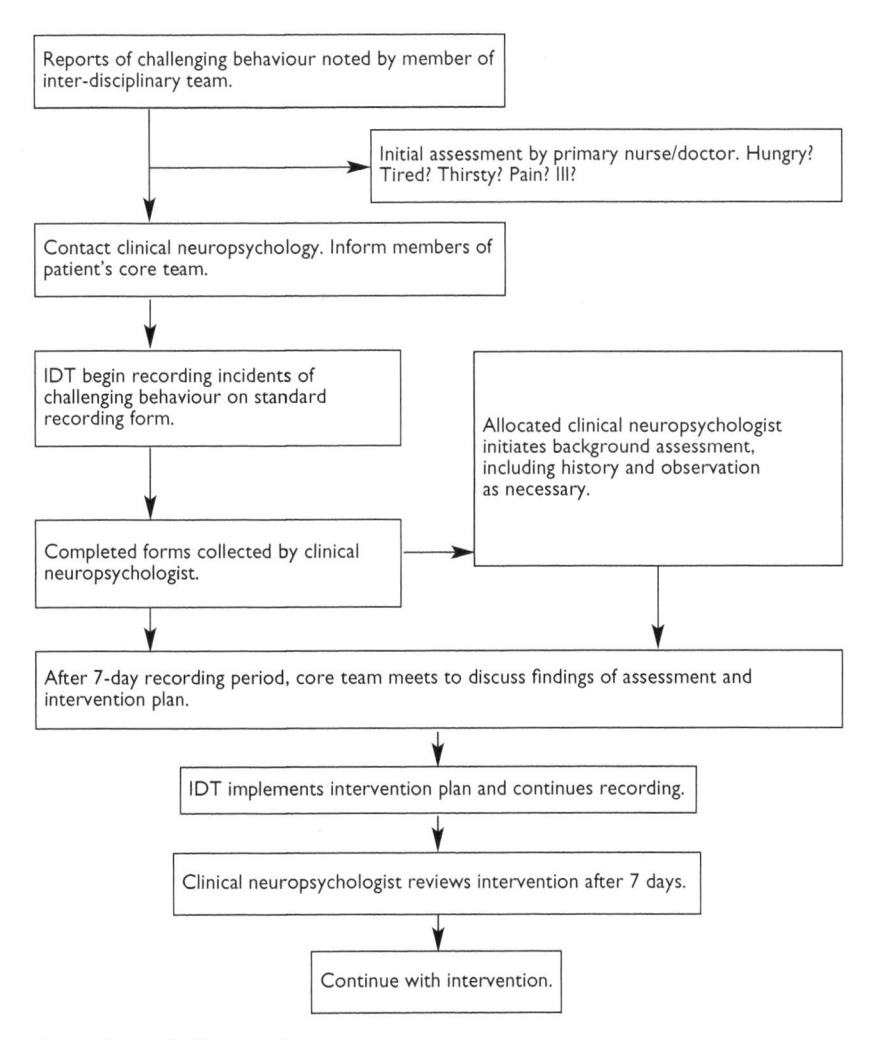

```
┌─────────────────────────────────────┐
│ Reports of challenging behaviour    │
│ noted by member of                  │
│ inter-disciplinary team.            │
└─────────────────────────────────────┘
         │         ┌──────────────────────────────────────┐
         │────────▶│ Initial assessment by primary        │
         │         │ nurse/doctor. Hungry? Tired?         │
         ▼         │ Thirsty? Pain? Ill?                  │
┌─────────────────────────────────────┐└──────────────────────────────────────┘
│ Contact clinical neuropsychology.   │
│ Inform members of patient's core    │
│ team.                               │
└─────────────────────────────────────┘
         ▼
┌──────────────────────────┐
│ IDT begin recording      │
│ incidents of challenging │      ┌──────────────────────────────┐
│ behaviour on standard    │      │ Allocated clinical           │
│ recording form.          │      │ neuropsychologist initiates  │
└──────────────────────────┘      │ background assessment,       │
         ▼                        │ including history and        │
┌──────────────────────────┐      │ observation as necessary.    │
│ Completed forms          │─────▶└──────────────────────────────┘
│ collected by clinical    │
│ neuropsychologist.       │
└──────────────────────────┘
         ▼                                    ▼
┌─────────────────────────────────────────────────────────────────┐
│ After 7-day recording period, core team meets to discuss        │
│ findings of assessment and intervention plan.                   │
└─────────────────────────────────────────────────────────────────┘
                               ▼
          ┌──────────────────────────────────────────────┐
          │ IDT implements intervention plan and         │
          │ continues recording.                         │
          └──────────────────────────────────────────────┘
                               ▼
          ┌──────────────────────────────────────────────┐
          │ Clinical neuropsychologist reviews           │
          │ intervention after 7 days.                   │
          └──────────────────────────────────────────────┘
                               ▼
                  ┌────────────────────────────┐
                  │ Continue with intervention.│
                  └────────────────────────────┘
```

Figure 2.2. Challenging behaviour pathway.

organic brain injury or a secondary psychological reaction to their brain injury. A fairly typical case is detailed below.

A case example

> A sixty-five-year-old gentleman attended a university teaching hospital neuro-triage clinic for a day assessment. He had been referred by his GP, who essentially posed the differential diagnostic question of depression

Challenging behaviour recording chart

Name:

Date: Time:

        Please complete this chart as soon after the incident as possible

Description of behaviour:

Location:

Others present:

Environment
(tick all that apply)

Noisy ☐	Crowded ☐	Hot ☐	Quiet ☐
Empty ☐	Cold ☐		

Other:

Precipitating events (i.e. what happened just before the behaviour?)
(tick all that apply)

End of therapy session ☐	Task started ☐	Family/friends visited ☐
Start of therapy session ☐	Task ended ☐	Review meeting ☐
Rest period ☐	Drug round ☐	Personal care ☐

Other:

Consequences (i.e., what happened just after the behaviour?)
(tick all that apply)

Stopped task ☐	Moved to different room ☐	Ignored ☐
Offered break ☐	TV/radio turned off ☐	Offered food or drink ☐

Discussed impact of behaviour ☐

Other:

Completed by

Name:

Department:

and/or dementia. The clinic offered a psychiatric state evaluation, a physical neurological examination, and a reasonably detailed cognitive examination conducted by a clinical neuropsychologist. His wife had attended the beginning of his triage appointment with him. She did not report any particular problems with memory or cognition in her husband, but felt that he had become somewhat fussy and obsessive around the house since his retirement and that he was less tolerant with his grandchildren and would often withdraw to another room when family visited. All of this she felt was out of character. The gentleman's performance on assessment was consistent with his scholastic and vocational history when he was seen by the neuropsychologist. Towards the end of the assessment, he complained of feeling hot and thirsty and was asked if he would like some water. The neuropsychologist left the consulting room to get some water. On his return, he was surprised to find that the patient had removed all his clothes with the exception of his boxer shorts. The client was reassured and encouraged to re-dress and the examination was concluded. It was customary for the clinicians involved in the triage to meet at the end of the day and discuss the patients assessed. Each discipline reported their findings and suggested formulations. The psychiatric registrar reported the client had recently retired and that his change in mood might be adjustment-related. The neurologist had found no focal signs, with the exception of some difficulty on a hand movement task. The clinical neuropsychologist fed back the pre-morbid-consistent test performance, but noted the client's unusual behaviour—much to the surprise of his colleagues. The neuropsychologist suggested that the behaviour could have been due to an inability to regulate impulses. Subsequent neuroradiological investigation revealed a fronto-temporal dementia. In this clinical case, behaviour, not initial medical examination or psychometric test results, had been the strongest clinical indicator.

The complex interplay of organic and so-called "non organic" factors is often debated in clinical and medico–legal practice. However, in everyday clinical practice, endlessly seeking definitive evidence of the relative contributions of such factors could easily bog you down. To quote our old friend Winnicott (1965), your assessment just needs to be "good enough" to pick up the range of things affecting your client's life. Use that information to formulate a treatment plan with the client to prioritise which cognitive and psychological issues to tackle first (e.g., you might need to work on mood first and then tackle memory, or tackle both at the same time).

One area that has received a great deal of attention (particularly within medico–legal claims) is that of post-concussion syndrome. Whatever the clinical debates regarding post-concussion syndrome, it is broadly accepted that mild organic dysfunction is not uncommon in both in the early days and the first few months following mild/minor head injury. During this time, both new psychological features can develop and pre-existing ones can be reactivated. In some cases, the post-concussion syndrome symptoms can persist. When the syndrome does persist, for some individuals the psychological features will entirely account for the symptoms. In others, it is the organic features that account for the symptoms (King, 2003). It is important to point out that similar symptoms, but with different aetiological processes, might present in different cases and possibly within a single individual at different times following a head injury. For example, when a patient begins to doubt the possibility of recovery, or when, as many have argued, issues surrounding compensation claims are present, self-doubt, low mood, and anxiety can be major factors. In the vast majority of cases, post concussion syndrome is unlikely to be at either end of the psychological or organic continuum. What is important is that clients who present with persisting and disabling post-concussion syndromes receive individualised formulations of their particular problems in order to facilitate rehabilitation.

There is a range of differential diagnostic questions after critical life events such as brain injuries. Clients can present with adjustment difficulties, mood disturbance, and, on occasion, serious post-trauma mental health issues such as psychosis, severe depression, and anxiety disorders (such as post-trauma stress). It is also important to remember that some of the early medical and rehabilitation interventions can be highly traumatising themselves, and that effect can be particularly distressing for clients who might have no recollection of their accident or of how they have sustained their injuries. The possibility of post-trauma stress in relation to treatments is frequently overlooked.

Dual and multiple diagnoses

Experienced readers will be only too familiar with a caseload of highly complex clients who bring not only two, but sometimes three or more additional diagnosable areas of clinical focus. Each of these difficulties such as substance misuse, alcoholism, anxiety, depression, post traumatic stress disorder (PTSD) are challenging enough to services in their own right. Mix them up with volatile difficulties brought by the acquired brain injury, then you have often got a pretty explosive mix that is exhausting for the practitioner, deeply worrying for families, but, most importantly, isolating and confusing for clients.

A dual diagnosis, or set of additional diagnoses, could include almost anything. As well as the difficulties described above, one could easily include additional neurological difficulties, such as dementia or multiple sclerosis, and any chronic or acute medical condition, such as diabetes or heart attack. It would be impossible to cover all of these additional difficulties, so we have chosen to focus mostly on the Axis 1 disorders as described by the *DSM-IV* (American Psychiatric Association, 2000), that is, the usual suspects of depression, anxiety, personality problems, drugs, alcohol, and pain, as our main points of focus.

Multiple diagnoses: a case example

> Robert. How many of you have somebody who is like Robert on your caseload? Robert is a twenty-two-year-old unemployed male living in a socio-economically deprived area in the North West of England. His home circumstances are extremely volatile; his mother has her own mental health difficulties—principally depression. He has long verbal arguments with his mother and sister and they are threatening to throw him out. He had an extremely poor education and had periods of refusing to attend school. He briefly did well in a specialist educational establishment where he was able to form a strong bond with the headmaster. He began to do well and to consider vocational qualifications. However, in his mid-teens he became involved with substance abuse (cannabis and cocaine), which led to him being expelled from school. He began to drink heavily and became involved in a fight outside a pub, during which he was knocked unconscious and sustained a traumatic head injury.
>
> Following the traumatic brain injury, Robert attempted to re-start his life of substance abuse. However, he quickly found that he could not "hold his drink" and became extremely violent whenever he drank; he did, however, resume taking cocaine and cannabis. After briefly seeking support from the community brain injury service, where the "headmasterly" relationship was rekindled with the consultant neuropsychologist, Robert

began not to attend appointments and became extremely erratic. He was arrested for assault . . .

The type of challenges that Robert presents to us in the case history set out above will be all too familiar for many of us. He is extremely difficult to engage, we have a brief window of involvement before he "disappears", falls between services in a journey towards police, courts, and possible imprisonment. He is somebody with whom, as a clinician, you can spend lots of time on the phone, talking to him, liaising with his family, talking to services, setting up appointments, and waiting in vain. At this stage in his life, he can only seem to disappoint.

What does the literature tell us about dual/multiple diagnoses?

For the past twenty to thirty years, there has been a burgeoning descriptive literature looking at the long-term consequences of significant traumatic brain injury. From the early works of Brooks and others (e.g., Brooks, Campsie, Beattie, & McKinlay, 1986; Brooks, McKinlay, Symington, Beattie, & Campsie, 1987), mood disturbance leads to poorer rehabilitation outcome, increased functional disability, reduced employment, probable increase of divorce, and increased carer burden. While there is clear agreement that *DSM-IV*'s Axis 1 difficulties do exist in significant proportions post traumatic brain injury, there is a singular lack of agreement on the sorts of prevalence rates that one might expect. Prevalence rates appear to range from under ten per cent to over eighty per cent (Hibbard, Uysal, Kepler, Bogdany, & Silva, 1998). As both Hibbard and collaborators and also Bowen and colleagues (e.g., Bowen, Chamberlain, Tennant, Neumann, & Conner, 1999; Bowen, Neumann, Conner, Tennant, & Chamberlain, 1998) confirm, a great deal of the variability is probably down to the ways in which prevalence rates are recorded and both the assessment measures and the type of recording that is undertaken. These can range from clinical judgement to carer report to self-report questionnaires. Even within the self-report questionnaires, there are concerns about confounds such as motor symptoms in measures such as the Beck Depression Inventory and cognitive confounds in the Hospital Anxiety and Depression Scale (e.g., I feel more slowed down). Looking at individual studies, some report that having a pre-existing substance abuse or mood disorder or mood symptoms can increase the likelihood of psychiatric difficulties (e.g., see Brenner et al., 2008 on a study of US veterans). Other studies, however, suggest that having no pre-existing psychiatric or substance abuse history can increase the likelihood of psychiatric difficulties after brain injury, for example, Hibbard, Uysal, Kepler, Bogdany, and Silva, 1998.

Comprehensive literature review articles of pain (Nampiaparampil, 2008) and substance misuse (Parry-Jones, Vaughan, & Cox, 2006) report similarly ambivalent relationships between these variables and traumatic brain injury.

What, then, can the clinician make from the morass of ambivalent findings?

1. Recognise that the literature is useful but might not always be totally transferable to your situation. It is true to say that much of it is developed from US military veterans, those that attend trauma centres, and that the presentations investigated are often mixed with PTSD. While it is important that we can and should call for a greater UK-based literature, the issues are not so absolutely different that we cannot tell anything from the predominant literature. The literature reviewed gives a clear indication that significant numbers of people you will see in an ABI population will additionally have significant other problems. It would be good to have a greater UK data, but let us not be precious about it.
2. It is important to get familiar with the review literature. Over the past decade or so, significant comprehensive database-style reviews (Cochrane) have addressed issues of multiple diagnoses. Interested readers would do well to look at reviews on depression (e.g., Fleminger, Oliver, Williams, & Evans, 2003), anxiety (e.g., Allgulander, 2010), pain (e.g., Nampiaparampil, 2008) and substance misuse (e.g., Parry-Jones, Vaughan, & Cox, 2006).
3. Within traditional research paradigms, many of the associated findings are weak trends. Although there are a number of consistent findings, such as higher base rates within ABI populations of psychiatric disorder (e.g., Corrigan & Deutschle, 2008), pain, and substance misuse than the general population, there are often few strong associations with traumatic brain injury and ambiguous findings (possibly because milder traumatic brain injuries get more psychopathologies).

Why is this? There are the usual limitations of research in acquired brain injury. Clear results are concealed/minimised by the heterogeneity of the populations: that is, within the usual definition of acquired brain injury lies a plethora of different conditions having an impact on a variety of people with different backgrounds. This is undoubtedly true. However, a review by Bjork and Grant (2009) on substance misuse alerts us to the fact that the research process in many studies actually excludes people with dual diagnosis (Slewa-Younan et al., 2008). Further, the research that focuses on ABI often excludes substance misuse or people with psychiatric problems, as these problems "confound" the area under question. As a parallel, researchers looking at the cognitive effects of illegal substances will specifically exclude ABI. In many ways, the published research does not always reflect the reality of clinical working in the real world; you cannot necessarily assess someone and then refuse to treat them because they have more than one diagnosis![2] Additionally, clients might acquire these additional diagnoses during the course of our work with them, despite our best efforts, and once a relationship has been established, it is much harder to terminate.

4. The co-morbidity is real. Studies such as Williams, Cordan, Mewse, Tonks, and Burgess (2010) looked at 197 UK young offenders and found forty-six per cent had a traumatic brain injury. Over thirty per cent of that population had more than one traumatic brain injury and this was often correlated with a violent offence, as well as substance misuse and psychiatric problems. Further, in the US literature, Sacks and colleagues (2009) report up to fifty per cent of a population using a drug and alcohol services in New York had six plus or minus two blows to the head. They recommend, as the traumatic brain injury can often be missed, the use of sensitive tools. It also worth noting that underlying drug or alcohol use or offending behaviour can often be masked by the severity of the disability or close supervision that people experience when in a rehabilitation unit (Bjork & Grant, 2009). However, when out in the community, "where there is a will there is a way". For example, from my own experience (GN) I am aware of a wheelchair-dependent substance abuser who is regularly able to obtain cannabis through the postal system.

5. The pre-morbid history of someone is informative and predictive; unfortunately, across each of the additional diagnoses that this section focuses on, there is a pretty stable finding that an ABI does not necessarily stop a client from resuming their psychiatric or substance misuse career and might even exacerbate it.
6. Trauma is a moderator. Having PTSD or being involved in a trauma increases your risk of a co-morbid condition if you also have a traumatic brain injury.

What can we do about it?

From the above, we feel that the following is necessary.

- Have sensitive screening tools across specialities that allow you to pick up significant brain injury as well as the co-morbid psychiatric and pain conditions.
- Develop joint working protocols across specialities. This would limit the experience of clients being jettisoned by one service because they happen to have the other diagnosis.
- Develop clear client and family information about the specific issues and difficulties associated with having an ABI and alcohol (e.g., Brain Injury Rehabilitation Trust's (BIRT) excellent leaflet, *Alcohol Following Brain Injury*, 2011; Brown & Thompson, 2011) and cannabis.
- There is a strong need to develop clear adapted treatment guidelines to help work across specialities and for people with dual diagnosis (e.g., British Geriatrics Society, 2011). Substance misuse treatment guidelines can also be adapted along the lines shown in Chapter Three in this volume.
- There is a need for more research in the area. We know this is a hoary old chestnut, but it is true, not least in respect of the need to have a greater UK dataset that reflects UK NHS environmental conditions.

Feeding back assessment results

Feeding back and reporting the results of neuropsychological assessment is a core part of the process of assessment. Yet, it is often overlooked or neglected, and, accordingly, the potential for delivering feedback in a collaborative way that fosters engagement and develops the therapeutic relationship can be missed. It can be helpful to establish early on with the client the most helpful way of feeding back assessment results. During testing, it is helpful to clarify that it is not possible to give the results of the assessment at the end of the session, and that it can take some time to objectively score and formulate the results of an assessment. In considering feedback of results, three components need to be given attention: the purpose of the feedback, the audience to which the feedback is directed, and the approach and mode in which the feedback is given. Gorske and Smith (2009) offer a comprehensive model for conducting neuropsychological assessment feedback, based on the principles of motivational interviewing and Rogerian counselling, that some readers might find useful.

Discussing the results of an assessment, whether with a client or team might fulfil a number of purposes. At the most basic level, it is the client's opportunity to receive the results of the assessments that they have expended considerable effort in completing. At another level, it represents an opportunity to raise awareness of a client's cognitive problems, particularly valuable where there are issues associated with reduced insight. It can be used to highlight a person's residual strengths, since too often feedback focuses exclusively on a person's weaknesses and difficulties, potentially reinforcing appraisals of loss and engendering a sense of hopelessness. Furthermore, discussion of results from the assessment presents an opportunity to discuss the rationale for the intervention that will follow. Having a greater understanding of the rationale for intervention is likely to foster greater engagement and subsequent generalisation of therapeutic gains to other environments.

It is possible that assessment results might need to be communicated to a range of different audiences, including the patient, his/her family, the multi-disciplinary rehabilitation team, and other professionals. Common considerations for each of the above is to ensure that the results are communicated in a way that is understandable, with as little use of jargon as possible. Crucial to meeting the needs and expectations of all is that the information is communicated in a straightforward way. Rather than making statements such as, "there was evidence of impairment in immediate verbal recall", comments such as "might have difficulty remembering new information" are likely to be more accessible. The probable functional impact of impairments identified through assessment should be highlighted (but placed in perspective), and there should be discussion of the impact these impairments could have for both rehabilitation and day-to-day functioning. For example, this could include noting that a person's memory difficulties might be reflected in everyday life as forgetfulness, and that the use of written lists to support physiotherapy sessions, or a written checklist to organise performance on functional tasks, is recommended.

It is important to pay attention to the mode in which feedback is delivered. Results are often given verbally, but written summaries might be required to support retention of relevant information. Not surprisingly, there is a body of research suggesting that brain injured clients struggle to recall the content of hospital and primary care consultations (e.g., McKinstry et al., 2011). However, as the McKinstry research group points out, even those without brain injury can have limited recall of such discussions, particularly when multiple and complex issues are being discussed. Recall is better, however, for non-brain-injured clients in more relaxed primary care settings if topics are discussed sparingly and simply. Although standard neuro-rehabilitation practice would guide you to backing up oral discussions routinely with additional written material, McKinstry and colleagues (2011) suggest further larger-scale research needs to be carried out to confirm such an assumed beneficial effect in clinical consultations.

Following the feedback session, a letter might be written to the patient, summarising the results and the discussion that took place about them, highlighting strengths, impairments, and recommendations for managing these problems. However, anyone who has ever provided a patient with assessment feedback will know that this is often far from straightforward. For many reasons, our clients can find honest feedback difficult to accept, and we might find ourselves bordering on an "argument" where each party tries to convince the other of the "truth" of the situation. It can be helpful in your post-assessment feedback summary letter to factually draw attention to such areas of disagreement between the therapist and the client (e.g., if a client has been unaccepting of the conclusions you have drawn); this offers a non-challenging way of opening up further conversations about these areas of possible conflict and the possible reasons behind the disparity.

Using standard forms to communicate feedback to the rehabilitation team can be a helpful way of summarising a large amount of information in a succinct manner, an example of which is shown in the boxed text below.

Example of summary report for neuropsychological assessment

Clinical neuropsychology assessment summary

This document summarises the results of a preliminary screening assessment and, as such, the results reported here are provisional.

Name: Date of assessment:

DOB: Assessed by:

NHS No: Job Title:

Summary of results

Estimated premorbid intellectual ability:

	Clear evidence of impairment	Evidence suggestive of impairment	Grossly normal	Not assessed
Memory Vision Language Speed of thinking Executive skills				

Further testing required: YES/NO
If yes, areas to be assessed:

Comments:

Mood assessment

Distress thermometer rating: /100

Identified concerns:

1.

2.

3.

4.

(continued)

Plan
1.
2.
3.
4.
Implications for rehabilitation
If you have any queries please contact the Department of Clinical Neuropsychology on:
Summary completed by:
Name:
Job title:
Date:

Conclusions

Neuropsychological assessment represents a broad area of clinical enquiry, drawing upon many sources of data, and requires considerable skill to integrate and interpret in a clinically meaningful way. Ultimately, the purpose of neuropsychological assessment is to inform the rehabilitation of our clients. Good rehabilitative practice is to examine cognition in its very broadest sense, by including observation and recording of the behavioural, emotional, social, and functional presentation of individuals who have suffered brain injury and/or neurological illness.

Critical to the assessment process is obtaining a detailed history of the patient, qualitative observation of their functioning and the data available from neuroimaging and other clinical and diagnostic procedures. This chapter has attempted to give a flavour of how clinical neuropsychologists deploying models of brain–behaviour relationships, assessment skills, and formulation can help determine the cognitive and/or neuro-behavioural functioning of individuals following brain injury or neurological illness with a view to informing their ongoing rehabilitation.

Notes

1. We recommend the novice clinician learn as much as they can about these by visiting friendly radiology departments.
2. Although, of course, such active substance misuse might well make any attempted rehabilitation pointless and be a *de facto* exclusion criteria for your service.

References

Allgulander, C. (2010). Morbid anxiety as a risk factor in patients with somatic diseases: a review of recent findings. *European Neurological Journal*, 2(1): 31–39.

American Psychiatric Association (2000). *Diagnostic and Statistical Manual of Mental Disorders, 4th edn (DSM-IV)*. Washington, DC: American Psychiatric Association.

Bjork, J. M., & Grant, S. J. (2009). Does traumatic brain injury increase risk for substance abuse? *Journal of Neurotrauma*, 26: 1077–1082.

Bowen, A., Chamberlain, M. A., Tennant, A., Neumann, V., & Conner, M. (1999). The persistence of mood disorders following traumatic brain injury: a 1 year follow-up. *Brain Injury*, 13: 547–553.

Bowen, A., Neumann, V., Conner, M., Tennant, A., & Chamberlain, M. A. (1998). Mood disorders following traumatic brain injury: identifying the extent of the problem and the people at risk. *Brain Injury*, 12: 177–190.

Bowen, M. (1980). Key to the use of the genogram. In: E. A. Carter & M. McGoldrick (Eds.), *The Family Life Cycle: A Framework for Family Therapy* (p. xxiii). New York: Gardner.

Brain Injury Rehabilitation Trust (2011). Alcohol Following Brain Injury. Leaflet, electronic version: www.birt.co.uk/images/BIRT%20-%20 Alcohol%20Following%20Brain%20Injury.pdf. Accessed 27 May, 2011.

Brenner, L. A., Harwood, J. E., Homaifar, B. Y., Cawthra, E., Waldman, J., & Adler, L. E. (2008). Psychiatric hospitalization and veterans with traumatic brain injury: a retrospective study. *Journal of Head Trauma Rehabilitation*, 23(6): 401–406.

British Geriatrics Society (2011). Use of antidepressants following acquired brain injury. Electronic version: www.bgs.org.uk/index. php?option=com_content&view=article&id=311%3Aantidepressantsabi&catid=42%3Acatclinguidelines&Itemid=107&limitstart. Accessed 27 May 2011.

British Psychological Society (2009). Assessment of effort in clinical testing of cognitive functioning for adults. Electronic version: www.bps.org.uk/sites/default/files/documents/assessment_of_effort_in_clinical_testing_of_cognitive_functioning_for_adults.pdf. Accessed 21 December 2011.

Brooks, N., Campsie, L., Symington, C., Beattie, A., & McKinlay, W. (1986). The five-year outcome of severe blunt head injury: a relative's view. *Journal of Neurology, Neurosurgery, and Psychiatry, 49*: 764–770.

Brooks, N., McKinlay, W., Symington, C., Beattie, A., & Campsie, L. (1987). Return to work within the first seven years of severe head injury. *Brain Injury, 1*: 5–19.

Brown, P., & Thompson, J. (2011). Brain injury, drugs and alcohol. Electronic article, Brain Injury Rehabilitation Trust: www.birt.co.uk/content.asp?page_id=616. Accessed 27 May 2011.

Chaytor, N., Temkin, N., Machamer, J., & Dikmen, S. (2007). The ecological validity of neuropsychological assessment and the role of depressive symptoms in moderate to severe traumatic brain injury. *Journal of the International Neuropsychological Society, 13*: 1–9.

Christie, N., Savill, T., Buttress, S., Newby, G., & Tyerman, A. (2001). Assessing fitness to drive after head injury: a survey of clinical psychologists. *Neuropsychological Rehabilitation, 11*(1): 45–55.

Coezter, R. (2010). *Anxiety and Mood Disorders following Traumatic Brain Injury: Clinical Assessment and Psychotherapy*. London: Karnac.

Collicutt-McGrath, J. (2007). *Ethical Practice in Brain Injury Rehabilitation*. Oxford: Oxford University Press.

Corrigan, J. D., & Deutschle, J. J (2008). The presence and impact of traumatic brain injury among clients in treatment for co-occurring mental illness and substance abuse. *Brain Injury, 22*(3): 223–231.

Coughlan, A. K., Oddy, M., & Crawford, J. R. (2007). BIRT Memory and Information Processing Battery. Horsham: BIRT.

Delis, D. C., Kaplan, E., & Kramer, J. H. (2001). *The Delis–Kaplan Executive Function System*. San Antonio, TX: Harcourt Assessment, The Psychological Corporation.

Emerson, E. (2001). *Challenging Behaviour: Analysis and Intervention in People with Severe Intellectual Disabilities*. Cambridge: Cambridge University Press.

Fleminger, S., Oliver, D. L.,Williams, W. H., & Evans, J. (2003). The neuropsychiatry of depression after brain injury. *Neuropsychological Rehabilitation*, 13(1–2): 65–87.

Gill-Thwaites, H., & Munday, R. (1999). The Sensory Modality Assessment and Rehabilitation Technique (SMART): a comprehensive and integrated assessment and treatment protocol for the vegetative state and minimally responsive patient. *Neuropsychological Rehabilitation*, 9: 305–320.

Gorske, T. T., & Smith, S. R. (2009). *Collaborative Therapeutic Neuropsychological Assessment*. Springer: New York.

Gurd, J., Kischka, U., & Marshall, J. (2010). *The Handbook of Clinical Neuropsychology* (2nd edn). Oxford: Oxford University Press.

Hibbard M. R., Uysal, S., Kepler, K., Bogdany, J., & Silver, J. (1998). Axis I psychopathology in individuals with traumatic brain injury. *Journal of Head Trauma Rehabilitation*, 13(4): 24–39.

King, N. S. (2003). Post-concussion syndrome: clarity amid the controversy? *British Journal of Psychiatry*, 183: 276–278.

Lezak, M. D., Loring, D.W., Hannay, H. J., & Fischer, J. S. (2004). *Neuropsychological Assessment* (4th edn). [[CITY, STATE]]: Oxford University Press.

McGoldrick, M., Gerson, R., & Shellenberger, S. (1999). *Genograms: Assessment and Intervention*. New York: Norton.

McKenna, P., & Warrington, E. K. (1983). *Graded Naming Test*. Windsor: NFER-Nelson.

McKinstry, B., Watson, P., Elton, R. A., Pinnock, H., Kidd, G., Meyer, B., Logie, R., & Sheikh, A. (2011). Comparison of the accuracy of patients' recall of the content of telephone and face-to-face consultations: an exploratory study. *Postgraduate Medical Journal*, 87: 394–399.

Nampiaparampil, D. E. (2008). Prevalence of chronic pain after traumatic brain injury: a systematic review. *Journal of the American Medical Association*, 300(6): 711–719.

Odhuba, R. A., van den Broek, M. D., & Johns, L. C. (2005). Ecological validity of measures of executive functioning. *British Journal of Clinical Psychology*, 44: 269–278.

Parry-Jones, B. L., Vaughan, F. L., & Cox, W. M. (2006). Traumatic brain injury and substance misuse: a systematic review of epidemiology and outcomes research (1994–2004). *Neuropsychological Rehabilitation*, 16(5): 537–560.

Prangnell, S. J., & Dean, D. (n.d.). The role of appraisals in predicting post stroke emotional distress. Manuscript in preparation.

Sacks, A. L., Fenske, C. L., Gordon, W. A., Hibbard, M. R., Perez, K., Brandau, S., Cantor, J., Ashman, T., & Speileman, L. A. (2009). Co-morbidity of substance abuse and traumatic brain injury. *Journal of Dual Diagnosis*, 5: 404–417.

Shiel, A., Wilson, B. A., McLellan, L., Horn, S., & Watson, M. (2000). *Wessex Head Injury Matrix*. London: Pearson Assessment, The Psychological Corporation.

Slewa-Younan, S., Baguley, A. J., Herisenau, R., Cameron, I. D., Pitsiavas, V., Mudaliar, Y., & Nayyar, V. (2008). Do men and women differ in their course following traumatic brain injury? A preliminary prospective investigation of early outcome. *Brain Injury*, 22(2): 183–191.

Strauss, E., Sherman, E. M. S., & Spreen, O. (2006). *A Compendium of Neuropsychological Tests: Administration, Norms and Commentary* (3rd edn). Oxford: Oxford University Press.

Vanderploeg, R. D. (Ed.) (1999). *The Clinician's Guide to Neuropsychological Assessment*. Mahwah, NJ: Lawrence Erlbaum.

Warrington, E. K., & James, M. (1991). *The Visual Object and Space Perception Battery*. London: Pearson Assessment, The Psychological Corporation.

Wechsler, D. (2010). *Wechsler Adult Intelligence Scale Version Four*. London: Pearson Assessment, The Psychological Corporation.

Wechsler, D. (2011). *Test of Premorbid Functioning*. London: Pearson Assessment, The Psychological Corporation

Williams, W. H., Cordan, G., Mewse, A. J., Tonks, J., & Burgess, C. N. W. (2010). Self-reported traumatic brain injury in male young offenders: a risk factor for re-offending, poor mental health and violence? *Neuropsychological Rehabilitation*, 20(6): 801–812.

Wilson, B. A., Alderman, N., Burgess, P. W., Emslie, H., & Evans, J. J. (1996). *Behavioural Assessment of the Dysexecutive Syndrome*. London: Pearson Assessment, The Psychological Corporation.

Winnicott, D. W. (1965). *The Family and Individual Development*. London: Tavistock.

CHAPTER THREE

Therapy and engagement

*Stephen Weatherhead, Rudi Coetzer,
Audrey Daisley, Gavin Newby, Giles Yeates,
and Phillippa Calvert*

*Introduction: dilemmas, theory, and
adapting practice* (Rudi Coetzer)

One of the most entrenched uncertainties of brain injury rehabilitation is whether psychotherapy is possible and/or is effective for the clients we work with. Psychotherapeutic needs and goals are often aspired to in treatment plans, despite many rehabilitation professionals wondering how to do it and whether it works. Most brain injury rehabilitation professionals will concede, at least in part, that cognitive rehabilitation is effective and that it can result in favourable, ecologically valid outcomes. But is psychotherapy perhaps more smoke and mirrors as opposed to evidence? In these times of financial limitations, if evidence is defined as extensive data from randomised controlled trials, then yes, there is perhaps very little of this type of evidence. But we should not forget that the same caveat applies to large areas of brain injury rehabilitation interventions. However, if evidence is to include the emerging findings from case reports, qualitative studies, and other methodologies, then psychotherapy probably has a robust role in augmenting other brain injury rehabilitation initiatives. This takes on particular relevance when we look beyond the cognitive and physical impairments associated with brain injury and include the emotional difficulties and associated behavioural changes that can accompany brain injury.

For some psychological difficulties, diagnoses (e.g., anxiety and depression) and some models of delivery (e.g., cognitive–behavioural therapy), there is an emerging evidence base of effectiveness. Although emotional difficulties are common co-morbid symptoms of brain injury, can psychotherapy really be useful to clients with a condition or diagnosis where one of the most prevalent symptoms include cognitive impairment and there is no known physical "cure"? The answer, fortunately, is almost certainly yes. One of the main reasons psychotherapy can be helpful is that for many people with brain injury, their emotional difficulties more generally represent a complex process of adjustment to a long-term neurological condition. There are, unfortunately, no "quick fixes" for this. Clearly, psychotherapy has a potentially important contribution to make to clients' attempts to work towards adjustment.

When working psychotherapeutically with brain-injured people, it is important to consider how clinical practice might need adapting for this population (Coetzer, 2010). Psychotherapy is a complex endeavour even under the most optimal conditions. With specialist populations, psychotherapy practice must frequently be adapted to best meet their often singularly unique needs. For example, engaging the person and making sure a therapeutic relationship develops is one of the fairly universal tasks throughout most psychotherapy processes. With certain clinical populations, this might generally be more complex than with others. It might take extra effort or awareness of potential obstacles, to adjust the clinician's approach to pursue this objective more effectively. Hence, to some extent, successful engagement relies fairly heavily on both practical adjustments to a therapist's approach, and managing internal clinician factors.

Each clinical area has its own "do's and don'ts", or particular characteristics which tend to influence practice. Working psychotherapeutically with clients who have a brain injury commonly presents practitioners with many unique challenges. Judd and Wilson (2005), in a qualitative study, reported some of the obstacles encountered by clinicians during psychotherapy interventions for clients with acquired brain injury. According to these authors, some of the more frequent practitioner-reported difficulties included memory problems and negative reactions (Judd & Wilson, 2005). These and other difficulties common to many forms of acquired brain injury, including poor attention, distractibility, impairment of executive control function, poor insight, apathy, and language difficulties often require the practitioner to be creative in adapting processes and strategies.

Generic therapy skills are just as important in brain injury rehabilitation work, but some specific adaptations might be useful with this population, as listed below.

- Practitioners need to be aware of the pace in sessions:
  ○ go slowly
  ○ focus on the present while maintaining an understanding of the contribution of the person's individual history.
- Help clients to gain perspective on reality, and try to assist them to derive a sense of meaning or purpose after brain injury.
- Be honest and empathic with patients (adapted from Prigatano, 1999).

The importance of therapists continually considering their clients' pre-morbid history cannot be overemphasised. History colours presentation. Knowing the client's history, and knowing it well, facilitates engagement, formulation, and re-formulation over time. How impairments and associated difficulties present in the individual can be affected to a great degree by the person's pre-injury history, personality, and other factors, including social and cultural phenomena. Clearly, many factors potentially contribute to individual clients' presentation after acquired brain injury. However, whether this always represents a fundamental change from how the person was before the injury remains open to debate. Indeed, Yeates and colleagues have made a powerful argument against biological factors being the sole determinant of change after brain injury (Yeates, Gracey, & McGrath, 2008). How can these points inform clinical practice?

For most psychotherapeutic work intended to address adjustment after acquired brain injury, it would be essential for the psychotherapist to have a robust understanding of the client's background. Besides being invaluable for initial diagnoses and subsequent formulation, it also communicates a real commitment to knowing the person, rather than only focusing on the symptoms and difficulties stemming from the individual's injury. This can help make the person feel understood and valued, consequently facilitating and preserving engagement. It also has many other obvious benefits, not least the identification of potential risks. For example, without an understanding of pre-morbid factors and personality, it would be difficult for both therapist and client to identify exactly what has changed and work towards increased self-awareness and adjustment. Or, as another example, identifying and capitalising on pre-existing personality characteristics, such as stoicism, can lead to long-lasting and effective change. Any therapist who is familiar with a client as a whole person, and not only their injury and resulting symptoms, perhaps also has an advantage for preserving engagement or re-engaging clients.

Theoretical background

Can theoretical models provide clinical direction when working psychotherapeutically with these clients, who often pose many challenges, or may be difficult to engage? There are many different schools of psychotherapy and theoretical models underpinning different therapists' respective approaches to delivering psychological therapy. Unsurprisingly, as a result, there seems to be little consistency in approach. To counter this difficulty, it might sometimes be useful to have as a starting point a more trans-theoretical approach to understanding people with brain injury and their individual presentation. Orlinsky and Howard (1995), over several years, developed and refined their generic model of psychotherapy. This model's unique feature is that it outlines the six characteristics thought to be shared by most, if not all, of the different psychotherapies.

Orlinsky and Howard's (1995) model is, in essence, a research theory and, as such, transcends specific schools of psychotherapy. The purpose of this model is to identify and describe the more generic facets of psychotherapy practice. These characteristics or facets of the psychotherapeutic process individually represent several different variables, which operate at the same time (Orlinsky & Howard, 1995). The facets described in Orlinsky and Howard's generic model of psychotherapy include:

1. The therapeutic contract.
2. Therapeutic operations.

3. The therapeutic bond.
4. Self-relatedness.
5. In-session impacts.
6. The phases of treatment made up by sequential events within, and also between, sessions.

Here is a brief description of each facet identified by Orlinsky and Howard (1995). The therapeutic contract refers to the roles of both patient or client and the therapist. It includes practicalities such as the length of sessions and duration of treatment, as well as the therapist's treatment model. Therapeutic operations in psychotherapy constitute the client presenting information to the clinician. In response, the psychotherapist evaluates this information to determine which technical intervention could be indicated for the individual client. It is a two-way process, and the client actively co-operates. The therapeutic bond is the relationship that develops during psychological therapy. It is manifested by each of the parties' investment in their respective roles, as well as the personal rapport that develops between them over time. The self-relatedness of people refers to how people respond to themselves during interactions with others and the environment. This facet includes clients' self-awareness. The in-session impacts in psychotherapy include emotional relief and insight experienced by clients, among others. More generally, Orlinsky and Howard (1986) highlighted the import role expressing emotion during psychotherapy has. Finally, the sequential events that form the phases of treatment in psychotherapy (Orlinsky & Howard, 1995) can be thought of as events during sessions that combine over both time and sessions. These combine to ultimately represent the phases of psychotherapeutic interventions.

The different schools or systems of psychotherapy are too many for all to be included here. Furthermore, psychotherapy is not a static field and new systems or approaches are continually evolving. The main psychotherapy systems, which most therapists will be familiar with, are outlined in established texts such those by Bongar and Beutler (1995) and Dryden (2007). Some examples include psychodynamic therapies, behaviour therapy, existential approaches, experiential therapies (including Gestalt, client-centred, and existential therapies), the many formats of cognitive therapy, including cognitive–behavioural therapy (CBT), integrative or eclectic psychotherapies, group-based psychotherapies, and all the different family therapies (Bongar & Beutler, 1995). More recent developments include, for example, combining mindfulness approaches with cognitive therapy (Williams, Teasdale, Segal, & Kabat-Zinn, 2007) and new developments in behaviour therapy, for example acceptance and commitment therapy (Hayes, Strosahl, & Wilson, 1999).

Many of these psychotherapy systems or approaches, for example, CBT, have been successfully adapted and fairly extensively used for different clinical populations. This includes the adaptation of CBT to assist people with brain injury also. These systems or schools of psychotherapy have a much more specific focus on technique than that of a trans-theoretical approach such as the generic model of Orlinsky and Howard (1995). However, even if discarding a transtheoretical approach in favour of more specific psychotherapy systems, there does appear to be recurrent universal psychological themes when working with brain-injured people. These themes are usually phenomenological in nature, and can be important for practitioners working in brain injury rehabilitation to be aware of.

Psychotherapy models applied to brain injury rehabilitation tend to follow a general algorithm of successive themes, or temporally unfolding stages. These "milestones" include the initial assessment and formulation, followed usually by psycho-education and a subsequent or co-occurring increase in self-awareness, with a culmination in emotional expression and adaptation (e.g., Coetzer, 2006; Ben-Yishay & Diller, 2011; Klonoff, 2010). Each stage potentially has a multitude of individually determined qualitative characteristics. For example, several authors have highlighted the emotion of grief as part of the process of adaptation after brain injury, and the complexities surrounding self-awareness and understanding of losses associated with acquired brain injury (Coetzer, 2006; Kaplan-Solms & Solms, 2000; Klonoff, 2010). Indeed, irrespective of theoretical model or psychotherapy system, this struggle to come to terms with loss, with simultaneous problems of awareness, probably frequently lies at the heart of a large proportion of psychotherapy endeavours with people who have suffered acquired brain injury. Despite the many models and theories we have at our disposal, many of our clients' difficulties do not always fit neatly with our academic knowledge base.

Fortunately, there are also additional sources of knowledge and inspiration other than academic theories and models for the aspiring psychotherapist to consider and potentially learn from. These include the visual arts, literature, films, and philosophy, to mention but a few. Art and literature provide an informal, uncensored (by academic or scientific constraints) view on the human condition. Many clinicians are aware of this, and their approach to psychological therapy in brain injury rehabilitation has been influenced accordingly. For example, Klonoff (2010) describes the use of films and films during psychotherapy. The arts often provide rich metaphors that can be used in psychotherapy. For example, Ylvisaker, McPherson, Kayes, and Pellett (2008) describe the use of personally salient metaphors with clients to facilitate engagement, exploring of identity, and goal setting in rehabilitation. These authors also point out the important role of metaphors in compensating for memory problems. Photography is another example of how the arts can potentially help to inform and develop the thinking of the psychotherapist. Photography is very much about observation, perception, and creativity, essential skills to psychotherapy also. For example, the famous photographer Henri Cartier-Bresson is credited with what has been labelled "the decisive moment", clearly a concept that has potential application to psychotherapy also, in particular with regard to patient insight and therapist timing of responses, including interpretations. Photography can also "hold" metaphors, as above. For example, the fourth author (GN) has recently worked with a male brain injured client who created a portfolio of images to represent his psychological and physical pain. The high quality of the portfolio not only gave the client an enormous sense of pride and self-fulfilment in a work of art that drew praise, but also affirmed his internal reality of pain and helped his partner have some sense of the intensity of his distress.

Finally, it is important to consider issues related to service delivery and configuration. The role of clinical pathways can be useful in raising rehabilitation professionals' detection rates of emotional difficulties associated with acquired brain injury, as well as provide an outline structure for the contribution psychological therapies can make to patient care in this regard (Coetzer, 2009). A simple pathway would include identification of anxiety and depression in the context of brain injury, including a consideration of potentially significant cognitive impairment. It also should include the provision of psychoeducation and family therapy, as well as a structured approach to reviewing clinical outcomes. In the UK, with the recent initiative intended to "Improve Access to Psychological Therapies" (IAPT), including, for example, for people with stroke,[1] clinical pathways might have an important contribution to make. Whereas more general theories of psychotherapy can provide guidance to the therapist with regard to the technical delivery of therapy, pathways can, at a more strategic level, raise awareness and influence service configuration and development. Ultimately, though, at the everyday "coalface" of clinical practice, it is the adaptations to actual technique that can be invaluable for engaging individual clients.

Adaptations to clinical practice

With regard to clinical techniques, it can often be more productive to consider general adaptations to practice in the first instance, before looking at modifications to specific techniques. When considering the combination of cognitive, physical, behavioural, and emotional difficulties some patients often face, there are some more generic adaptations that can be made to the practice of individual psychotherapy (Coetzer, 2006, 2010). These adaptations include, but are not limited to:

- shortening sessions;
- making use of memory aids such as session summaries or audio recordings;
- reviewing notes at the start of sessions;
- limiting the number of (therapist) responses during the consultation;
- always considering the role potential problems of self-awareness in limiting the patient's capacity to work towards better self-knowledge and understanding (Coetzer, 2006).

Many of these adaptations, which are discussed in a bit more depth below, in addition to making the techniques more appropriate to this population, can greatly facilitate the actual process of engaging people with acquired brain injury (Coetzer, 2010).

One of the most useful, and often overlooked, strategies is to consider using shorter sessions. Although shortening sessions might feel counterintuitive to many psychotherapists, there are potentially some real benefits to this strategy for some clients. Shorter sessions can help to minimise the potential negative effects of fatigue or poor attention, which often prove to be significant barriers to the successful engagement of some clients. Fatigue or poor attention might, under certain circumstances, present as irritability or agitation during sessions. Furthermore, to counterbalance shorter sessions, the total number of sessions may be increased and more widely spread out over time. This strategy often proves to be helpful in facilitating the long-term processes of emotional adjustment and the development of more accurate self-awareness.

Most professionals working in brain injury rehabilitation will know that, for many people, adjustment can be painfully slow and that it requires much more time than is generally available in time-limited programmes. Prioritising total length of time of follow-up over the number of sessions in this way might also communicate to patients that there is a "safety net" that will support them if they have a setback. It can also be an important strategy for developing the therapeutic relationship to a depth that might ultimately prove much more productive for pursuing emotional adjustment. Lengthening the period of time between follow-up sessions could also help with generalisation, as there is likely to be increased opportunity for psychological work in an ecologically valid environment—for example, via homework assignments.

Some of the more practical (often environmental) adjustments that can be made to psychotherapy practice include the following. The importance of ensuring a noise-free room or treatment environment to limit distractions during psychotherapy consultations should not be underestimated. Many people with brain injury can become quite irritable or agitated where there is noise or distraction causing information processing problems. This, for obvious reasons, can have a negative effect on engagement and development of the therapeutic relationship. Some people with brain injury also tend to value the predictability and security, in as much as it is possible to arrange, of course, of being seen in the same room every time. Many services ignore the importance of a friendly and welcoming reception area. The role of this environment and the people who staff it cannot possibly be overstated. There are many potential benefits, including a reduction in agitation or aggressive behaviours, clients feeling valued, and facilitating engagement in people who have often had "more than their fill" of hospital environments and, as a result, do not attend (DNA).

Many adaptations to clinical practice are intended to compensate for cognitive impairment common to brain injury. The most frequently encountered is perhaps strategies to compensate for memory problems, for example, recording sessions in one form or another. Another very powerful technique to overcome, or at least minimise, the effects of poor memory, is for the therapist to make use of metaphors. Personally salient information appears to be easier for clients to identify with and remember, rather than overly complex technical explanations. Other strategies include starting sessions with a summary (ideally, directly from clinical notes) of the previous session to check what the client has remembered and also to ensure integration or continuity of the themes that make up the overall psychotherapeutic process. Limiting both the number and length of the therapist's verbal responses can help to maximise the potential for accurate understanding. This strategy might also help to prevent distraction due to concentration problems, or memory lapses, during sessions (as opposed to between sessions).

At least some strategies should be employed to try to overcome the "Achilles' heel" of many brain injury rehabilitation programmes: the tendency for poor generalisation of gains made in rehabilitation environments to the world where clients live their everyday lives. The same nettle, of course, applies to psychotherapy with this population. Some of the following strategies and adaptations to clinical practice can be employed by the therapist to try to increase the chances for generalisation of gains and insights made during sessions to the world outside the consultation room.

- The clinician may use Socratic questioning or role reversal to check for client understanding, for example, at the end of sessions or when discussing results from neuropsychological testing.
- Providing written information for the client to take home, for example, with regard to homework assignments or general information about acquired brain injury and its likely consequences, can sometimes facilitate generalisation. This approach, of course, also functions as a compensatory strategy for memory problems or a way to increase insight or self-awareness. These ideas are extended via the use of SMS texting and email in Chapter Ten, by Newby and Coetzer, in this volume.
- Where indicated and mutually agreed, clients can ask a friend or relative to help with the implementation of, for example, home-

work assignments. Nevertheless, despite the use of these and other compensatory strategies, many experienced therapists are regularly humbled by the very real difficulties related to poor generalisation when clients unintentionally, often due to poor self-awareness, "talk the talk, but don't walk the walk" in psychotherapy.

A particularly salient issue to ensuring engagement relates to the emotions both client and therapist experience during psychotherapy. The emotions clients experience in response to the clinician (transference) and vice versa (countertransference) come with the territory that is psychotherapy. This is included under in-session impacts in Orlinsky and Howard's (1995) model. From a pragmatic viewpoint, this almost certainly lies at the heart of many of the obstacles to effective engagement in psychotherapy with people suffering from acquired brain injury. Therapists need to be constantly aware of potential countertransference issues unique to working with this population. These include, for example, feelings of frustration, irritation, anxiety, or thoughts that change is impossible. Often, the therapist's countertransference could be a valuable clue to what happens in the client's interpersonal contact with others also, and so provide rich in-session material for exploration during psychotherapy. However, at other times, countertransference might actually be much more a function of therapist issues. It is always important to differentiate where countertransference stems from. Accordingly, even the most experienced psychotherapist working with brain-injured people should have regular and timely access to appropriate supervision to discuss these potential dilemmas. Failing to address this can adversely affect the therapeutic relationship, or prevent engagement in the first instance.

Finally, while these and other adaptations to psychotherapeutic practice for people with acquired brain injury can often be useful, it should, of course, be kept in mind by all therapists that sometimes, despite our best efforts, adjustments to process, and personal commitment, our clients might not benefit from psychotherapy as an approach to, or component of, their rehabilitation. Psychotherapy is simply not the approach of choice for some clients. Brain injury rehabilitation is complex enough, and psychotherapy particularly so, not to have to be burdened with dogma. It is, perhaps, also a sign of professional maturity in clinicians who can recognise that some problems simply do not have solutions. Indeed, it is perhaps a fair point to assert that those who fail to develop this clinical wisdom are possibly at increased risk for professional burnout.

The same case from different perspectives

So far, I/we have discussed some of the theoretical aspects of psychotherapy in brain injury settings, as well as providing some tips on potentially useful adaptations to therapy. In order to "bring it to life" a bit, what follows is a case study that presents familiar aspects to many psychological therapists working with people who have an acquired brain injury.

The same case is considered from a number of different therapeutic models, in a relatively "pure" form. Obviously, it is not feasible to cover a significant number of the huge range of models available to clinicians. We have selected cognitive–behavioural therapy, psychoanalysis, narrative therapy, systemic therapy, and cognitive analytical therapy. The orientations chosen inevitably reflect our own interests, but, more than this, we have selected a range which we hope captures some of the main schools of therapy, new and old, to give a flavour of how they may be applied with people who have an acquired brain injury.

When writing these sections, we have been very cognisant of how each approach has its own concepts, and, to some extent, a unique language. Often, the language used can feel very appropriate to the disturbing and devastating experiences that follow brain injury. However, the concepts and associated language can, at times, feel inaccessible to readers unfamiliar with the approach. Therefore, we have done our best to minimise the use of jargon as much as possible.

Case study

> *Diagnosis and clinical history*: Lisa is a forty-seven-year-old single parent of two children, Ben, aged thirteen, and Meg, aged eleven. Two years ago, Lisa was diagnosed with a subarachnoid haemorrhage (SAH) erupting from a left fronto-temporal arteriovenous malformation (AVM). Surgical intervention was successful, although there remains some uncertainty about prognosis.

Rehabilitation and resettlement: Lisa had a four-month stay in hospital, during which her mother moved into Lisa's house to look after Ben and Meg. Following a series of short home-stays, Lisa was discharged home. She was discharged with a support package of twice-daily visits to help with medication and symptom management. A referral was made for further input to support with family tasks.

Her mother stayed with the family for the first two weeks, and then moved back to the south. The transition period was very difficult; Lisa and her mother had some intense verbal disagreements, primarily about differences in their views on how to care for Ben and Meg. A brief excerpt of an observed disagreement follows:

Lisa: I'm OK now, just let me get on with looking after my kids.

Mum: You're not OK, you can't look after yourself properly, never mind the kids.

Lisa: They're my kids and I'll look after them my way. You've always been like this, you think you know how to do everything best!

Mum: I'm just trying to help, I've been here all the time while you were in hospital, and I'm not going until I know you can manage. You're too bloody stubborn to let me help. You were like this before you went into hospital, and now it's even worse.

Lisa: I can do it. I'm fine, just leave me alone!

The conversations often then repeated this same pattern of Lisa demanding that her mother leave her alone to manage the children, and her mother insisting that Lisa could not manage.

Clinical presentation: The community ABI service accepted the referral for case management and neuropsychological input. An initial assessment highlighted that Lisa and her family were concerned to varying degrees about the cognitive and behavioural sequelae of the brain injury. Lisa presented with significant prospective memory problems, as well as retrospective episodic memory loss, stretching back approximately eighteen months. She was easily fatigued, and struggled severely with initiation and self-monitoring. She also developed diabetes and hypothyroidism.

On one-to-one discussion, Lisa appeared to have some insight into her difficulties, reporting that she's "got a crap memory now, and gets tired a lot". She brought out a diary, which she was using as a memory aid. However, on further inspection, it was crammed with information, and had little functional application. She had also missed a number of medication doses, and had not attended for a blood test in relation to her diabetes. These missed schedules were despite prompts being in place in the form of an alarm on her watch, and notes on the calendar.

Lisa's children came in part way through the session, and she was completely appropriate in setting boundaries for their play in a different room. However, she seemed not to show any inhibition in the topics she would discuss in front of them, and, on a number of occasions, was prompted by the ABI team members to consider speaking about some of the topics when the children were not present.

Lisa was a warm, engaging person, with a good sense of humour. There was a consistent pattern of her having some limited insight into her difficulties. Often, she would say something was a minor problem, but, on further investigation, it proved to be much more pervasive (e.g., memory deficits). On a personal level, it felt as if Lisa was something of a "tortured soul". She seemed to be hiding an inner pain, with humour. This particularly came to light when discussing relationships. She became a little upset, saying that she wished she had "a decent man", adding that she "wasn't getting any younger". However she quickly turned this glimpse of unhappiness into a joke about her age, followed by a change in subject.

Family background: Lisa is the middle of three sisters. She describes herself and her younger sister (Jo) as being quite competitive and independent. She says her older sister, Sarah, is less competitive and much more sensible. Lisa had a number of previous unsuccessful relationships, describing herself as "always picking bad lads". When she was 17–19 years old, she was in a relationship in which she was the victim of prolonged domestic violence. Her current boyfriend has sporadic involvement in her life, and her family object to his presence. The children's father has no contact with them, through his own choice.

Lisa's father died when she was fourteen. She describes him as very driven; he worked hard, was very successful in business, and a keen sportsman. Her mother looked after the family, and did not work. Lisa and her mother always had an unsteady relationship: at times they were the best of friends, but they would also have frequent arguments.

Cognitive–behavioural therapy (CBT) (Rudi Coetzer)

Many authors have reported on the potential usefulness of CBT in this population, particularly because it is a highly structured psychotherapy which can be fairly easily adapted as needed for a range of difficulties (Bradbury et al., 2008; Gracey, Oldham, & Kritzinger, 2007; Gurr & Coetzer, 2005; Kahn-Bourne & Brown, 2003; Lincoln et al., 2000; Manchester & Wood, 2001; Rasquin, Van de Sande, Praamstra, & Van Heugten, 2009; Williams & Fleminger, 2003). Perhaps unsurprisingly, then, CBT is the most widely used psychological therapy used in brain injury rehabilitation settings in the UK (Wilson, Rous, & Sopena, 2008). Nevertheless, there are obvious limitations and difficulties with CBT as an approach, not least the issues of possible bi-directionality existing between thoughts and feelings (it is almost certainly not correct that emotions always originate from thoughts) and a failure to address emotion at a deeper psychodynamic level, among many others.

In the case study contained in this chapter, from a CBT perspective, Lisa appears to present with thought patterns, or schema, which, in part, might predate her acquired brain injury. These schemas or beliefs appear to include over-generalisation, negative self-evaluation and possibly cognitive rigidity or perfectionism associated with competitiveness. Since her acquired brain injury, these patterns might have been accentuated by automatic negative thoughts: for example, about her age and ability to settle down. These might further negatively affect her self-concept. The cognitive difficulties associated with acquired brain injury could also make a person like Lisa less able than in the past to "think things through" and reduce the potential for emotions "running away" with her. Moreover, it appears that, to some degree, there might also be a contribution to her presentation associated with subtle problems with self-awareness (see Figure 3.1 for a diagrammatic representation of these patterns).

Potentially, the main aims of CBT in this case would be to provide Lisa with an understanding of how her thought processes can, under certain circumstances, influence how she feels, and, accordingly, affect her level of engagement in meaningful activities: in particular, how automatic negative thoughts might undermine participation in interpersonal activities. CBT as an approach might also, almost by default, augment any compensatory strategies offered as part of Lisa's cognitive rehabilitation. For example, there appears to be a potential role for memory compensatory strategies to increase her functional independence. To some extent, Lisa has already started with this, using a diary, for example. However, there is some evidence of general disorganisation when Lisa tries to apply compensatory strategies. It is here

```
┌─────────────────────────────────┐
│     Thought patterns/schema     │
│   • Over-generalisation         │
│   • Negative self-evaluation    │
│   • Cognitive rigidity          │
│   • Perfectionism               │
│   • Competitiveness             │
└─────────────────────────────────┘
                 │
                 ▼
┌─────────────────────────────────────────────────────┐
│               Precipitating factor                   │
│ Acquired brain injury = less able to think things through │
└─────────────────────────────────────────────────────┘
                 │
                 ▼
     ┌───────────────────────────────────┐
     │ Negative automatic thoughts based │
     │  around age and "settling down"   │
     └───────────────────────────────────┘
           ↗                    ↖
┌──────────────────────┐   ┌──────────────────────┐
│ Limitations on self- │◄─►│ Tendency for emotions│
│ awareness/           │   │ to "run away" with her│
│ self-monitoring      │   │                      │
└──────────────────────┘   └──────────────────────┘
```

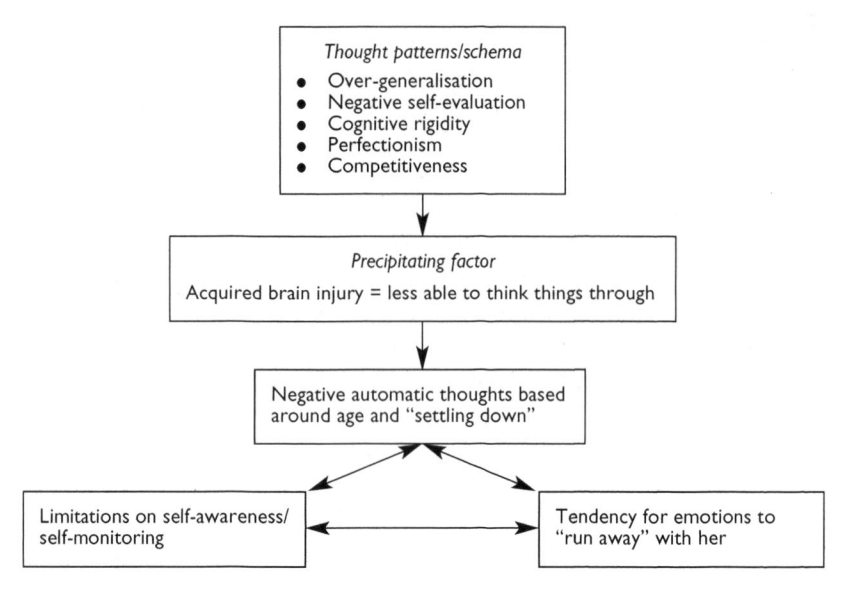

Figure 3.1. Diagrammatic formulation.

that CBT might help to provide an overall structure, or additional "scaffolding", which may be particularly useful if it transpires through neuropsychological testing that she has executive problems.

CBT, in Lisa's case, as with many other people with acquired brain injury, has the potential to facilitate participation in meaningful activities. For example, behavioural activation, including the setting of goals and objectives, form a core component of CBT—in effect, the "B" of CBT. In Lisa's case, ensuring participation would not only have the intended aim of increasing ecologically valid outcomes, but, true to the behavioural component of CBT, also have a function to improve low mood and negative self-concept. Behavioural experiments might also have the potential to increase Lisa's confidence. The general skills fundamental to CBT could also have an inoculation effect for Lisa, in that they might provide her with the tools to better manage future anxieties or vulnerability to low mood. In view of her pre-morbid history, this relapse prevention function of CBT is perhaps of particular relevance. CBT, similar to all other therapies, has the psychotherapeutic potential to facilitate Lisa progressing through some of the universal stages of insight, coming to terms with, or defining at an existential level, the meaning of acquired brain injury and working towards adjustment. CBT merely provides the "language", or a more concrete tool or systematic strategy, to work towards these phases when Lisa is emotionally ready to proceed. This can be no bad thing for many clients with acquired brain injury.

Neuropsychoanalysis (Giles Yeates)

A neuropsychoanalytic formulation is based on certain assumptions and has several aims. It assumes that, for every loss or impairment of an aspect of mental functioning following brain injury, there is a corresponding emergence of more developmentally primitive emotional responses (Kaplan-Solms & Solms, 2000). This is based on psychodynamic ideas around internally competing and conflicting mental processes—some top-down and controlling, others bottom-up—that are emotionally driven and less influenced by external reality. The aims of such a formulation are to fully integrate a neuropsychological profile, historical biographical themes in a person's life, their subjective experience and emotional response to the injury, and, finally, the interpersonal process within the therapeutic relationship. As with any other good psychological therapy in the context of brain injury, standard psychodynamic practice can be adapted to compensate for cognitive deficits (see examples in the journal *Neuropsychoanalysis*).

Based on the case details provided for Lisa, this approach will proceed by identifying a problem list from a psychodynamic perspective, summarising the main historical and biographical themes, outlining the formulation, and indicating the probable direction of intervention.

Problem list

1. The objectively identified *physical and cognitive impairments* noted in the case description and the limitations of her strategy use (e.g., diary and use of alerts and reminders).
2. Lisa's *relationship to these difficulties*: some partial awareness is evident, alongside a tendency to minimise these and their impact in her life (there seems to be a sense of a tension between (1) and (2): Lisa is neither blissfully unaware of them nor wholly and explicitly organised by their presence in her life).

3. Importantly, Lisa's *experience of psychological distress* and her attempted solutions to manage this seem to be helpful only to a point.
4. *Relationships*: tension is evident in the interrelationships between Lisa and her mother, and the mother's relationship and role with the two children. The absence of good enough romantic relationships in Lisa's life is also significant.

Historical and biographical themes

Little information is provided on family and interpersonal life prior to the death of Lisa's father, and it is unclear what Lisa's position among her two siblings stood for in this family. However, the passing of her father when Lisa was fourteen can be read as marking a shift in Lisa's relationship with her mother, entering into a more conflictual pattern that has lasted to this day and shows itself mostly in times of stress and trauma. The loss of the father seems to have some relevance to Lisa's choice of romantic partners thereafter (relationships that are marked by emotional distance and lacking intimate connection, interspersed by Lisa "going it alone"), and the parallels of Lisa's age at the time of her father's death and the age of her children (particularly the son) in the current context of her post-injury struggles seems important.

Neuropsychoanalytic formulation

The biographical themes are seen as the "subjective and interpersonal palette" through which the consequences of the brain injury are expressed and given meaning, but also influence themselves. The first step of the formulation is to link the current emotional experiences (both in and on the edge of awareness), defences (Lisa's ways of managing these emotions), and neurocognitive deficits, in the context of current social and historical influences. A diagram of this formulation is presented in Figure 3.2.

The core of the formulation is a triangle of conflict (following the useful visual heuristic provided by Malan, 1976), comprising hidden feeling, anxiety, and defence. This pattern seems to be evident in Lisa's self-experience and her experience in relation to significant others, including clinicians. Her subjective experience of people (e.g., her mother) intruding and interfering in her life, judging her, and not

THERAPY AND ENGAGEMENT 85

Historical factors

– Early relationships with parents and siblings
– Family responses to loss of father, renegotiation of family relationships, what gets talked about (Lisa's age at time of loss and her subsequent identity positioned within wider family response)
– Continuing organising role of father's (*idealised?*) identity in the family following his death

⇩

Continuing psychological conflict throughout adult life

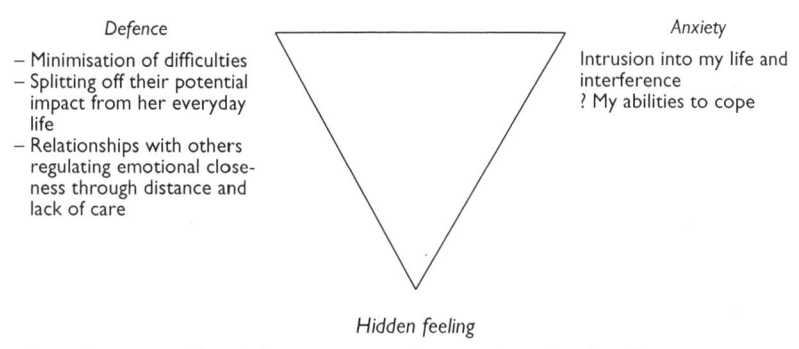

Defence

– Minimisation of difficulties
– Splitting off their potential impact from her everyday life
– Relationships with others regulating emotional closeness through distance and lack of care

Anxiety

Intrusion into my life and interference
? My abilities to cope

Hidden feeling

– Loss of containing figure (who is energetic, achieves goals, etc.) and grief
– Loss of a particular aspect of self in presence of containing figure
– Absent external figures and bad internal objects

⇩

Injury and unconscious meaning of impairments

Impairments represent lost qualities and attributes identified with father and already lost in her life

⇩

Maintaining cycle post injury

Need to realise delayed intentions and goals in prospective memory and planning operations

– Cognitive failure (in eyes of self and children) = loss of containing faculties and identity
– Not tolerable, pushed out of immediate awareness
– Identity and problem solving not updated
– Struggling part of self remains split off and does not communicate with publicly presented self

– Executive impairment (initiation, monitoring)
– Reduced arousal from fatigue
– Minimisation of deficits and impact reducing attentional focus on intentions/goals
– Minimisation precluding collaboration with rehabilitation technicians
– Minimisation reducing arousing/alerting alarms and calendar entries

GOAL NEGLECT

– memory slips, missed appointments

Figure 3.2. Neuropsychoanalytic formulation for Lisa.

allowing her to get on with it on her own terms, are undoubtedly true in one sense. But the motivations for her wishes and, perhaps, the particular sting of the intrusive experience can be seen to derive from other feelings outside of conscious awareness.

Lisa's anxieties would be considered claustrophobic in nature psychoanalytically.

A hypothesis can be formed about the loss of a containing figure in Lisa's life, her father, and her emotional response to this as a young teenager in need of emotional containment as she stands at the doorway to adulthood. Using a psychoanalytical approach derived from Melanie Klein and object relations theory (see Hinshelwood & Zarate, 2006, for an introduction to these ideas), this external loss would be thought about as having a corresponding loss of an internalised representation and relationship, fused with emotion—an internal object. This loss seems not to have been worked through, perhaps as a result of her age and a wider pattern of family response to the loss (unknown to the author at this point). What follows in Lisa's life appears to be a striving for autonomy and independence alongside repeated involvement with her sense of unkind, absent, and withdrawing relationships. The loss of the good paternal object, perhaps increasingly idealised posthumously, seems now to be subsumed under an ever-present bad, neglecting object. It may be explored if Lisa's romantic choices occur within an oscillation of idealisation of new lovers (preventing discretionary decisions about their suitability), followed by a subsequent neglect of her own needs. Furthermore, it could be equally likely that these relationships might break down through a combination of the other partner withdrawing and Lisa's own distancing when a male figure gets too close, because of the risk of emotional investment and potential further loss.

It is hypothesised that there is a defensive quality to these decisions, in that such partners would serve her well in not accompanying her to a closer recognition of her emotional responses to her father's death, and intense feelings of loss and grief (hence, perhaps, the potency of the historical contact and disagreements with her mother). It appears that prior to the injury, instances of disappointment or difficulty seem to be only momentarily acknowledged, then minimised and put aside before returning to an ideal of "soldiering on" by herself, able to cope. A return to distanced isolation seems to be similar to the emotional distance that characterises her experiences within romantic relationships. This experience of self and relating (repeating switches between idealising and a negative relationship) is considered within the Kleinian view to prevent integration of feelings and representations, and so preclude a working through of emotional responses elicited by the loss of her father.

The brain injury produced losses of embodied vitality through fatigue and diabetes and cognition—difficulties realising goals, holding on to important memories (both anterograde memories of intentions and retrograde memories that would have included important moments in her children's lives). The parallel between losses of goal accomplishment, success, and competency and the loss of a father who was positively characterised by his ability to do all of these things is noteworthy. This would be seen psychoanalytically as a life trigger that potently reactivates those hidden feelings of loss through its similar themes, and so would trigger the same anxieties and defences.

This is, indeed, what the clinicians find themselves negotiating, a mixture of partial acknowledgements of new difficulties that intrude into Lisa's life post-injury, and defensive minimisations and attempts to create distance from those who want to think seriously about these problems (clinicians and mother). The loss of a goal-accomplisher and threats to a competent mother identity in the eyes of her children, alongside lost memories of moments of contact with them, is all disturbing information for Lisa and unlikely to be held in mind for long enough. Her children, and, in particular, the important male figure of her son, approaching her own age at the time of her father's death, will only make these feelings and internal relationships more poignant.

There is an unfortunate fit of these emotional dynamics with Lisa's dysexecutive problems (initiation, prospective memory, and error monitoring) and fatigue, which interact to over-determine and amplify the neuropsychological goal neglect problem (Duncan, Emslie, Williams, Johnson, & Freer, 1996) and monitoring of her behaviour in front of her children. Dysexecutive difficulties can often be usefully formulated within emotional and interpersonal goal-directed sequences (Yeates et al., 2008). As a result of these factors, the resultant cognitive slip and its consequences is further minimised and Lisa's post-injury identity is not updated in any way, her struggling post-injury self split off and deprived of internal dialogue with other parts. The role of a rigid, idealised pre-injury identity and narrative structure to scaffold anxieties and give some sense of coherence in those who are judged to lack awareness has been noted elsewhere (Yeates, Henwood, Gracey, & Evans, 2006).

Lisa's response to suggested strategies would also be formulated using the triangle of conflict. Her diary use seems to reflect an idealised attempt to get everything down, but this is not guided by a neuropsychologically informed process that is suitable for her particular impairments (as this would have required several sessions of thinking about her needs in detail). Alerts and reminders are set, calendar entries written, but not acted upon. A procedural flaw in reminder setting and response to alerts (e.g., effectively setting the alarm, being in the room when the alarm activates, not being distracted between the alarm activation and the initiation of the activity) must be initially ruled out, in addition to a perceptual or attentional deficit precluding the noticing of a calendar entry. Beyond this, a hypothesis of resistance to these strategies must be explored with recourse to the formulation above. The resistance might be directed to the clinicians who suggested the strategy (and what they stand for), the implications of permanent strategy use for her sense of self and self in the eyes of others, or a combination of these factors (Yeates, Gracey, & McGrath, 2008).

This formulation would be intended for use primarily by the clinical neuropsychologist to guide assessment and intervention, and only parts of this would be shared in the moment with Lisa. Obviously, this formulation is presented on the information available from the case study and subject to revision as the therapy progresses. In particular, psychodynamic approaches are sensitive to the "devil in the detail" and seemingly random or unusual elements in the client's self-report and relationship with the therapist. A small detail could either substantiate or revise the emerging formulation. Finally, a postmodern approach to psychodynamic formulation is advocated here: tentative ideas that are offered as such and are eventually judged as more or less useful as a function of the experiences that they give meaning to, in particular those disturbing and confusing aspects of mental life that do not neatly fit into approaches based on common sense and rationality.

Suggested intervention

The initial aim of the therapeutic process would be to gather more information to explore the above hypotheses, and Lisa would be asked about her relationship to her sisters and mother in the immediate months and years following her father's death. Dreams would be feasible topics and sources of information within this model. A range of psychodynamic techniques, therapy formats, timescales for intervention, and treatment philosophies are available to use. In the spirit of this book, and in the context of a clinical neuropsychology application within an NHS community brain injury team, an approach is suggested here that is both time-limited (Malan, 1976) and integrated within team practice.

Individual sessions would be offered with Lisa to map out the triangle of conflict as it occurs in the room, and in response to the psychologist's questions about injury consequences. Phrases such as "do you notice when we start to talk about x, you do y"; or "you seem to find the topic of z most difficult to hold on to?" would be used for this purpose. The therapist's use of his or her own emotional reactions (countertransference) to Lisa would be a key part of both assessment and intervention (e.g., "Lisa, I'm feeling that when I bring this up you would rather I not be here"; or "I'm feeling a huge urge not to discuss these very important issues with you every time we meet ... what does that raise for you?"). The aim would be to facilitate an experiential understanding of all points of the triangle of conflict for Lisa, including, ultimately, the hidden feelings, in the moments in which they occur. However, a visual formulation of the triangle might be useful in the context of her cognitive impairments, and, with her permission and collaboration, shared with the team to support them to help Lisa notice these patterns when they occur in other sessions (Yeates et al., 2008).

Joint sessions with the children and Lisa's mother could be usefully informed by this formulation, to explore wider ideas and anxieties held by the family and transmitted across generations since the father's death. A key additional question would be how Lisa's mother is coping with these post-injury losses for her daughter following the loss of her husband. Similarly, in future years, couples therapy support for Lisa if she embarks on a new romantic relationship could benefit from these ideas.

Finally, the use of cognitive rehabilitation strategies and compensatory aids would feature in this form of therapy—the use of diary and alerts would be re-explored. However, the meaning of each particular strategy, and the impact of the therapeutic relationship on its introduction, would be explored with Lisa in depth, to support her acceptance and use of such (Yeates, Gracey, & McGrath, 2008). Once negotiated and accepted, Lisa's intentions from each therapy session (e.g., to try and have a different conversation with her mother, to try not to cope with feelings through distancing others) would be supported through the use of effective diary entries (probably brief and structured), problem-solving frameworks and alerting or cuing procedures using mobile phones, computer calendars or pagers (for detailed suggestions, see Yeates et al., 2008).

Narrative therapy (Stephen Weatherhead)

Narrative therapy (NT) is referred to as a "storied therapy" because it is built on the premise that we live our lives according to the stories, discourses, and narratives that have built up over time. These narratives are influenced by a range of societal, social (including family, friends, and other relationships), and individual discourses. These all merge to form our dominant values and identity or identities.

Our lives are constructed by the language we have available to us, and through which we make sense of our experience. The language we use as individuals (whether as a professional or a layperson) is iteratively developed through relationships (White & Epston, 1990). If we become defined by thin narratives (i.e., lacking in context, richness, and diversity), then problems develop from which we can see no escape.

In the context of NT, the role of the therapist is to help unpick the stories on which problems are built. Looking at problems in this way requires paying attention to the discourses and narratives that are present in relation to the problem. Exploration of the different levels at which these narratives exist is necessary. This exploration can be done explicitly with the person one is working with, or implicitly through the questions asked and the language used by the therapist.

Defining the problem

The initial challenge in NT within brain injury work is defining what "the problem" is. The effects of a brain injury can be so pervasive that they disrupt every aspect of a person's sense of self (Myles, 2004; Nochi, 1988).

Often, during narrative therapeutic conversations in brain injury, it can be helpful to capture ways to define the general complexity of life after a brain injury in a personally meaningful way. "The warehouse of responsibilities" was one such way of capturing an important aspect of life with a brain injury for a group of men that GN and I have worked with in the past (Weatherhead & Newby, 2011). This generalised view of a set of difficulties might well be a good place to start for Lisa, when looking at how to create a life that is not as heavily defined and dictated by the brain injury.

For Lisa, the problem might be the general impact of the brain injury, or any of the specific "cognitive and behavioural sequelae" referred to in the case example. For example, she might prefer to focus on "the crap memory", "the anger" that interferes with her relationship with her mother, or "the unhappiness" that was alluded to.

Mapping the problem

It is important to gain a rich understanding of a person's narrative. Two useful techniques with this process in NT are "externalising the problem", and "thickening the narrative".

Externalising the problem

A core premise of NT is that the person is not the problem; rather, the problem is the problem. This is perhaps one of the easiest techniques in a brain injury setting: for example, one would refer to "the brain injury" rather than "your brain injury". A way of embedding this is to define the problem, give it a name, and get to grips with its characteristics. With Lisa, I would be interested in hearing how the brain injury has influenced her relationships with others, particularly her children and her mother. The emphasis would be on disentangling her sense of self from the brain injury. Questions asked to begin this process might include:

- What effect has the brain injury had on your view of yourself?
- What are your views on your relationship with the brain injury?
- If you could interview the brain injury, what questions would you ask?
- In what way does the brain injury interfere with your view on life?

Thickening the narrative

Narrative therapists often speak of developing an "experience-near" understanding of the problem. For Lisa, one would seek to explore how the problem influences her life on a day-to-day basis, what are the positive and negative aspects of it,[1] and how it relates to her own values, beliefs, and intentions (as indicated by some of the questions above).

This also builds on the externalising process, by encouraging the person to position themselves in relation to it. For example, Lisa states that she has "got a crap memory now, and gets tired a lot". If this were reframed in NT terms, one could think of the problem along the lines of a radio interference metaphor, interrupting the signals to Lisa's memory and fatigue. This would present an opportunity to discuss other forms of signal interference relating to cognitive, behavioural, and general functioning. It would also present an opening for discussing other signal interferences that Lisa has experienced.

Wider discourses

Typing "severe brain injury" into any internet search engine, as Lisa or her family might well do, primarily brings up sites relating to compensation, charity, and news reports of celebrity injuries. For the general public, the result can be inaccurate beliefs, misconceptions, and inappropriate labels (Swift & Wilson, 2001). Often, the content of such sites encourages a dichotomous view of brain injury being something that one either recovers from quickly or that destroys one's life. There are many people who sit somewhere in between this false dichotomy; they are living with what has commonly become known as a hidden disability.

It would be difficult to predict another person's preconceptions of any issue, so I am not going to do so with Lisa's case. We do not know what Lisa's pre-morbid experience or knowledge about brain injury was, or what information she has sought since her injury, but it would be important to consider some of these issues with her, and ensure she has a good understanding of the neurological aspects of her specific injury.

Family discourses

It is likely that Lisa's current narrative is heavily influenced by her experiences of growing up, being the middle one of three sisters, the death of her father while she was a young teenager, and an "unsteady" relationship with her mother. It might be useful to see what Lisa thinks about these relationships and how they relate to the different levels of discourse on narratives such as gender. Gender roles often come with strong narratives, and it might be important to Lisa. Particular areas for exploring this in relation to Lisa's experience might be in reference to her comments about her previous boyfriend's aggression, as well as parenting and families (Figure 3.3).

The intervention

All the factors discussed above are likely to be influential in feeding the dominant narrative for Lisa in relation to the brain injury (as shown in Figure 3.3). When it comes to developing an NT intervention, as with most therapies, it begins from the moment you enter into

Society and ABI
– Misperceptions
– Inaccurate beliefs and labels
– False dichotomy

Family and social narratives
– "Unhappiness"
– Difficult parental relationships
– Victim of abuse

Personal views
– "Crap memory"
– "Anger"
– "Tired a lot"
– Parental role important

CURRENT BRAIN INJURY NARRATIVE

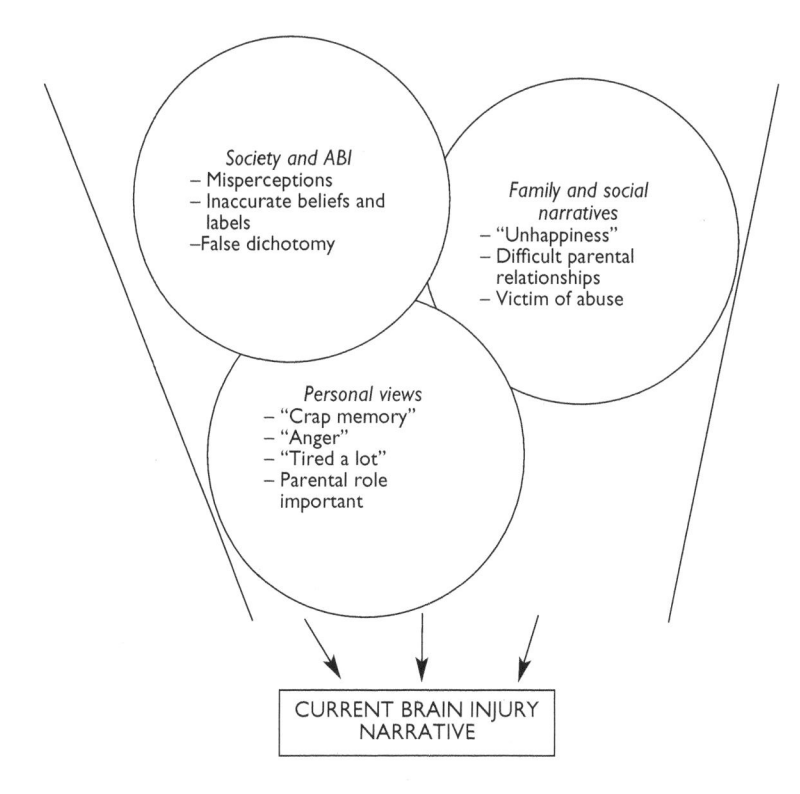

Figure 3.3. Exploring Lisa's narratives.

conversation with the person. The questions one asks, the language one uses, and the way one relates to those involved all form part of the process. Specific aspects for exploration here, in what can reasonably be framed as the intervention, include re-membering conversations, unique outcomes, re-authoring conversations, and definitional ceremonies/documents.

Re-membering conversations

It is often said that to connect with the concept of "re-membering", it can be helpful to think of our life as a members' club. The process of re-membering facilitates discussions about who is important in a person's life, what influence they have, to what extent, and what values are shared with them. If I were working with Lisa, I think one of my first areas to explore would be things such as:

- Who does she think about most frequently?
- What are her most salient memories of those people?
- What do/would they say about the problem and her response to it?

This would present an opportunity to reflect on people with whom she is in immediate and regular contact, as well as her father, and previous partners. The purpose of these conversations is to give Lisa the control over which narratives are dominant in her life, and how those narratives affect her relationship with, and response to, the problem.

Unique outcomes

These are examples of when the problem was less dominant. Thickening the stories around these exceptions introduces context and richness over previously thin descriptions. For example, being a single mother who has incurred a brain injury presents a significant challenge. Despite memory, fatigue, initiation, and self-monitoring problems, Lisa is still observed being "completely appropriate in setting boundaries" for her children.

It would probably be a very useful process to explore Lisa's narratives about herself as a parent, and highlight examples of when the neuropsychological sequelae of the brain injury were not wholly defining. There are exceptions to her "crap memory", and other difficulties, otherwise she would not be able to independently parent her children at all, even with the support from family services.

Re-authoring conversations

Re-authoring conversations are ways of further developing a rich understanding of a person's narratives. The aim of them is to facilitate awareness of "the bigger picture". White (2007) defines two "landscapes" to map in a person's narratives. The idea is that conversations with Lisa would look at how she made sense of the world, in terms of her knowledge, value weightings, and understandings (landscape of identity), and how this interacted with the tangible events and circumstances of her life (landscape of action). These processes would be discussed in tandem, and be related to Lisa's past, present, and preferred future identity and action. For example, Lisa was a very active person prior to her injury, but suffered from fatigue afterwards. Therefore, we might discuss the importance of physical activity to her, and the part it plays in her self-concept. Then we could consider ways in which she could remain active, while being mindful of her physical limitations (i.e., what action could she take to strengthen her preferred narrative?).

Definitional ceremonies/documents

Over time, it is hoped that NT would help build up a picture of the brain injury and reduce its influence. This would be reinforced through definitional ceremonies (if appropriate and useful) such as celebratory parties, video diaries, or meetings with other people who have experienced a brain injury. Therapeutic documents can also act as useful reinforcements for the gains that have been made. These can be anything from a postcard that reminded a person of their professed values and beliefs, to a detailed letter, email, or mission statement for life.

Obviously, as with every aspect of NT or, indeed, any therapy with a person who is experiencing cognitive difficulties, the presentation of such documents, as well as therapeutic sessions, should be pitched at the right level for the person at the heart of the intervention, where possible using their own language. In conclusion, as Hogan (1999) states in her case discussion: "Narrative therapies suggest that co-authoring processes that privilege the language of people with neurological and communication barriers can be a rich source of new terrain to explore . . ." (Hogan, 1999, p. 25).

Systemic therapy (Gavin Newby and Audrey Daisley)

Systemic approaches attempt to understand and address an individual's difficulties within the context of their relationships. Emphasis is placed on understanding the processes and interactions that take place within a family (such as its patterns of communication and its dominant belief systems), the mutual influence of people within the system, and the wider cultural context. Problems, from a systemic perspective, are seen as fundamentally interpersonal, and so interventions focus on relational change. This section illustrates a systemic approach to Lisa's situation.

Obviously, we are biased, but we use systemic ideas because we have seen how they "free up" both professionals and clients and their families to address seemingly intractable and complex problems. They encourage clients and their families to move away from the passivity of the medical model to develop meaningful, creative, and self-generated solutions to their problems and, in doing so, foster a sense of mutual support and shared resilience. Given that acquired brain injury (ABI) can lead to life-long problems with problem solving and flexibility, systemic ideas can provide families with a positive framework in which to successfully manage future challenges.

In common with many modern systemic practitioners, we have adopted a third-order postmodernist approach with this case (see Dallos & Draper, 2005 for a review). To truncate a hugely complex literature, the approach essentially asks the therapist to step away from trying to be the expert who knows everything and "does unto the passive family". A third-order postmodernist approach recognises that people and families define themselves (and to some extent are "held prisoner") by their own meanings, language, and experiences. The role of therapy, as such, is for therapists and family to work together to developed shared understandings and solutions rather than imposing the expert view.[2]

This would begin with two assumptions: first, we would be open-minded, curious, and do our best to avoid any prior assumptions or prejudices about Lisa's situation. Second, we would abrogate the "expert" position—that is, that we are the experts, know everything, and "do unto" Lisa. We would hope this makes us open, friendly, curious, and ready to listen to what Lisa and her system tells us. We would invite her to attend with her "family"; for most people, this involves their close relatives but others will also include friends and significant others in their system.

The presenting issues

Within systemic practice, assessment, formulation, and intervention are seen as intertwined, indistinct processes which take the form of creative, exploratory, and collaborative conversations with families. At the heart of this is the "deconstruction" of the presenting problems, as this both "exposes the story and analyses what the story is maintaining" (Winek, 2009, p. 27). We would already have some initial curiosity about Lisa's ABI in the context of her relational world, but, as the "not-knowing" therapist, we would take these thoughts to initial contacts and begin gently to explore their veracity to elaborate or exclude them.

Similar to other approaches, we would begin by focusing on the presenting problems (e.g., seeking information about what issues the family members are concerned with, the history and extent of these difficulties, and their understanding of why problems are continuing); throughout this exploration, systemic approaches emphasise the importance of the therapist listening out for how the people involved are discussed in relation to the problems described. We would, therefore, want to pay particular attention to the following.

- How the problems are talked about (are they described as Lisa's or the family's?)
- Are there differences in how family members view the issues, and who allies with whom and about what?
- To whom are problems most obvious (e.g., who in the family is most likely to notice that Lisa has not taken her medication).Who is most concerned about her?

- When do the problems seem to affect relationships between people in the family *and* when do family issues seem to affect Lisa's problems?
- We would also be interested in times when the ABI *does not* seem to interfere in Lisa's life (e.g., when she can remember an appointment).

Systemic approaches actively encourage families to discuss these apparent "exceptions", as they can open up the possibility that the problem is not as all-encompassing as might first appear, can suggest that some competent aspects of the pre-injury person remain, and, thus, might instil hope for further improvement (as such, the discussion of "exceptions" is both a useful assessment and intervention technique).

It would also be helpful for us to attend to Lisa's family's constructions or explanations of the problems described. Dallos and Stedman (2006, p. 81) note that individuals typically "hold contrasting beliefs which encapsulate and maintain the patterns of relationships within the family". In Lisa's case, we might be interested in the family's understandings and beliefs about her cognitive problems (their everyday impact on Lisa—particularly on her parenting abilities—and why they are continuing), as it is common for relatives to misattribute these difficulties to "personality" or motivational factors (e.g., initiation difficulties can be misconstrued as laziness or unwillingness on the part of the injured person). Such erroneous beliefs can have significant relational consequences for the people involved, as relatives can become angry and withdraw from the injured person, who, in turn, can feel confused and unsupported.

While psycho-educational interventions go some way to counter simple misunderstandings, they cannot always adequately address the relational impact of strongly held family belief systems. In Lisa's case, possible misunderstandings about her cognitive problems might be further complicated by contextual factors, such as longer standing family beliefs about her as a person. In this context, we would also want to understand the family's views on how needs are communicated and recognised, and their position in relation to offering, seeking, and accepting help—from both within and outside of the family.

We would find it helpful to have a visual portrayal of Lisa's family and wider system in the form of a genogram or "family tree" (See

THERAPY AND ENGAGEMENT   99

Figure 3.4). This is used not only to map the facts about family members, but also to gain an idea of the nature and quality of relationships and their wider context and connections. In particular, genograms can help families to identify sources of support that they might not have considered, or to prompt discussions of familial resilience and strength, which can provide a more positive relational framework in which to contextualise the current problems. We would encourage the reader to be creative in using genograms; one can use them to identify gaps in our knowledge and understanding (hence, the frequent use of question marks in Figure 3.4) and to speculate about relationships. Importantly, genograms are typically "works in progress" where information can be added or deleted as hypotheses are proved, disproved, or changed not only by therapists, but by the other participants in the session.

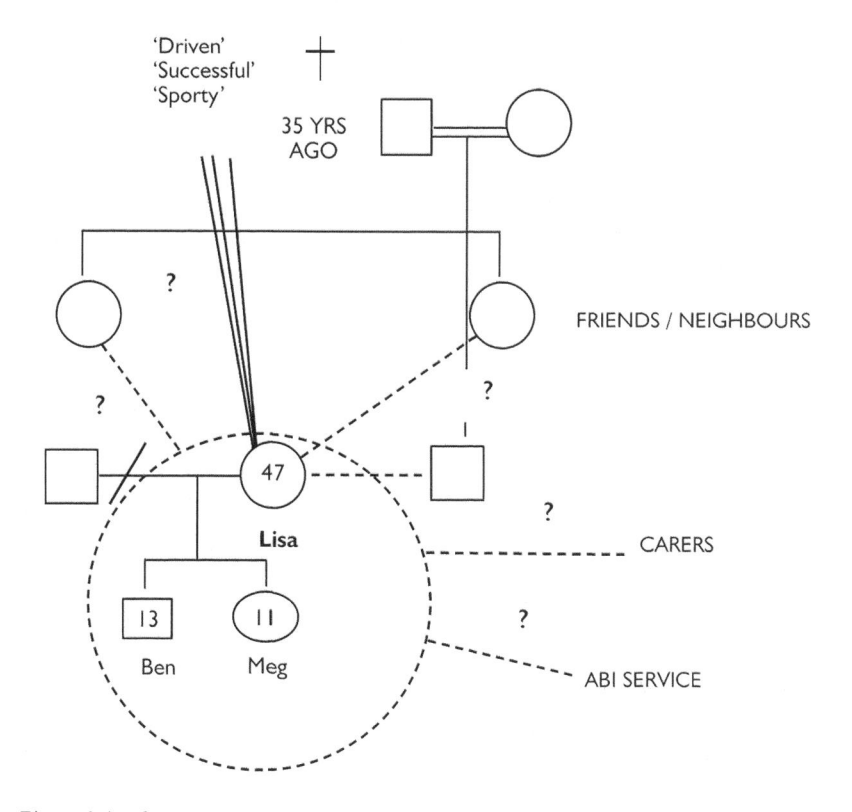

Figure 3.4. Systemic genogram of Lisa and her context.

In Lisa's case, we might be curious about her position and standing within her systems before the haemorrhage. As the middle one of three sisters (and with her father dying when she was a teenager), we might wonder if her birth position historically led her to feeling unheard (perhaps prompting her to seek affirmation from relationships with young men in a relatively uncritical manner, and in which she seemed to not have been valued or became a victim of abuse). We might speculate that moving "South" was, in some way, an escape from them, and now, whether the return "home" (placing her back in their support) is met with some ambivalence, resulting in her attempting to resist their input.

The genogram might also prompt us to speculate about whether any family interactions or dilemmas were created over the issues of parenting. Lisa's illness might present her own mother with an opportunity to re-engage with Lisa and her grandchildren in a way not possible prior to the illness; Lisa might experience this as unfamiliar or unwelcome, seeing it as a challenge to her own parental competency and personal independence, thus creating resistance. It might be helpful to explore Lisa's experiences as a lone parent (perhaps usefully done within the context of a conversation about her own mother's experience, who, like Lisa, cared for her children alone) as this might offer a framework of previous competency against which Lisa can safely talk about herself as a parent with an ABI (a neglected topic within neuro-rehabilitation. Please see Rachel Skippon's Chapter Twelve, in this volume, for further detailed discussion).

Other important network variables, such as friends and professionals, can be usefully included in the genogram: for example, it would be helpful to explore gaps in services, previous agency involvement, and the role of friends, and discuss who has been helpful to Lisa and why.

Testing out systemic hypotheses/developing working formulations

Within systemic practice, the use of reflecting teams (i.e., a group of consultants who view the family session and make comments on the processes and interactions they observe) to share formulations with the family is commonplace; however, we acknowledge that this resource might not be available within most ABI services. In our experience, it is perfectly possible to work with families without having to use two-way mirrors and a reflecting team. An in-room supervisor model can work well, whereby two therapists work in the room with the family, one acting as the direct interviewer and discusser while the second therapist sits slightly removed from the therapeutic horseshoe and either drops in comments to the therapist in earshot of the family, or they both break into a direct conversation, also in front of the family, at an agreed time. This allows the two therapists to speculate on hypotheses and dynamics and for the family to then comment on what they have heard. In our experience, this can really free up situations, elucidate very strongly felt feelings, and help families to develop clear and shared modes of working together.

In order to develop a working formulation, information from the family conversations and the genogram are drawn together to try to understand what family relational patterns are being maintained by the account of the current problems that is given. For Lisa and her family, our formulation might focus on opposite themes of dependence *vs.* competence and help seeking *vs.* acceptance of support, and what these concepts mean for their relationships. We might offer our view that the account of Lisa's current ABI problems that we are being given are of her denying the extent of her difficulties and portray her as being unaccepting of help and of pushing the family away. This account appears to maintain a pattern of Lisa and her family not being able to support each other at difficult times, and seems to position Lisa as the headstrong and obstinate family member in this situation. This account serves to align the family against her and, in turn, position Lisa such that she continues to resist their input (a problem-maintaining pattern of interaction).

Systemic approaches encourage families to consider alternative explanations for the problems they are facing. In this vein, we might share with the family a hypothesis that reframes Lisa's refusal to accept help being as a result of her being fearful of being judged by family and services as "not coping", or as not being a "good enough" mother. We would encourage discussions to expand this theme in the light of the significant losses she has experienced as a result of the ABI, difficult past relationships, and recent family criticism of her current parenting skills. We would, perhaps, want to build upon earlier conversations about their differing views on seeking, accepting, and offering help, as we have speculated that independence in the family was an important factor for Lisa and that requiring help would be challenging. Helping the family to air such differences and disagreements facilitates the development of new understandings and explanations for difficulties and (via reflective reframing of family conversations) alternative solutions can be collaboratively generated.

Systemic interventions

Systemic interventions, like systemic formulations, are exploratory—there are no right or wrong answers to a family's difficulties. The aim is to enhance their sense of joining together against the problems they are facing in ways that work for them, to reduce negativity and blame and to instil hope that issues can be resolved.

Based on our tentative formulation of Lisa's difficulties, intervening at the level of family beliefs might be helpful. Offering different perspectives on those beliefs might support Lisa and her family to talk about how the ABI symptoms have been affecting her parenting skills, in a less blaming and guilt-provoking way, possibly facilitating discussions of new ways in which she could be offered, and accept, help. Specific work tasks with the family might include modelling less emotional forms of communicating with Lisa about these sensitive issues, allowing the family to take risks with Lisa—for example, taking responsibility for child-care, or perhaps rebalancing communication styles. For example, if Lisa found it difficult to be heard in family interactions, it could be the role of the therapist and in-room supervisor to enable the family to hear Lisa's feelings.

In addition, individual sessions with Lisa might be helpful to explore further her ideas about what constitutes a good parent and what being "brain-injured" means in order to reveal the dominant familial, societal, and cultural discourses that might have shaped her beliefs about these issues. Together, we would hope that these interventions might produce change in other areas, such as family interactions with Lisa, as well as their perceptions of her. This could support Lisa to consider accepting help with fewer feelings of defensiveness and fear.

We might also want to raise awareness of family life-cycle theory (Carter & McGoldrick, 1989), speculating that Lisa's family life-cycle stage now almost exactly mirrors that of her family of origin: her elder child, son Ben, is approximately the same age as she was when her father died. Lisa might well be extremely cognisant of her feelings and sense of loss of her own father and might be worried about her children having to face life without either parent or a stable father figure. Work here might focus on establishing extensive commitment of the extended family to provide parenting should anything untoward happen to Lisa, alongside some individual work with Lisa for an accurate understanding of her actual risk of re-bleed.

At a systemic level, we would wish to engage with Lisa's wider context; it can, therefore, be helpful, where possible, to include other important members of the system, such as the GP or social worker. For Lisa, it might be helpful to widen the circle of support around her, by working alongside organisations such as Headway, local parenting groups, and perhaps individual counselling for Lisa herself.

Cognitive analytic therapy (Phillippa Calvert)

What is cognitive analytic therapy?

Cognitive analytic therapy, or CAT for short (said as the word rather than spelling out the acronym in individual letters), is an integrative psychotherapy developed by Anthony Ryle (Ryle & Kerr, 2002). The approach suggests that we develop ways of relating to, and interacting with, others, and ourselves, through our relationships. The individual is seen as a social being that cannot be separated from their social interactions or culture (Dunn, 2002). Our experiences and interactions help us develop ways of getting our needs met as well as managing and responding to our emotions. These patterns are then repeated throughout our lives and in our various relationships, a process that has been likened to procedural memory (Dunn, 2002). Unfortunately, some of these patterns can be problematic and, while they help us to manage our emotions and needs, the patterns can limit our responses and ability to adapt to different situations. If we consider how individuals with an acquired brain injury (ABI) can struggle with cognitive flexibility and shifting from one response to another, CAT could help to conceptualise these difficulties by integrating the CAT model with neuropsychological understandings (Yeates, Gracey, & McGrath, 2008).

The process of CAT

The approach emphasises empowering the individual to become aware of unhelpful patterns and, in turn, be able make choices and exit from these patterns. The therapy involves three stages, known as the three Rs: Reformulation, Recognition, and Revision. As with any psychotherapeutic approach, there are some key concepts in CAT. Some of these will be highlighted while referring to Lisa's case. For a more in-depth discussion and glossary, see Ryle and Kerr (2002).

The first "R": reformulation

In CAT, the process of gathering information and developing an understanding of the person's difficulties is called reformulation rather than formulation. This is an acknowledgement that people will already have an idea or formulation about what is happening and why. The process of reformulation aims to validate an individual's difficulties while identifying how these might have developed in a non-judgemental and non-blaming way.

When working with Lisa, it would be important to consider her "zone of proximal development" (ZPD). This refers to what a person is currently able to do or tolerate. The therapist would aim to work within Lisa's ZPD and help to develop or widen the zone at her pace. Working outside the ZPD could result in Lisa feeling de-skilled, invalidated, worthless, and frustrated, all of which are not conducive to the therapeutic aims. The concept of ZPD could also be used to formulate the notion of insight after a brain injury. Lisa has demonstrated some insight into her difficulties by talking about her "crap memory" and "getting tired a lot", but appeared to be underestimating the extent of her difficulties. The reformulation process could help Lisa to explore these difficulties and develop her understanding and insight.

The first few sessions are used to consider different areas of the person's life, their life experiences, and how they have learnt to cope and manage in the world. In Lisa's case, it would be important to pay attention to her recent experiences and those prior to the brain injury. A family tree, or genogram, is often used, as well as plotting out a life timeline including significant events and people. Typically, the reformulation stage involves writing a reformulation letter and developing a sequential diagrammatic reformulation (SDR) often referred to as "a map" of the patterns involved in the person's difficulties. Both are developed in collaboration with the individual, and the SDR will be revised throughout the process. It is important to use the client's language and terminology throughout the sessions, while breaking down descriptions they might use into specific feelings and patterns of behaviour. For example, if Lisa said "I feel bad", it would be important to identify whether this perhaps meant upset and anxious, or if she stated "it's just a mess", this could be explored and agreed to mean "I try to sort out the problem but won't ask for help even if it means getting it wrong".

The reformulation process involves identifying reciprocal role procedures (RRP). An RRP is a pattern of interacting and relating to others and ourselves which have been repeated throughout our lives. They consist of *reciprocal roles* (RR) and *procedure*s. Reciprocal roles consist of two poles and are thought to originate mainly from relationships with parents or significant care-givers, but can develop through other significant relationships. An RR can be healthy or unhealthy. Reformulation tends to focus on the unhealthy RRs, as these are involved in the individual's ongoing difficulties; however, it can be important to acknowledge the healthy RRs. Figure 3.5 shows an example of an unhealthy reciprocal role. This would be described as rejecting to rejected.

Traditionally, exploring a person's history and past relationships is a key task within CAT, as it helps to identify RRPs and develop a compassionate understanding of their difficulties in the context of their lives. When working with an individual after a brain injury, this process might help to identify patterns that are interfering with their adjustment, or to accepting input from health professionals (Rice-Varian, 2011). The extent to which this is possible with someone after

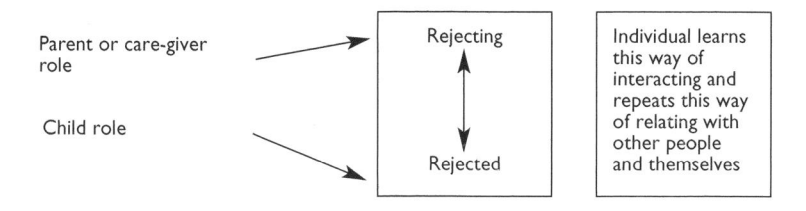

Figure 3.5. Example of an unhealthy reciprocal role.

a brain injury will depend on the individual and how the injury has affected their personality and memory.

Lisa described an "unsteady relationship" with her mother, and I would wonder with Lisa, how she felt during their interactions. For example, Lisa could feel criticised or attacked. These descriptions could indicate an RR of criticising to criticised, or attacking to attacked. It would then be important to listen for similar descriptions in Lisa's other relationships, such as the one with her first serious boyfriend that involved domestic violence. Noticing how Lisa describes her recent experiences in relation to her health issues would be important, as Lisa might demonstrate a similar relational pattern to the brain injury. This, in turn, could predict how she reacts to the consequences of her brain injury, which might be in a similar way to when she was arguing with her mother.

It would be important to explore Lisa's relationship with her father and attend to her descriptions of him. It is likely that this would identify another RR. From the description in the case study, there are indications that her father strove to be successful, and, as a "keen sportsman", was perhaps competitive. I would wonder whether Lisa was expected to strive and, while she may value being competitive, this might be in response to spoken and unspoken demands, perhaps indicating a demanding to striving RR. Lisa's description of wanting to find a "decent man", and the sporadic involvement of her boyfriend might indicate a neglecting to neglected RR. This might then be repeating both in her relationship with her children and in her relationship with herself. For any RR identified, the accompanying procedure must also be explored.

A procedure describes the individual's thoughts, beliefs, behaviours, and actions of others that result from an RR. These procedures are defined as goal-directed and describe coping patterns that were helpful in the past, either by getting an individual's needs met or by helping to manage emotions, but have now become problematic. There are three types of problematic procedures which would be targeted in therapy:

1. *Snag*: when an individual sets out in pursuit of a particular goal or aim, but ends up abandoning it.
2. *Trap*: like a vicious circle, or self-reinforcing thoughts and behaviours.

3. *Dilemma*: a false dichotomy or choices that are polar opposites. Either I do this, or I do that. Either choice results in difficulties for the individual.

Procedures can be intrapersonal, interpersonal, or a mixture of both. One potential procedure for Lisa might involve a pattern of not looking after herself. This could have occurred prior to the brain injury, but might have been magnified due to her cognitive impairments. For example, as a result of feeling neglected (one end of the RR), Lisa might aim to protect herself by hiding away. However, this results in her not looking after herself either physically or emotionally, leading her to the neglecting end of the RR. This is now potentially exacerbated by her memory problems and missing appointments for her diabetes and hypothyroidism. Currently, others might then get annoyed, such as her mother, resulting in arguments, which Lisa might experience as the other attacking and/or criticising her. Part of Lisa's SDR might, therefore, look like Figure 3.6.

Colours and pictures can be helpful when developing the SDR. For example, Lisa could use a magnifying glass to signify that there are times when her cognitive impairments magnify her pre-morbid patterns, or a stop sign when they make it a lot more difficult for her to follow a previous pattern.

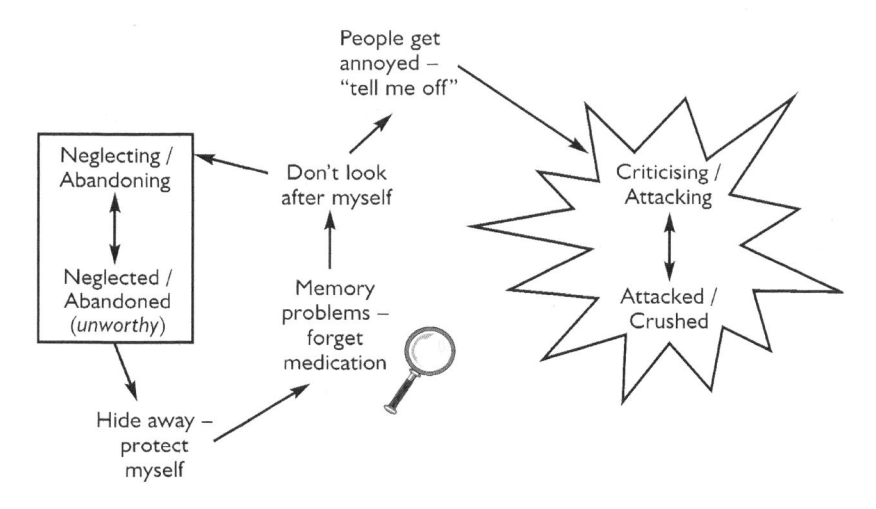

Figure 3.6. Hypothetical part of Lisa's "map".

Ordinarily, the reformulation letter is developed first, followed by the SDR. Depending on whether Lisa found prose or diagrams easier to follow, and whether her cognitive profile suggested her auditory or visual processes were stronger, I might start to map out with Lisa what she is describing. This might help Lisa connect to the descriptions offered in the reformulation letter. The SDR as a whole could then be completed. It would be interesting to note whether Lisa tended to talk about her cognitive difficulties, physical difficulties, such as the fatigue or diabetes, or her family relationships. This will help to identify which problems are the most salient for Lisa and what she would like to focus on. Examples of reformulation letters can be found in Ryle and Kerr (2002).

The second "R": recognition

The SDR is used to identify which area the client would like to focus on in the first instance. The client is encouraged to recognise when a target problem procedure (TPP) occurs by using monitoring sheets and discussions in the ensuing sessions. In Lisa's case, it would be important to consider her cognitive impairments and agree how to help her recognise when a pattern was occurring. It might be beneficial to share the SDR, or parts of it, with her family, other health professionals, and carers, but only with Lisa's permission. It may be that Lisa could use technology to support her with these tasks.

The aim of recognition is to help the individual become more aware of their patterns in the moment, thus allowing for more opportunity for them to use "exits" from these patterns. During this process, and similarly in the other stages, it is important to be mindful of enactments between the therapist and client. An enactment is when a reciprocal role and procedure happen during an interaction between the individual and the therapist. These help to identify what happens in the individual's relationships, which the therapist helps the client reflect on. In Lisa's case, she might try to please the therapist, hoping they will look after her, but end up feeling disappointed. Or, if challenged, she might experience this as criticising, resulting in her feeling attacked and not good enough.

Such an interaction can result in a rupture, a point in the therapy when the individual can become angry, feel rejected, or perhaps criticised by the therapist. This often results in the person missing a session or trying to end therapy. If handled skilfully, a rupture can help the therapist and individual to develop their understanding of the individual's current relationships and move towards a healthier RR, such as understanding to understood.

The third "R": revision

The final stage involves helping the individual to identify "exits" from the patterns. These exits might involve developing new skills, or utilising existing ones. The exits allow the person to develop alternative responses and coping strategies that are more helpful and adaptive. Ryle emphasises integrating any tools or techniques from other approaches that could help the client and therapist to consider and implement changes (Ryle & Kerr, 2002). In Lisa's case, it would be important to utilise techniques from neuropsychological rehabilitation, such as memory strategies and fatigue management, as well as more traditional psychological therapy techniques to help her reduce her distress.

These "exits" are added to the SDR that the client keeps to help her continue to think about her patterns and how to change them. As the client finds a new way of relating to others and themselves through the therapeutic relationship, this new RR is also added to the SDR, along with the procedures and benefits associated with it. Lisa's process in therapy and her utilisation of such exits, including the challenges, would be summarised in a goodbye letter. Finally, it would be helpful to discuss with Lisa the pros and cons of recruiting others to help her use these exits and strategies, and continue to review them at follow-up sessions after the main period of input has ended.

Overall conclusion and synthesis

Neuropsychotherapy is an emerging area, which presents clinicians with a broad range of philosophical and practical challenges, such as how to capture its efficacy, and what adaptations should be made to particular models in order to make them meaningful to someone with cognitive deficits. However, it is important for us to rise to these challenges in order to meet the psychological needs of the people with whom we work.

In order to bring neuropsychotherapy to life in this chapter, we took the approach of formulating the same clinical case from different perspectives. We hope that this has illustrated the strengths, possibilities, and challenges of using "mainstream" approaches in brain injury settings. Often, these approaches require some adaptations, as discussed in the introduction. However, what they show is that brain injury does not have to be a diagnosis of exclusion when it comes to accessing psychological therapy.

All of the approaches presented here (and those which are not), have something to offer to the brain injury setting. Many have particularly salient aspects, for the individuals and systems with which we work. However, they share the common recurring theme that ABI does not just affect the individual sufferer. Its devastating effects can ripple through relationships, friendships, families, work, and the wider community, and beyond. It is not always necessary to work with these different levels in all cases, but to ignore them would be to the detriment of the individual who has incurred the injury.

Similarly, it is not always necessary for a person who has experienced an injury to engage in therapy. Indeed, in some situations, the injury itself can be a prohibitive factor. However, to ignore psychological therapy as a consideration is to ignore a vital aspect of a person's rehabilitation: their psychological wellbeing. This, in itself, can be one of the biggest predictors in a person's recovery. Consequently, psychological therapy is as important as assessment, in many cases more so.

Notes

1. It is important to avoid "totalising" descriptions of any issue. A totalising description is one that defines it in wholly positive or wholly negative terms.
2. The interested reader is referred to the works of Anderson and Goolishian (1988, 1992) and Gergen (1991), and the excellent summaries found in Dallos and Draper (2005).

References

Anderson, H., & Goolishian, H. (1988). Human systems as linguistic systems. *Family Process*, 27: 371–393.

Anderson, H., & Goolishian, H. (1992). The client as the expert: a not knowing approach to therapy. In: S. McNee & K. Gergen (Eds.), *Therapy as a Social Construction* (pp. 25–39). London: Sage.

Ben-Yishay, Y., & Diller, L. (2011). *Handbook of Holistic Neuropsychological Rehabilitation: Outpatient Rehabilitation of Traumatic Brain Injury*. New York: Oxford University Press.

Bongar, B., & Beutler, L. E. (Eds.) (1995). *Comprehensive Textbook of Psychotherapy. Theory and Practice*. Oxford: Oxford University Press.

Bradbury, C. L., Christensen, B. K., Lau, M. A., Ruttan, L. A., Arandine, A. L., & Green, R. E. (2008). The efficacy of cognitive behaviour therapy in the treatment of emotional distress after acquired brain injury. *Archives of Physical & Medical Rehabilitation*, 89(Suppl. 12): S61–68.

Carter, B., & McGoldrick, M. (Eds.) (1989). *The Changing Family Life Cycle: A Framework for Family Therapy* (2nd edn). Boston: Allyn and Bacon.

Coetzer, R. (2006). *Traumatic Brain Injury Rehabilitation. A Psychotherapeutic Approach to Loss and Grief*. New York: Nova Science.

Coetzer, R. (2009). A clinical pathway including psychotherapy approaches for managing emotional difficulties after acquired brain injury. *CNS Spectrums*, 14(11): 632–638.

Coetzer, R. (2010). *Anxiety and Mood Disorders Following Traumatic Brain Injury: Clinical Assessment and Psychotherapy*. London: Karnac.

Dallos, R., & Draper, R. (2005). *Introduction to Systemic Family Therapy* (2nd edn). Maidenhead: McGraw Hill/Open University Press.

Dallos, R., & Stedman, J. (2006). Systemic formulation: mapping the family dance. In: L. Johnstone & R. Dallos (Eds.), *Formulation in Psychology and Psychotherapy* (pp. 72–97). London: Routledge.

Dryden, W. (Ed.) (2007). *Dryden's Handbook of Individual Therapy* (5th edn). London: Sage.

Duncan, J., Emslie, H., Williams, P., Johnson, R., & Freer, C. (1996). Intelligence and the frontal lobe: the organization of goal-directed behavior. *Cognitive Psychology*, 30: 257–303.

Dunn, M. (2002). Cognitive analytic therapy. In: W. Dryden (Ed.), *Handbook of Individual Therapy* (4th edn) (pp. 266–293). London: Sage.

Gergen, K. (1991). *The Saturated Self*. New York: Basic Books.

Gracey, F., Oldham, P., & Kritzinger, R. (2007). Finding out if "The 'me' will shut down": successful cognitive–behavioural therapy of seizure-related panic symptoms following subarachnoid haemorrhage: a single case report. *Neuropsychological Rehabilitation*, 17(1): 106–119.

Gurr, B., & Coetzer, B. R. (2005). The effectiveness of cognitive–behaviour therapy for posttraumatic headaches. *Brain Injury*, 19(7): 481–491.

Hayes, S. C., Strosahl, K. D., & Wilson, K. G. (1999). *Acceptance and Commitment Therapy. An Experiential Approach to Behavior Change*. New York: Guilford Press,

Hinshelwood, R. D., & Zarate, O. (2006). *Introducing Melanie Klein*. London: Icon.

Hogan, B. (1999). Narrative therapy in rehabilitation after brain injury: a case study. *NeuroRehabilitation, 13*: 21–25.

Judd, D., & Wilson, S. L. (2005). Psychotherapy with brain injury survivors: an investigation of the challenges encountered by clinicians and their modifications to therapeutic practice. *Brain Injury, 19*: 437–449.

Kahn-Bourne, N., & Brown, R. G. (2003). Cognitive behaviour therapy for the treatment of depression in individuals with brain injury. *Neuropsychological Rehabilitation, 13*: 89–107.

Kaplan-Solms, K., & Solms, M. (2000). *Clinical Studies in Neuro-Psychoanalysis. Introduction to a Depth Neuropsychology*. London: Karnac.

Klonoff, P. S. (2010). *Psychotherapy after Brain Injury. Principles and Techniques*. New York: Guilford Press,

Lincoln, N. B., Husbands, S., Trescoli, C., Drummond, A. E. R., Gladman, J. R. F., & Berman, P. (2000). Five year follow up of a randomised trial of a stroke rehabilitation unit. *British Medical Journal, 320*: 549.

Malan, D. (1976). *Individual Psychotherapy and the Science of Psychodynamics*. Oxford: Butterworth-Heinemann.

Manchester, D., & Wood, R. L. (2001). Applying cognitive therapy in neurobehavioural rehabilitation. In: R. L. Wood & T. M. McMillan (Eds.), *Neurobehavioural Disability and Social Handicap Following Traumatic Brain Injury* (pp. 157–174). Hove: Psychology Press.

Myles, S. (2004). Understanding and treating loss of sense of self following brain injury: a behaviour analytic approach. *International Journal of Psychology and Psychotherapy, 4*(3): 4587–504.

Nochi, M. (1988). "Loss of self" in the narratives of people with traumatic brain injuries: a qualitative analysis. *Social Science & Medicine, 46*(7): 869–878.

Orlinksy, D. E., & Howard, K. I. (1986). Process and outcome in psychotherapy. In: S. L. Garfield & A. E. Berglov (Eds.), *Handbook of of Psychotherapy and Behavior Change* (pp. 311–383). New York: Wiley.

Orlinksy, D. E., & Howard, K. I. (1995). Unity and diversity among psychotherapies: a comparative perspective. In: B. Bongar & L. E. Beutler (Eds.), *Comprehensive Textbook of Psychotherapy* (pp. 3–23). Oxford: Oxford University Press.

Prigatano, G. P. (1999). *Principles of Neuropsychological Rehabilitation*. New York: Oxford University Press.
Rasquin, S. M., Van de Sande, P., Praamstra, A. J., & Van Heugten, C. M. (2009). Cognitive–behavioural intervention for depression after stroke: five single case studies on effects and feasibility. *Neuropsycological Rehabilitation*, 19(2): 208–222.
Rice-Varian, C. (2011). The effectiveness of standard cognitive analytic therapy (CAT) with people with mild and moderate acquired brain injury (ABI): an outcome evaluation. *Reformulation*, 36: 49–54.
Ryle, A., & Kerr, I. B. (2002). *Introducing Cognitive Analytic Therapy: Principles and Practice*. Chichester: John Wiley.
Swift, T. L., & Wilson, S. L. (2001). Misconceptions about brain injury among the general public and non-expert health professionals: an exploratory study. *Brain Injury*, 25(2): 149–165.
Weatherhead, S. J., & Newby, G. J. (2011). The warehouse of responsibilities: a group for survivors of a brain injury. Institute of Narrative Therapy: Papers & Resources, Web-based article: www.theinstituteofnarrativetherapy.com/Papers%20and%20resources.html. Accessed 29 May 2012.
White, M. (2007). *Maps of Narrative Practice*. London: Norton.
White, M., & Epston, D. (1990). *Narrative Means to Therapeutic Ends*. London: Norton.
Williams, M., Teasdale, J., Segal, Z., & Kabat-Zinn, J. (2007). *The Mindful Way through Depression: Freeing Yourself from Chronic Unhappiness*. New York: Guilford Press.
Williams, W. H., & Fleminger, S. (2003). Neurorehabilitation and cognitive–behaviour therapy of anxiety disorders after brain injury: an overview and case illustration of obsessive–compulsive disorder. *Neuropsychological Rehabilitation*, 13(1–2): 133–148.
Wilson, B. A., Rous, S., & Sopena, S. (2008). The current practice of neuropsychological rehabilitation in the United Kingdom. *Applied Neuropsychology*, 15(4): 229–240.
Winek, J. L. (2009). *Systemic Family Therapy: From Theory to Practice*. New York: Sage.
Yeates, G., Hamill, M., Sutton, L., Psaila, K., Gracey, F., Mohamed, S., & O'Dell, J. (2008). Dysexecutive problems and interpersonal relating following frontal brain injury: reformulation and compensation in cognitive analytic therapy (CAT). *Neuropsychoanalysis*, 10: 43–58.
Yeates, G., Henwood, K., Gracey, F., & Evans, J. J. (2006). Awareness of disability after acquired brain injury (ABI): subjectivity within the psychosocial context. *NeuroPsychoanalysis*, 8: 175–189.

Yeates, G. N., Gracey, F., & McGrath, J. C. (2008). Biopsychosocial deconstruction of "personality change" following acquired brain injury. *Neuropsychological Rehabilitation, 18*(5/6): 566–589.

Ylvisaker, M., McPherson, K., Kayes, N., & Pellett, E. (2008). Metaphoric identity mapping: facilitating goal setting and engagement in rehabilitation after traumatic brain injury. *Neuropsychological Rehabilitation, 18*(5/6): 713–741.

CHAPTER FOUR

Social consequences and social solutions: community neuro-rehabilitation in real social environments[1]

Howard F. Jackson and Gemma Hague

Introduction

Brain injury rehabilitation, like travel plans, comes in many formats and permutations, but all have an end destination. Rehabilitation's end destination, in the very broadest sense, is to increase independence and facilitate adjustment. This chapter looks at the challenges of working with clients with acquired brain injury (ABI) and of developing effective rehabilitation programmes in community settings. In particular, we draw the reader's attention to the gulf between theory and practice, at both a clinical and a social policy level. It is recognised that the richness and variety of human experience brings with it its own challenges, and that personalisation of rehabilitation is necessary if it is to address the needs of the client with ABI. This chapter is a reflection of our clinical experiences and approaches to addressing such challenges with clients with ABI in a specialist service and the neuropsychological principles underpinning this specific approach.

The effects of a brain injury and their rehabilitation inevitably involve consideration of various factors including:

- the areas of the brain impaired;
- the developmental and personal history of the brain at the time of injury;
- the environment, lifestyle, and demands on the individual;
- the circumstances of the injury and the individual's perception of the injury and associations;
- the events and experiences since the injury;
- the coping strategies used by the ABI person and their supporters;
- the availability and accessibility of appropriate rehabilitation frameworks.

However, within this complex array of uncertainties, some common issues emerge that are pertinent to the majority of ABI cases and which can help to guide the development of many rehabilitation services. Neuropsychological rehabilitation after ABI might be described as a process of increasing the ability to solve problems, remain organised and focused, selectively remember relevant events, and engage in independent strategic behaviour while participating in tasks valued by the culture (in increasingly varied contexts, with gradually expanding domains of content) and with systematically decreasing support from others.

As we progress through childhood, one would normally experience guidance from adults gradually reducing in line with increasing abilities, competences, and functioning. Putting it simply, the more we show we can do things and do them in a manner that is acceptable to the supervising adult, the more those adults step back and let us get on with things. In addition to developing cognitive competencies, each child develops coping strategies such as increased organisation/ management of their environment, behavioural routines, timetabling, self-prompting, goal setting/commitments and skills that increase their effectiveness. These coping strategies are initially guided by the parents/teachers/siblings, and later managed and developed by the child himself as he wrestles for control (sometimes constructively and sometimes destructively). The degree of control relinquished by parents (ideally) is in tune with their child's ability to cope, both in terms of ability and in terms of the development of their coping strategies. All of this seems a little obvious as a framework for successful learning and skill development, yet the same logic is rarely applied to clients with ABI. We suggest that similar principles should underpin effective neuro-rehabilitation. How to do this is discussed by considering the rehabilitation setting, the expertise of the rehabilitation team, and the approaches employed in working with individuals across community settings. A final aim of this chapter is to consider the infrastructures that should be provided for effective post acute brain injury rehabilitation. We start by considering areas of human functioning that are often affected by ABI and become particularly relevant when considering neuro-rehabilitation approaches in the community.

Cognitive functioning

As discussed throughout this book, ABI can result in a range of cognitive impairments associated with primary and secondary consequences of the injury. While the effects (and outcome) can be very varied, there are some aspects of cognition that can become particularly challenging for the individual and the system around them as they attempt to re-establish former roles, responsibilities, and relationships. In particular, we focus your attention on the complex area of executive functioning.

Disorders of executive function are generally manifested by emotional lability, irritability, rigidity, apathy, defective behavioural initiation, carelessness, poor judgement, and inappropriate social behaviour. Lezak (1983) has described the problem as a serious impairment in starting, switching, and stopping behaviour. This results in a decrease in spontaneous behaviour, productivity, initiative, and self-control, while at the same time increasing perseveration, impulsiveness, and disinhibition. However, while there are some qualitative similarities and neuro-anatomical overlaps, impairments of executive function should be distinguished from those of social cognition, which more specifically relates to cognitive processes underpinning social interactions. Executive function can be conceptualised as consisting of four primary areas (Lezak, 1983).

1. Formulating goals.
2. Planning/problem solving.
3. Carrying out the plan.
4. Effective performance.

Luria (1973) stated that all human activity begins with an intention directed toward a goal. When our ability to conceptualise our desires and needs before acting is impaired, the result is impulsive action with little thought of the potential consequences, or automatic and perseverative responses to environmental stimuli. The individual with executive dysfunction is often unable to formulate goals. It just does not occur to the person to do anything, resulting in an inability to initiate action that might resolve the situation. Many clients with executive dysfunction are capable of performing a task, but will not engage in the activity unless directed in a step-by-step manner.

Planning requires an ability to generate options, consider the consequences of those options, make an appropriate choice, and develop a framework or cognitive map to direct the activity. In addition, the capacity to sustain attention and to view oneself and the environment objectively is critical to effective planning and problem solving (Lezak, 1983; Prigatano, 1986). The inability to initiate a plan is often described as a decrease in, or absence of, motivation and can present as a significant challenge in neuro-rehabilitation. The client might be referred to as lazy, emotionally disturbed, or malingering (Lezak, 1983) when, in fact, the individual might lack the ability to identify the sequential steps to plan an activity. These individuals are often impulsive when solving problems. They act immediately without analysing options and often the option selected is the same, regardless of the problem at hand. They perseverate and apply the same poor solution that leads to further failure. These clients might be virtually immobilised by their inability to plan and effectively solve problems, or at other times appear highly impulsive and chaotic.

Translating an intention or plan into a productive and purposeful activity requires the ability first to initiate, switch, and stop action in an orderly fashion. The lack of initiative is a difficulty frequently observed by the families of clients with ABI. Without being given specific and concrete instructions or direction, the ABI survivor might lack the cognitive skills to know how or when to carry out goal directed activity (Prigatano, 1986). These individuals might demonstrate difficulties in abstract reasoning. The cognitive skills required to carry out complex action might not be present without cues and routine procedures. In structured settings, they can follow direction, but, again, they can become chaotic or immobilised when left to use self-direction.

In meeting a client with ABI, deficits in executive functions are often not immediately apparent in casual conversation or, indeed, during the course of a highly structured interview setting at a first meeting between the ABI client and a professional. This is a particularly important consideration when assessing an individual with a severe ABI in the community. Frequently, clients with disorders of executive functioning appear cognitively intact (Vogenthaler, 1987). Such clients generally perform well on neurological as well as neuropsychological examination, especially when provided with a structured setting (Lezak, 1982; Prigatano, 1986; Vogenthaler, 1987).

Younger pre-adult clients with an ABI might function adequately in school settings, since these are highly structured. The seriousness of any executive deficits then become apparent only after graduation/leaving school, when they subsequently fail to make a successful transition to the roles required of them as adults. At this point, the young adult's inability to direct and regulate behaviour can seriously interfere with community adjustment. This coincides with the continued maturation of the frontal system of the brain across adolescence, and the associated neuropsychological development of executive and social cognition functions. This helps to explain why, despite a clear history of significant trauma to the head during infancy or early childhood, many young adults only present to clinical services (or, often, the criminal justice system) as they reach late adolescence and early adulthood with significant behavioural challenges (also referred to as the "sleeper effect"). In our experience, such delays in identifying problems can often lead to practitioners neglecting the early trauma as a possible casual factor and can trigger inappropriate diagnoses and intervention.

As we grow up into adulthood, the number of additional responsibilities increases, especially those that require us to interact within an increasingly complex social environment. In order to do this, we need to have the ability to monitor our behaviour and its effects on our environment and then self-correct and self-regulate. Clients with executive dysfunction often do not perceive mistakes, are impaired in their processing of social cues (Jackson & Moffat, 1987; McDonald & Flanagan, 2004), and, thus, do nothing to correct their behaviour. They can often discuss their errors but still do nothing to remedy a problem. These clients frequently lack awareness of their strengths and deficits, resulting in unrealistic self-appraisals. Their deficits in self-awareness result in their not perceiving errors in performance. They fail to perceive or understand social cues and might be unable to be self-critical (Lezak, 1983). Such deficits make it difficult for these patients to profit from their experiences. Frequently, clients with an ABI, as a consequence of executive and social cognition impairments, will misread social situations, do not understand consequences of their behaviour, and misinterpret feedback. This decreased ability to self-regulate behaviour often results in socially inappropriate remarks and behaviour.

The inability to regulate behaviour or inhibit impulses is often referred to as a "disinhibition syndrome". The disinhibited ABI client will act before thinking. They tell you exactly what they think, are frequently demanding, and are non-compliant with rules or schedules. This results from a chain of behaviours that begins with poor perception of social cues and is maintained and exacerbated by poor judgement, faulty behavioural goal direction, and defective monitoring and self-correction in the emergence of aggressive outbursts. And it is this combination of executive function and social cognition impairments that can, in many cases, result in poor social, recreational, and occupational outcome after ABI, perhaps more so than physical disability *per se*.

An individual's impaired ability to perform executive functions will result in certain failure in the community where the demands exceed their capabilities. In addition, these deficits often lead to social isolation and lack of social support systems. Friends and family become less tolerant of the individual's behaviour (Brooks, 1984). Unfortunately, poor insight and awareness of such problems can lead to individuals being unable to recognise core support needs and rejecting opportunities of support and service interventions. When considering this in the context of other neuropsychological problems, such as memory deficits after severe ABI, it is not surprising to know that many individuals will miss outpatient appointments or decline assessments or interventions, particularly without direct support to connect with such activities. Furthermore, individuals will readily report that they are experiencing few problems and, indeed, might confirm to the practitioner that they do not need any rehabilitation or support. Unfortunately, many assessment frameworks often focus upon such interactions in isolation and often conclude that the individual does not have any presenting need or desire to engage in any further input, resulting in individuals being discharged from the service. This is often in the face of overwhelming evidence from family and friends of significant challenges for the individual (or the system around them) in their everyday interactions and activities. Unfortunately, it can be many years later before individuals access appropriate rehabilitation.

It is essential to describe dysexecutive functioning from the outset as a neuro-behavioural syndrome comprising integrated cognitive, behavioural, and personality changes. Too often, clinicians rely on standardised performance tests of executive functioning that can, by their very nature, exclude those functions we are most interested in assessing. (See also Chapter Two, by Jones and co-authors, in this volume.) Furthermore, often the array of tests used can be limited to assess in depth such a complex system as that of executive control functions. The conclusions that can be drawn from these test data without reference to everyday functioning are few. There is much literature on the importance of venturing away from traditional assessment frameworks in assessing an individual with ABI and instead assessing the individual in the real world (see Manchester, Priestly, & Jackson, 2004 for a more detailed review), including the world of interpersonal functioning.

A social world

One client of ours once stated that he preferred to communicate with silicon-based life forms (computers) rather than carbon-based life forms (people). When asked why, he showed considerable insight when he replied, "You don't have to guess how the computer will respond, it waits until you are ready and it responds as expected." When we consider behavioural problems, they rarely involve issues with objects; they almost invariably involve people and social situations (although when objects start being unpredictable like people, then all of us can become angry, confused, and sometimes "lose the plot"). As such, in addition to executive functioning, social cognition becomes an important consideration in understanding a client with an ABI and, therefore, developing suitable interventions.

Social judgements require us to consider ourselves abstractly within the situation of the other person (including past experiences), evaluate or predict our own affective responses and thoughts, and infer from this process of introspection the other person's internal influences. Such aspects of cognition are rarely explicitly, or even implicitly, assessed during formal neuropsychological evaluations. The ability of the ABI client to make introspective judgements, compare these with the behaviour of others, and make inferences with respect to the internal states of another is not an area generally assessed. In this respect, rehabilitation therapists will need to be aware of the difficulties clients have with social inference. Interactions, therefore, need to be more overt and direct. Often, we need to be concrete with the client and state the obvious. Innuendo, abstract communications, analogies, and the like should, in many instances, be kept to a minimum. This is actually quite difficult to do and takes a little practice.

It is mainly from these social–cognitive functions that moral values and social rules emerge. Intersubjectivity allows for the development and implementation of empathic processes, moral evaluations, and socially skilled interactions. Indeed, social cognitions not only require introspective or intersubjective evaluations, but also comparison of the observed behaviour with moral standards and social rules. It is through the interactive triadic comparison of others, self, and social/moral rules that we develop our own social and self identity (Tajfel, 1982). Unfortunately, a brain injury can upset this delicate equilibrium.

Within the social environment, we develop a sense of self that is based, at least in part, on our roles and responsibilities within our social networks. Gracey and colleagues (2008) explored how individuals make sense of their self, and the changes experienced, following an ABI. Social and practical activities and the meaning awarded to their experiences in such activities were fundamental in driving their sense of self or identity. Markus (1983) refers to identity as self-schema that is a knowledge structure about the self derived from past experience serving to guide and organise information relevant to the self. Identity, therefore, provides an anchor or frame of reference by which to choose particular responses, understand the self, and predict one's own response in a given situation and the likely efficacy of that response. To some extent, self-awareness and identity is abstract self-knowledge. They involve cognitive processes of integration of disparate sources of information about the self and the self's relationship to the world. As we have mentioned previously, consistency and predictability are important components for psychological wellbeing. Identity forms the basis for this continuity and congruency.

The ABI client, in many cases, is a victim when some or all of these components that play a part in forming, maintaining, and modifying identity are impaired. The external circumstances that are used to reaffirm the positive qualities of both personal and social identity are changed. Social contacts are lost and the social status of the ABI victim is dramatically altered. Constructs of important personal qualities, such as athletic, intellectual, or social ability, are threatened. In some cases, the identity construct itself might have been directly damaged due to retrograde amnesia (loss of pre-morbid memories). However, in most cases, such loss will be minimal, leaving behind a sense of self which is grossly different from that after the brain injury and which strikes deep at the central core of identity constructs. The ability to call upon the identity constructs and apply them to different circumstances is likely to be dysfunctional after brain injury, again due to impairments in executive functioning. The cognitive ability to accommodate and assimilate new experiences is also impaired. Thus, psychological adjustment in the ABI population is a major challenge. It is understandable, therefore, that many clients avoid contact with other people who have suffered an ABI.

This conflict between old self-constructs and current abilities commonly causes a barrier to engaging the client in rehabilitation and can be one of the core issues in psychological denial. Presenting brain injury rehabilitation to the client as a treatment with which they need to collaborate is often resisted, since it challenges the pre-morbid sense of self that is often fiercely defended. Thus, engaging people in brain injury rehabilitation must also consider and overcome the client's need to defend pre-morbid self-identity. Such resistance can be considerably lessened if you can find a way of presenting rehabilitation as a set of approaches that will help them improve areas in their world that are now difficult following their ABI and will not unduly challenge their fragile self-identity. Rehabilitation can be presented as "developing work skills", or "resuming areas of responsibilities", rather than an imposed treatment that accentuates their perception of themselves as a brain injured person.

It is through the processes of hypothesis investigation and then integrating this information into existing belief schema about the world and the self that individuals are able to function in complex social systems. Research suggests that even individuals with severe amnesia generate cognitive hypotheses (although often erroneously) and respond rigidly to these hypotheses irrespective of the consequences of their behaviour. As such, a simple behavioural approach that solely manipulates the consequences of the behaviour seems unlikely to be effective. Verbal mediation of the behavioural contingencies is clearly important. This can take the form of developing intentions, goals, and plans. Verbal self-instruction and use of diaries and planners can help maintain the direction of the behaviour.

It is evident that the coping strategies that are adopted by individuals have a significant impact on both their emotional life and their everyday functioning. Furthermore, both the trauma of the brain injury and its aftermath are likely to have a significant impact on the individual's coping strategies. Recent research has found that different coping styles after brain injury are not influenced by the severity of the injury or the nature and extent of the residual cognitive impairments, but have a significant impact on subjective complaints (Wolters, Stapert, Brands, & van Heugten, 2011). To some extent, this translates to how a person copes after a brain injury, as manifested through the phenomenology of complaints, determines what can be done, or what they present as their rehabilitation goals. Which can be, shall we say, tricky . . .

Ho hum, nothing can be done

The ever-present challenge for brain injury rehabilitation is to develop effective strategies that enhance executive system functioning and make community living and gainful activity (ideally employment) a realistic goal for clients. Since executive dysfunction results in difficulty in interpersonal relationships, or not even recognising that there are, in fact, difficulties, we have focused our treatment primarily upon social competence training and secondarily upon functional activity training and generalisation skills. Before effective rehabilitation programmes can be developed, it is evident that the concept of rehabilitation needs to be better understood and, almost certainly, myths about when/how this is effective need to be challenged.

Historically, brain injury rehabilitation initially focused on restoration of ability, and this involved attempts at retraining of cognitive abilities directly through a series of exercises (e.g., Sohlberg & Mateer, 1989). While there is some evidence that direct retraining can be effective to some extent in the early stages of recovery and also in younger people whose brains are still developing, such direct retraining is now widely accepted to be of very limited effect and generally limited to the specifics of the task with little generalisation into everyday life. In particular, this concept of brain injury rehabilitation has led to the notion that there is a critical period in the recovering brain, beyond which no further interventions can be effective. Add to this the biological reductionist view that, since neurons do not regenerate like other cells in the body, there was nothing that could be done above the mere passage of time, and for a long time brain injury rehabilitation was neglected.

It is generally accepted that performance on neuropsychological tests of cognition show an initially rapid improvement that gradually slows down and eventually "plateaus". This is generally in line with the timeline for physical recovery. While there is some debate about the time it takes to plateau, the conclusion is that there is a critical time for recovery and, thereafter, future improvements are unlikely. In general, the view was that the longer the time between the injury and the assessment, the less likely specialist brain injury rehabilitation would be considered. For some areas of functioning, rather than a plateau, there is evidence for deterioration. Family members and close friends can provide very valuable information with regard to the changes observed in the client and their history. There are certain neuropsychological devices, such as the modified Katz social adjustment scale (Jackson, Hopewell, Glass, Ghadiali, & Warburg, 1992) (hereafter referred to as the acquired brain injury–Katz adjustment scale (ABI-KAS)), that can promote understanding of such changes. Similarly, the informant's version of the *Behavioral Rating Index of Executive Functioning—Adult Version* (BRIEF-A; Roth, Isquith, & Gioia, 2005) provides important information about executive functioning in everyday life, whereas other performance tests are likely to prove insensitive (Manchester, Priestly, & Jackson, 2004).

There is considerable evidence regarding the late onset of a number of ABI sequelae that involves enduring physical problems such as epilepsy, fatigue, and pain, but also, importantly, psychological factors such as depression, anxiety, realisation of loss, and grief (Jackson, 1988). In our study of the neuropsychological changes after acquired brain injury (Jackson, Hopewell, Glass, Ghadiali, & Warburg, 1992), we noted that across an extended period of time (20+ years), rather than "plateauing", a number of neuropsychological variables increased for individuals with severe ABI but not for those with milder brain injury or those with traumatic injuries which did not involve the brain (i.e., spinal injuries).

Fleminger (2010) suggested three possible reasons for deterioration:

1. The client "gives up". After initial gains in the months or years after a severe injury, the patient becomes non-compliant with therapy and withdraws socially, and rehabilitation gains are lost. Fleminger (2010) suggested that this is possibly a consequence of the client's greater awareness of his very disabled state.
2. Psychosocial factors affect the client's recovery. Compared with clients who do well, clients who deteriorate have more problems with alcohol (both before and after the injury), have lower self-esteem, and are more likely to have been injured in an assault. Incidence of alcohol misuse is high among the ABI population and it is also highly associated with offending (see also Jones and co-authors' section on dual diagnoses in this volume). However, it is interesting to note the process by which alcohol misuse develops. One possible explanation is that the distress caused by the brain injury and its consequences leads to alcohol abuse as solace. Another is that the ABI person is impaired in terms of self-control. Other processes might relate to deterioration in the social network and social opportunities available to the client, bringing them more into contact with unhelpful social influences. Reduced opportunities to engage in a varied life of enriching activities and relationships, together with cognitive problems such as impairments in motivation and initiation, can often lead to a lack of activity and experiences of boredom, which, in turn, could contribute to unhelpful routines that might fill time and/or alleviate distressing emotional experiences.
3. Dementia might ensue. Clients who have sustained an ABI might be at increased risk for Alzheimer's disease or other dementias, or for a greater degree of age-related decline in cognitive function, most likely through an acceleration of the inflammation process (Sastre, Richardson, Gentleman, & Brooks, 2011). This has not

been a universal finding though, and is unlikely for the majority of cases (see Fleminger, Oliver, & Lovestone, 2003).

> According to Darwin's *Origin of Species*, it is not the most intellectual of the species that survives; it is not the strongest that survives; but the species that survives is the one that is able best to adapt and adjust to the changing environment in which it finds itself. (Megginson, 1963, p. 4)

There are other potential reasons why individuals with impaired executive abilities might deteriorate. We are all affected by changes in our lives to which we have to adjust and adapt. Most of these minor changes we can manage easily. Others, such as major life events, require considerably more emotional and cognitive resources to manage. Certainly, it is difficult to think of a more devastating life event than a traumatic brain injury, and the emotional and cognitive demands made on someone adapting to these changed circumstances cannot be understated. However, the same might be said of many other conditions. The difficulty that individuals with executive impairments have is managing change itself. A recurring theme is that changes in life, often only small changes (e.g., a change in the layout of the supermarket, or someone not returning a call, etc.) can be a challenge. Change makes demands on our memory for new information (a function likely to be impaired). Change makes demands on our problem solving and executive abilities to make adjustments, establish new routines, and re-establish a structure. If these executive functions are impaired, then responding to changes will prove difficult, create stresses, and result in ineffective coping and adjustment to the new circumstances.

As discussed, clients with impaired executive functioning often have difficulties initiating, organising a strategic plan, inhibiting impulsive responding, or following plans through. As a result, their actions often contribute to the destabilisation and destructuring of their external and internal (psychological) environments, further compounding the changes in their lives. To illustrate this process, one young geophysics PhD student who suffered a severe ABI returned to his studies shortly after being discharged from hospital. As part of his research project, he had developed a computer simulation to predict the movement of tectonic plates. His academic supervisor at the time reported that he had settled in quite well and, although a little slow, seemed to pick up on the work very well, remembering his studies and project well. As the student tried to improve and develop the computer programme, it became increasingly dysfunctional with every attempt to resolve the problems each change had caused. Eventually, the student had to abandon his PhD.

The above example is common for many people with executive impairments. Although they can function better in a structured environment, clients often contribute to the lack of a structure. Many will abandon regular sleep–wake cycles, ignore regular meal times, and fail to organise their home environments. More importantly, many will fail to set personal timetables, plans, or goals to guide their behaviour throughout the day, leading to long periods of inactivity and empty time. Such conditions will render them more vulnerable to over-responding to the immediate cues in their environment. They are easily distracted, impulsive, and intolerant of delay, uncertainty, and ambiguity. Others will perseverate with coping behaviours that are no longer valid or applicable to the changed circumstances. Many of these processes occur in the context of problems with insight for the client with severe ABI and, as such, there can often be limited recognition of such problems occurring in the first place.

It is worthy of note, at this point, to reflect on the natural developmental changes that are likely. The majority of ABI clients sustain their injuries at times in life when changes are at their most frequent. It is well documented that young men (and, to a lesser extent, young women) are at greater risk of suffering an ABI (Yates, Williams, Harris, Round, & Jenkins, 2006). It is in these adolescent and early adult periods of life that most people experience significant changes in their circumstances. Leaving home, going to college, developing new social networks, starting work, etc., are all significant life events creating major changes. At these stages in life, greater demands are made and less support provided by parents, teachers, and others, and the young adults are expected to organise themselves and be responsible for their own timetables and decision-making. Many who are unable to meet these challenges experience considerable emotional difficulties, social rejection, and their sense of loss becomes more acute (Jackson, 1988).

If it is psychological and social factors that generate deterioration, then this opens the possibility that such factors might also be used to generate progress and functional recovery long after biological recovery. The following example provides stark evidence that rehabilitative interventions can be effective many years after the acquired brain injury.

> In 2004, we assessed "Joe", a fifty-four-year-old blacksmith who suffered an ABI from an assault some twenty-six years previously. Pre-morbidly, there was no evidence of any psychiatric problems. He was resident at the time in a psychiatric nursing home, but had many different psychiatric hospital placements from which he was moved due to excessive aggression. Reports indicated increasing aggression. In 1993, attempts to support him in the community had failed, due again to his aggressive behaviour. He presented with marked disorientation, a pronounced left hemiplegia, dysarthric speech, and evidence of dyskinesia (the latter due to the use of antipsychotic medication). PRN medication was used often to manage his aggression. He presented with significant memory impairments typical of organic amnesia, with repetitive theming and frequent questioning. He had little or no insight. Nursing staff reported severe motivation problems and he invariably required prompting with regard to self-care activities. He was reluctant to engage in social or recreational opportunities offered to him. There was no incentive or behavioural reward programme available to him.
>
> Joe was admitted initially to the neurobehavioural residential programme at the Transitional Rehabilitation Unit (TRU), and a goal-orientated behavioural incentive and reward programme was introduced, targeting social behaviour, engagement, and self-care. A structured activity programme was developed that filled his day with vocational, domestic, and recreational activities. Staff used pre-emptive redirection scripts for signs of aggression. Also targeted for development were orientation, memory, and planning aids and routines. With behavioural stability, his medications were reduced and non-sedating alternatives were used. As Joe developed reliability in his routines, he progressed to TRU's Community Entry residential programme. As he became more reliable in his social behaviour, social activities were increased and expanded with longer-term opportunities. Joe has since been on several supported holidays, joined in community activities regularly, interacted well with the public, has considerable choice with regard to his activities, and requires less direct support. Sadly, Joe has not been able independently to use his external aids reliably, and, therefore, he continues to require some support to organise and structure his daily activities. His self-care has improved. He still tends to theme, but his breadth of conversation has markedly improved, as has his speech and language.

Aggression levels are low, although not extinguished, and are relatively easily managed. The majority of the time, Joe might best be described as a "grumpy old man", although he is respected and valued by his peers and he appears to enjoy a varied range of social and leisure activities with other people, including holidays to the USA—a far step from the sedated, isolated, and aggressive psychiatric patient in a locked ward.

The case of "Joe" provides an example where appropriate rehabilitation can still make a considerable difference even 20+ years after an injury and also, perhaps, gives testimony to the lost potential. Joe's progress, albeit remarkable, might well serve to emphasise the potential he could have had if he had been afforded a seamless pathway of rehabilitation that recognised the importance of structure and behavioural activation. At this point, it is important to point out that structure applies not only to the external world, but also to the psychological world. Joe remains limited in his ability to use external aids to structure his life, develop structured thinking and problem-solving routines, or adaptive habits in terms of maintaining the structure to one's world. It is certainly true that "old habits die hard" and "nothing predicts behaviour like behaviour".

The rehabilitation setting

One of the key elements in the evolution of neuropsychological rehabilitation has been the recognition of the importance of the context within which we function. In considering the plight of individuals with an ABI, it is equally important to consider the environmental factors as much as the injured individuals themselves. What types of environment can clients with an ABI function successfully in? This seems an important element in terms of discharge and post-hospital rehabilitation, and applies to both inpatient and outpatient environments. Perhaps an even more important question is, how can rehabilitation be designed so as to help the individual with ABI control their environment so that they can be successful?

It is apparent that isolated neuropsychological interventions are unlikely to be effective for all clients. Furthermore, often the family are the least well placed to deal with the demands of post acute brain injury rehabilitation. Some clients with an ABI often have an array of cognitive impairments, such as executive and memory problems, that render such "office-based" interventions ineffective. They have difficulty remembering the events in therapy or applying advice into their everyday life. These problems of maintenance and generalisation present serious barriers to rehabilitation and epitomise the importance of context and environment. Logically, it seems reasonable, therefore, for rehabilitation to be provided directly in the individual's home and community. This has several advantages. Not only are the problems of generalisation minimised, but also there is less disruption to existing supportive resources or existing adaptive coping systems and resources. It is often less anxiety provoking for the client to be rehabilitated in familiar environments and the rehabilitation is clearly more ecologically valid. However, in many cases, rehabilitation directly in the community is fraught with difficulties.

Home-based and local community-based rehabilitation is sometimes difficult to provide without it being intrusive to other members of the family. It is more difficult to maintain consistency of rehabilitation input in the home environment. It can sometimes be more expensive, due to travel costs and client, family, and rehabilitation staff disruption. Equally, not all home environments are benevolent for the ABI client, and this can be made worse by the stresses and demands on family members trying to cope with the challenges of behavioural problems. Under certain circumstances, there can be increased risks to the ABI client and others in the community: for example, when rehabilitation attempts to increase independence and social integration. Some families manage such risks by being over-protective or restrictive. While this might help to establish some structure and proactive risk management, it militates against the individual developing greater levels of independence and self-structuring.

Similarly, the family is often ill equipped to advocate for the brain-injured person. Miller (1993) has pointed out numerous reasons why families struggle to advocate. These include lack of experience, understanding, and expertise, personal stress in caring for the brain injured person, and lack of understanding of the behavioural and cognitive difficulties they are experiencing from their brain injured family member. Indeed, Miller notes that, in some cases, the family interprets the client's behaviour as "in some way deliberate, even spiteful, and could be controlled by the patient if he or she really wanted to". Indeed, Miller pointed out that this might actually be true in a minority of cases where the brain-injured person uses their disabilities and emotionality to manipulate the family for a host of secondary gains.

The family can also become a part of the problem. Many families react to aggressive outbursts with acquiescence and avoidance. They often report "walking on eggshells" in order to avoid confrontation and aggression. In doing so, they often reinforce aggression and confrontation, leading to an escalation, albeit not deliberately and often in the context of trying their hardest to cope with the situation at hand. Failed attempts to address the aggression might well result in further escalation. Other families report situations in which they appease the person with an ABI. Sometimes this can result in collusion with excessive drug or alcohol use to "sedate" the ABI person. Eventually, most families fracture (sometimes acrimoniously, sometimes with quiet detachment), leaving only one person (if any) to advocate and care for the ABI person. This person is likely to be ill informed, disillusioned with the health system, and suspicious of professionals. In addition, their enriched attachment to the ABI person is likely to be highly protective (and, in some cases, self-serving). Engaging key supporters in the rehabilitation process is, therefore, less likely the more isolated, stressed, and enmeshed they become. A more graded home re-entry through psycho–social rehabilitation environments would potentially include family and friends in the rehabilitation process in a more positive and dynamic manner.

The social and emotional dynamics of relationships within the family unit are often complex and can be strained further by attempts at rehabilitation. Indeed, many family members suffer from emotional problems as a consequence of caring for a person with ABI (e.g., Panting & Merry, 1972). Divorce and separation rates have been reported as being as high as forty-nine per cent during a 5–8 year period following brain injury (Wood & Yurdakul, 1997), although clearly this has not been a universal finding (Kreutzer, Marwitz, Hsu, Williams, & Riddick, 2007). Several studies have noted that it is the neuropsychological problems, especially behavioural problems, that cause the family the greatest distress (e.g., Brooks, Campsie, Symington, Beattie, & Mckinlay, 1986). Sadly, some studies have shown that neither family education nor a combination of education and behaviour management programme resulted in a reduction in stress experienced by family care-givers (Carnevale, Anselmi, Busichio, & Mills, 2002; Carnevale, Anselmi, Johnston, Busichio, & Walsh, 2006), although there were significant improvements in behaviour with the behaviour management programme. Often, home-based rehabilitation suffers from a lack of sheltered and supported vocational settings, and the tendency is to try to provide some structured activities via colleges. However, many colleges are not equipped to address the ABI client's cognitive and socio-behavioural problems and, furthermore, term times are of relatively short duration with long periods of holidays.

The rehabilitation team

Clearly, if rehabilitation is going to be context specific within a social milieu and provided across a range of settings with sufficient consistency, then the infrastructure of the rehabilitation team needs to be considered. At a practical and financial level, it is impossible to provide the intensity or rehabilitative support by professional clinicians alone. Indeed, a core problem for the client with an ABI is that he is often confronted with a confusing array of approaches and advice provided by clinicians from different disciplines (even when multi-disciplinary teams are communicating well). In order to provide rehabilitation contextually, in the here and now, with consistency, and across a variety of settings, it is necessary to develop brain injury rehabilitation coaches with generic skills and supervision by a trans-disciplinary team of clinical professionals from a range of disciplines (including clinical neuropsychology, speech and language therapy, occupational therapy, neuropsychiatry, and physiotherapy). The notion of a specially trained brain injury coach is described in detail by Jackson and Manchester (2001). More recently, the American Brain Injury Association has developed a programme of training front-rank rehabilitation staff to establish minimum standards of knowledge and experience for working directly with people with acquired brain injury, through its Certified Brain Injury Specialist programme, which is gathering momentum in Europe. However, this is a minimum standard that falls far short of that recommended by Jackson and Manchester (2001).

In addition to training and education, ABI rehabilitation coaches need regular supervision and support from clinical professionals and more experienced ABI rehabilitation coaches, both generally and specifically in terms of the case they are working together on.

However, the central role of the rehabilitation coach cannot be underestimated. A good ABI rehabilitation coach will be able to:

1. Support the client in sessions with clinical staff and translate recommendations and procedures into every day practice.
2. Have an understanding of the basic approaches and practical applications of neuro-behavioural rehabilitation, speech and language therapy, physiotherapy, occupational therapy and emotional management, cognitive behaviour therapies, common medical problems, first aid, drug and alcohol misuse in relation to ABI, and counselling in relation to ABI.
3. Be able to detect and resolve any inconsistencies in recommendations from different disciplines.
4. Have skills in training people with an ABI in goal setting, problem solving, self-evaluation, and risk assessment.
5. Have a good understanding and skills in antecedent interventions for people with an ABI.
6. Have skills in maintaining and making modifications to compensatory systems and aids for cognitive impairments.
7. Have a good grasp of structure and self-structure and the processes involved for the client in moving between the two.
8. Have a good understanding of the neuropsychological bases of paranoia, anxiety, depression, anger, and episodic dyscontrol, motivational loss, etc., and their management.
9. Have a good understanding of motivational approaches: for example, motivational interviewing techniques.
10. Know when to intervene to prevent failure and encourage when the individual is being successful.
11. Know how to be concrete, overt, selectively positive, and interact within the client's cognitive capabilities.
12. Have a basic understanding about denial/awareness and their management.

Managing risk is always important in brain injury rehabilitation work. This is salient to the work of the rehabilitation coach also. For example, working with a client who might be at risk within a particular situation requires the rehabilitation coach to anticipate the risk. The process of reviewing risks for planned activities with the client is a central core of providing safe but adventurous rehabilitation. Thus, a good coach should:

1. Identify the risk in advance. This can only be accomplished if the client has projected plans that the coach might be able to evaluate in terms of risk. This is also a prerequisite for the coach to be able to support the client in identifying the potential risk.
2. Suggest an alternative cognitive or behavioural response to that situation that might be used in future to greater effect.
3. Explore with the client, as far as possible, the positive consequences of the alternative response and negative consequences of their previous responses.
4. Role play the alternative response to establish procedural learning.
5. Develop and repeat a verbal mediation script to establish verbal mediation.
6. Plan with the client for help-seeking and when this might be necessary.

These inputs from the coach should be timetabled to ensure consistency and pre-emption but be flexible enough to allow for prompt intervention if required. A brain injury rehabilitation coach is clearly a skilled role, but, sadly, one that is unlikely to be recognised in the organisational structure (at least financially), and so we are dependent on those souls who live their lives in the support of others. The initial investment in developing Certified Brain Injury Specialists and ABI rehabilitation coaches is considerable, but can provide a cost-effective alternative for providing rehabilitation for many clients. The limitations of providing direct clinical therapies in isolation without contextual approaches must be recognised as a factor in order to improve the effectiveness of some rehabilitation models in the UK.

Structure and self-structuring

"Gardeners don't grow plants, they create environment where plants can grow".

It is generally agreed, but rarely objectified, that structure in the environment is beneficial to the person with a brain injury. Equally, however, the definition and core elements of structure are ill defined. Many people think of structure as being the imposition of restrictions. Several, although not all, aspects of lives are routine, predictable, and mundane. It is true that applying structure can be all these things, and that often this imposition of structure is in itself the rehabilitation. However, leading a structured life does not have to be that way and, within self-determined boundaries, many possibilities and opportunities remain.

We suggest that the core elements of structure are:

- clear and concrete with few ambiguities;
- consistent;
- predictable;
- planned and organised;
- within the capacity of cognitive ability;
- goal focused;
- active.

To apply these principles, the initial task is to get the client operational. By this, we mean interacting with their environment rather than avoiding or combating. A structured environment provides for this by setting goals and routines. It should be success laden, so that the client can counter their common experiences of failure and helplessness. Success should be overt and rewarded. Ideally, such rewards should be ecologically valid. Many behavioural reward programmes aim to provide clear behavioural targets with frequent and contingent reinforcements for small but celebrated gains. However, often the reinforcements used are not naturalistic (e.g. tokens, stars on a chart, etc., which lead to a larger reward such as a meal out or a visit to the cinema). While these behavioural programmes can be effective, often the "reward" means little to the client. Nevertheless, they can shape staff's behaviour to attend more to successes and less to failures, and it is appreciated that social praise and recognition are perhaps the most powerful reinforcers available. Furthermore, the development of these contrived rewards often simply underlines the individual's role as a client. We do not believe that people who feel badly about themselves make progress; those who believe in themselves and their abilities make progress. Therefore, it is our responsibility to create an environment in which people can feel good about themselves and their accomplishments and contributions, no matter how small.

There is no obvious reason not to use ecologically valid reinforcers, such as money (so long as it does not present a significant risk to the client). The principle is that the structured environment should be arranged in such a way that clients can earn what they get. No one feels good about being "cared for" over a long period of time. In fact, most of us become tyrants in such a situation, demanding more and more of the people around us while inwardly disliking ourselves. The good feeling of "earning" your way and taking pride in the effort and accomplishment is a basic ingredient to developing personal motivation and self-esteem. It also gives a clear message that it is the endeavours of the individual that are being rewarded and that it is their responsibility to manage their own wellbeing, rather than some carer or benevolent state.

Anchors

Nearly everyone establishes routines in their lives; when we sleep, when we rise, a morning routine and an evening routine, set mealtimes, etc. These provide anchors throughout the day to maintain a structure to our activities. Equally, nearly everyone organises their environment. We will keep things in set places (e.g., keys, coffee, clothes, etc.) and spend time maintaining this environmental organisation. Equally, we might set routines for more complex things, such as paying bills, planning our next day's activities, etc. These routine activities and events anchor and punctuate the day and week. Furthermore, since they are routine, they do not involve many demands on our executive abilities, such as generating ideas, planning, sequencing, or estimating. Applying these to the rehabilitation environment, as part of the established routine, contact with rehabilitation staff for orientation, planning, and review and reflection should be built in. Initially, such structured meetings will need to be frequent. In this way, the opportunity for frequent reinforcements can be assured and the demands of the next activity period can be limited.

Importantly, the antecedents of preparing to be successful, priming positive rational thinking, rehearsing strategies, and focusing attention on the specific tasks can be assured. Gradually, as the individual progresses, the time between orientation and reviews can be extended so that demands gradually increase and reinforcement frequency gradually fades. Structuring orientations and reviews in this way also demonstrates the importance of compartmentalising activities so that only one task is attempted at a time, or breaking tasks down into manageable segments. Often individuals with an ABI will be distracted and move on to another task without completing the task at hand. Others will not take rest breaks, but, rather, perseverate on the task to the point of exhaustion with ever-diminishing returns for their efforts. Learning to break tasks down into manageable units, pace oneself throughout the day, maintain focus on one task at a time, and stop, reflect, and plan are important routines that one needs to build into everyday functioning.

Scaffolding

In order to maintain this structure, strategies and compensatory systems for managing cognitive impairments are required. Compensatory external aids can provide the regular prompts for those with initiative problems, and reminders to remain within structure for those with memory problems. The use of a simple daily planner or diary to prompt initiation provides a level of independence for some clients. In the initial instance, this independence is provided by the rehabilitation coach, who prompts to the external aid rather than the behaviour, and gradually demands greater routine use of these aids.

Such external aids to structure go some way to establishing a relationship between activity and time of day. If the client is aware of time, associates certain activities with time, and allows the time to prompt certain plans, then they are less likely to need prompting from a family member or support staff. Furthermore, more impulsive and risky behaviours are likely to be reduced, since they are replaced by more goal-focused behaviours. The commitment to prearranged plans and the prompts from external aids reduces the number of response options and, hence, reduces distraction and the potential for impulsive reactions.

As well as structuring time and activities, thinking procedures can be structured as well. Developing routines and structures to solving problems can assist the client in reducing impulsivity, overly emotional reactions, inactivity, and helplessness. While maintaining a structure to their activities and environment is essential, unseen problems or changes in structure or natural transitions (e.g., moving house, a shop closing down, etc.) are almost inevitable. We would argue that it is these times that present the greatest challenge to clients, since they make greater demands on cognitive functioning, especially executive functioning. Clients often respond to such demands with irrational and impulsive decisions, or no response at all, or continue to attempt to maintain their routines and structure when these are no longer feasible.

To address problem solving, the client requires a well-rehearsed and structured strategy or formula that they can apply. This can take many forms, but a simple strategy for problem solving is POST (problems, options, selection, test). There are a number of rules that apply to this approach. First, it is important, where possible, for the individual to write out the problem and the steps in finding a solution in much the same way as one would write out a structured series of procedures in calculating a difficult multiplication. We have found the use of pre-printed POST sheets to be of some assistance in this regard. Second, it is always beneficial to seek benevolent assistance in performing the structured problem-solving approach. Problems should be defined in terms of the desired outcome, rather than just stating the problem. Options should be generated without evaluation initially, so as also to eliminate invalid, impulsive, or ineffective options. As many options as possible should be generated. Many people with ABI become stuck on the first idea that occurs to them and few alternatives are explored. Again, seeking benevolent help in generating options is an advantage. Selection should consider each option in turn, with consideration of whether this achieves the defined outcome, and possible negative consequences or excessive cost. Initially, the task is to eliminate those options that are invalid, not feasible, or present too great a cost or risk. From the remaining options, one or more can be chosen. It is necessary to change these options into goals and to set both a time and date to implement them and also to review whether they were effective or not. This structured step-wise approach to solving problems requires considerable practice and such practice needs to be guided, in this first instance, by rehabilitation staff.

What are the ways in which an individual can live life relatively successfully without excessive levels of "restrictive support"? It is our contention that post acute brain injury rehabilitation should involve the gradual transition from applying structure with the client to their self-structuring for themselves. Moving the control of action to internal self-regulation is central to many modern rehabilitation programmes (High, Sander, Struchen, & Hart, 2005; Wilson, Gracey, Evans, & Bateman, 2009). The process by which this transfer of locus of control is achieved, however, is less than clearly delineated. The gradual fading of rehabilitation alone is unlikely to be sufficient for the individual to maintain the gains made. A process by which the client gradually and contingently takes control and responsibility for successful rehabilitation interventions is required. This generally involves the client taking greater responsibility for their behavioural programme. It also involves the client in setting their goals and behavioural targets, evaluating performance realistically, and self-rewarding for success.

As well as fixed external cognitive aids, such as checklists, recipes, etc., there is a need to develop more interactive external cognitive aids that help manage problems, changes, and transitions. This frequently entails using more interactive aids, such as calendars, planners, diaries, and the like, where new information, choices, and goals can be entered into the aid. Obviously, the danger is that clients will neglect such decision making, goal setting, and planning, so it is important that there is a commitment to set times each day to focus on preparing and repairing the planner/diary. It is with these interactive external cognitive aids that solutions for testing can be timetabled. If used reliably, these interactive aids serve as prompts and reminders for many persons.

Goal setting

Life is not only about maintaining routines or solving problems. It is also about fulfilling ambitions, enjoyment, relaxation, and leisure. Often, clients fail to engage in these activities due to impaired initiative, avoidance, impulsivity, forgetfulness, and distractibility. To overcome these handicaps, it is important to set goals, record these goals, and make a commitment to following these goals through. Common problems after ABI in terms of goal setting include: setting unrealistic goals, goals that are non-specific and cannot be translated into positive action, or setting goals without specifying a time for action. Goal setting can be structured using the acronym S(pecific), (M)easureable, (A)chievable, (R)ealistic, and (T)ime-Bound (SMART). Although, initially, many people with an ABI will find it difficult to generate goals or evaluate them against these criteria, with repeated guided practice and setting routine times within their structure to address goal setting, progress can be made. Again, the interface between goal setting and interactive external aids such as planners, to-do lists, diaries, and calendars, etc., is important for these strategies to be effective at a functional level. Below is some guidance to help achieve this.

1. A commitment to, and reliability in, maintaining set routines and anchors.
2. Reliable use of checklists, orientation aids, and other external cognitive aids and anchors.
3. The reliable use of planning procedures, systems, and external aids.
4. The client's ability to reliably self-monitor mood and behaviour.
5. The client's reliability in seeking help appropriately.
6. The client's ability to manage emotional issues.
7. Ability and reliability in predicting possible problem situations and engaging in strategies for structured problem solving.
8. Ability and reliability in recognising early warning signs of deterioration and de-structuring.

It is on these areas that the focus of rehabilitation should be directed as the client prepares gradually to withdraw from rehabilitation. If it is the case that clients are able to function well in a structured environment and they have the capabilities to develop effective controls over that environment so as to structure it, then they will have greater capacity to influence their own lives, develop self-esteem, and develop social infrastructures to support themselves. Efforts to assist clients to develop the skills, habits, and strategies to become more independent, therefore, should focus on helping the client to build core foundations in structuring their world, thinking, and activities. Basic functions such as maintaining a reasonable sleep–wake cycle, diet, pacing, hygiene, morning routines, etc., need to be reasonably reliable.

Strategies for structuring future activities are important also. This involves planning and the setting of personal goals, both short term (tomorrow, later today) and longer term (this week, this month), being aware of possible risks in these plans, and making allowances for them. It also involves using strategies to maintain a structured lifestyle, such as seeking help, discussing problems with others, using external memory and organisation aids to keep to plans, following through with longer-term plans, ongoing monitoring of performance, making reflective evaluations of performance, and making adjustments while managing moods. The assessment of the individual's progress in developing self-structuring is a central issue for rehabilitation, although there are few standardised measures that capture this process. The "behavioural assessment of self-structuring" (BASS) (Jackson, please contact the first author for further details) is one measure that evaluates an individual's ability to self-structure various activities and tasks across everyday functioning.

Structuring meaningful roles and activities

As we have already discussed, self-identity and social identity is based, at least in part, on an individual's roles and responsibilities within the social network. This is shaped by the opportunities available to the individual (and those initiated and maintained by the individual) and by the interpersonal achievements, experiences, and rewards provided through the structure of their daily lives. Self-esteem can flourish in those circumstances, or, conversely, diminish in the absence of mastery, success, and achievement in the social environment. After a traumatic brain injury, clients are likely to experience considerable challenges in accessing and sustaining such experiences. Indeed, many clients can experience significant losses in these areas of their life as social roles, status, and opportunities shift in their social environment. As such, many clients are likely to experience significant challenges to their self-identity and their social identity, and this must be an important consideration in supporting clients following an ABI, although it is often understated within rehabilitation models.

Structuring with the individual a range of valued, meaningful, and purposeful activities that are routine, predictable, and manageable is extremely important. This can create positive momentum that reinforces and builds upon established routines of daily living and promotes opportunities for enriching experiences and interactions with others. However, this is much more likely to occur when sufficient planning, organisation, and pre-emption is provided through the rehabilitation coach, and structured to ensure the individual (and environment) is best prepared to provide predictable, successful, and errorless interactions between the individual and their environment. This, of course, also has to be provided in line with the individual's own wishes, goals, and abilities.

The challenge is to provide an effective framework that *enables* the individual and environment to compensate for typical neuropsychological problems of initiation, motivation, planning and organisation, self-monitoring, social inference, and problem solving, while promoting functional engagement in a given task. Activities might well be planned into a timetable, yet, in the absence of sufficient structuring, pre-emption, prompting, and review frameworks for the individual and their supporters, problems are likely to occur in spite of the individual's functional abilities. All too often, we see such frameworks leading to individuals disengaging from activities, or activities/interactions being withdrawn as risks (or behaviours) are deemed to be unmanageable in that setting, without sufficient attention to the broader variables that impact upon the success of that activity.

Vocational rehabilitation models can contribute to the structuring of meaningful activities, particularly when individuals are likely to have experienced significant losses in these areas following a severe ABI (see Onsworth & McKenna, 2004, and also Walsh's Chapter Eight, in this volume). Vocational rehabilitation models can fulfil various purposes. Primarily, they may be seen as placements to support an individual's skills and abilities on the pathway to employment and, where this is a realistic goal, can be effective and valuable in individuals gaining employment after rehabilitation (Malec & Basford, 1996). However, there is also recognition that it can be difficult to maintain employment as well as to secure employment for individuals with ABI (Ben-Yishay, Silver, Piasetsky, & Rattok, 1987). For many individuals, vocational rehabilitation programmes can promote other important outcomes, including positive experiences of mastery, success, wellbeing, and positive self-identity. Such supported placements can provide invaluable forums for transferring and rehearsing compensatory external aids and systems to promote increased autonomy and self-management. They can also provide an important source of consistent and adaptive social interaction and explicit social boundaries that can be particularly helpful for the individual with an ABI.

Work environments can provide structure and also the potential for developing self-structuring. They provide naturalistic activities that individuals with ABI can relate to without confrontation of their denial or impaired awareness. Sheltered work environments can provide social networks and opportunities that would allow for real-life neuro–psycho–social rehabilitation (e.g., social interaction skills, pacing, stamina and attention building, goal setting, problem solving, self-monitoring and evaluation, self-esteem, and the reconstruction of personal and social identity) as well as actual vocational activities themselves. Return to work initiatives generally tend to have high ecological and face validity, also for clients themselves.

> Dr P, a consultant cardiologist, was injured in a head-on collision with a bus, resulting in five months PTA with severe frontal contusions. Neuropsychological test results indicated reasonably retained IQ (circa 120) but severe executive impairments, impaired awareness, and severe motivational problems. He was admitted to TRU's neurobehavioural unit three years after his ABI, having been unsuccessfully managed in a number of other rehabilitation facilities. Early attempts at rehabilitation had been met with explosive aggression when asked to engage. Behavioural reinforcement programmes were ineffective, orientations and prompting resulted in abuse and, at times, physical aggression. He demonstrated a marked lack of awareness, severe lack of motivation, with reglect of personal hygiene and self-care. Engagement in any recreational activity was limited. Dr P would isolate himself in his room. Interpersonal behaviour was abrupt and dismissive and he refused to use any aids to orientate or organise himself. He was invited to apply for the post of Health Adviser. Following being interviewed, a job contract was provided with clear expectations of his duties, which involved regular health checks on staff, including taking blood pressure, interviewing regarding lifestyle (e.g., smoking, drinking habits, etc.). A rota of appointments was arranged with TRU staff by a nurse at TRU who served as his assistant. There was a marked improvement in his engagement, with regular attendance at his "job", improvements in his mood and behaviour, and improvements in his self-care.
>
> However, while he would use organisational systems in his role as Health Adviser, which he did religiously, he continued to refuse to use such aids and systems in his everyday life. He refused to engage with any behavioural targets, even when these were related to his job role. A radical approach was taken, in which his cognitive attributions were routinely addressed in initially frequent CBT psychology sessions and supported by

rehabilitation coaching staff. His behavioural programme was modified to place him in absolute control. He was asked to design and set his own daily timetable and behavioural targets (which he did, although they did not differ at all from those initially suggested), to evaluate his own performance, and reward himself (financial rewards). Surprisingly, his self-evaluations and self-rewards were, by and large, remarkably accurate. For this position, we supported Dr P to set his own personal goals. Aggression levels markedly decreased. Self-care improved (albeit only partially). Dr P began to socialise more and participate in communal activities, outings, etc. He progressed from the neurobehavioural programme to a commuity re-entry programme and was eventually discharged into the community.

The case of Dr P provides a clear example of how vocational activities that provide for a person's self-esteem and do not confront the person with their disabilities and loss of role can catalyse engagement in productive ABI rehabilitation. From this base of improved engagement, the basic building blocks of goal setting, self-monitoring, and developing coping aids and strategies can be developed.

Furthermore, by eliminating the conflict that can occur in being a rehabilitation client who feels controlled by others and emerging as someone taking personal responsibility, the barriers to engaging in rehabilitation can often be reduced. Dr P's case also provides an example of how behavioural incentive programmes that would otherwise have been motivating and rewarding were perceived as elements of control. It is clear, therefore, that, as with that found in Jackson and Bentall's (1991) study that demonstrated that cognitive schema changed the responses to contingencies of reinforcement in persons with severe amnesia, so, too, did Dr P develop a cognitive interpretation of the behavioural programme that rendered it impotent in changing behaviour. It is clear, therefore, that simple behavioural programmes (especially those based on predominantly reinforcement contingencies) might, in many situations, be ineffective if the individual's cognitive schema is not considered simultaneously.

Traditional psychotherapy

While traditional psychotherapeutic models of rehabilitation are not dismissed (see Chapter Three in this volume), their value for people with severe ABI is questioned without direct application and support within context-specific situations. Even people with severe cognitive impairments might be able to benefit from a range of "adapted" psychotherapies, such as anxiety management, anger management, cognitive behaviour therapies, and even training in problem solving and self-reflection, although it requires a move away from office-based interventions into more systemic approaches. Systemic interventions are often essential if clients with ABI are to overcome the barriers of impaired memory, attention, and executive functions that can render isolated sessional psychotherapies ineffective. In this sense, the clinician is well advised to move away from periodic and isolated psychotherapy approaches for emotional adjustment and cognitive difficulties (albeit that these are important elements in a comprehensive rehabilitation programme). Instead, they could embrace a systemic approach to help the client structure their environments, thinking, and plans, and to support the understanding and expertise of individuals.

There is wide recognition of the range of emotional problems that can be encountered following ABI associated with both primary and secondary consequences of the injury (see Williams & Evans, 2003). Processes underpinning emotional disturbance can be complex, involving executive control function and memory problems, reactions to losses and changes, and to increased predisposition to further significant life events. While recognition of these processes is clear in the literature, there is much less focus upon how such problems are effectively treated within clinical frameworks. It could be assumed that some emotional problems might be amenable to standard therapeutic approaches, including individual and group therapies, although two factors must be considered.

1. The ability of the client to manage the demands and processes associated with the content of the session, including having sufficient memory, information processing, coping strategies, and insight.
2. The ability of the client (and environment) to support the transfer of information, strategies, and goals to the relevant activities and interactions of daily living.

These factors can present considerable challenges in evaluating the effectiveness and suitability of traditional psychotherapies for clients with an ABI. Various adaptations to therapy frameworks have been described and positively evaluated, particularly for individuals with a mild to moderate ABI (Tiersky et al., 2005). These include use of visual aids, chunking of information, role-plays, and repetition of information. However, there is recognition of the limited number of research trials and, indeed, the difficulties in abstracting from research, given the heterogeneity of processes involved for the ABI population (Soo & Tate, 2007). While adaptations can certainly be made to the therapy environment to promote more successful management of information, transfer of such information can be a significant obstacle for clients with very severe ABI and the associated significant cognitive impairment that can occur. Unfortunately, this is too often ignored in planning appropriate interventions. A focus upon direct therapy in isolation is likely to neglect the core challenges facing many individuals when they are faced with events and problems that trigger or maintain emotional problems outside of the therapy context. It is at this time that support to implement therapeutic strategies and techniques becomes most effective and most needed. This reinforces the importance of providing effective training, supervision, and support for coaches who are most likely to be working with the client at these points in time.

Accessing post acute brain injury rehabilitation

Recent years have seen the development of more local ABI teams with the aim of following the client into the community from the hospital setting. However, this welcome development is limited, with poor coverage in many areas still and difficulties for some ABI teams (where they do exist) in resourcing neuropsychological rehabilitation. In addition to a paucity of expert resources, there are sometimes fewer social, vocational, and domestic situations where rehabilitation can be provided intensively and safely. In our opinion, this has, on occasion, led to a hotchpotch of services with less clear or effective pathways towards successful community re-entry for clients with ABI.

The organisational structures of health and social services for people with ABI often militate against them receiving and benefiting from rehabilitation. The division in funding between health care and social care causes considerable problems in securing seamless pathways back into successful functioning in the community, with apparently endless debates over whether the services provided are addressing health or social needs. There is often little preparation of the client and their families prior to discharge, and often little in the way of follow-up assessments that would provide for the early identification of neuropsychosocial problems and swift intervention to prevent secondary problems. The average time since injury that referrals are made to the Transitional Rehabilitation Unit (TRU) is about five years. In that time, most clients will have lost friends and supporters, and/or developed unhelpful coping strategies, such as avoidance, alcohol misuse, aggression, and offending. Recent studies on the UK prison population have identified a high prevalence of prisoners with a history of traumatic brain injury. Similarly, mental health services vary greatly in their understanding of traumatic brain injury and the appropriateness of the services they can provide.

In the first instance, the means by which a client with an ABI accesses post acute neuropsychological rehabilitation services is clearly important. Currently, only a small proportion of individuals with ABI are referred for post acute rehabilitation and then, in the majority of cases, only after many years of failure within the community. Despite the growing awareness of the nature and extent of handicaps caused by impairments to cognitive and social functioning to both clients and their families, the predominant treatment is often medical rather than psychological. Physical needs are given priority, and rightly so, perhaps, in the early stages. However, neuropsychological problems often cause greater burdens and handicaps to clients and their families. Currently, significant areas of the country have no access to neuropsychological rehabilitation (and, in some cases, even neuropsychological assessment). It is likely that many clients are being discharged without a reasonable assessment of their ability to function within the environment to which they are being discharged, or the environment itself. There are many reasons for this.

Among them are:

1. Assumptions that there is nothing that can be done.
2. Paucity of neuropsychological services and local expertise in some areas.
3. Insensitive and inappropriate methods used in assessing functioning after ABI.

4. Lack of insight by the client with an ABI.
5. Lack of knowledge by the supporters of the client with an ABI.
6. Poor integration of services and funding streams.

The US General Accounting Office report (1998) highlighted that those brain injury victims who have difficulty accessing services are those with cognitive impairments but without physical disabilities, since, in the USA, as in the UK, there is a bias towards physical disability in rehabilitation. In the UK, the report of the Royal College of Surgeons in 1976 included a forceful appendix castigating doctors for being too concerned with acute episodes of illness and not concerned enough with long-term disability. The US General Accounting Office also identified those individuals without advocates as being particularly vulnerable with regard to accessing rehabilitation. However, it should be acknowledged that, in the UK there have been significant improvements in brain injury rehabilitation since the 2000s (Royal College of Physicians and British Society of Rehabilitation Medicine, 2003).

Compounding this problem is the psychological difficulty many ABI victims have in returning to rehabilitation, having been discharged from hospital. This can be seen as a failure, often both by the client and their family, resulting in a resistance to engagement. It is sometimes also a function of poor self-awareness, especially during the early post acute stages. Another potential obstacle regards logistics—sometimes the person or their family simply do not have the means (e.g., transport in rural areas) to regularly access services available to them. To overcome some of these difficulties, a rehabilitation system and health/social services infrastructure that provided for graded and contingent pathways towards community re-entry would be more effective in reducing the deterioration in psychosocial and psychiatric problems seen after ABI and provide greater possibilities for progress.

ABI rehabilitation inevitably relies on an organisational infrastructure to be successful, or, indeed, available. Currently, health and social services need to develop pathways for clients with ABI that allow for assessment and intervention at different stages of recovery and in response to the variety of needs that occur at each stage in the pathway. In 2005, the UK government developed a blueprint for the management of long-term neurological conditions in the *National Service Framework for Long-term Conditions* (NSF for LTNC) that reflected this need for more psychosocial specialist ABI services, with rehabilitation extending into the community via interim specialist placements for more intensive rehabilitation within structured environments, including vocational, behavioural rehabilitation and cognitive rehabilitation services (Department of Health, 2005).

The client's experience of professional support is generally poor where the infrastructure for providing interventions and support is fragmented. Families often complain about the lack of support, education, advice, and input. They cite misinformation and absence of support after discharge from hospital. Under these circumstances, their trust in rehabilitation services and professionals generally is often low. Equally, the client is prone to suspiciousness, and they are less likely to seek or engage with rehabilitation. Early psychosocial rehabilitation has been found to improve outcome, although later rehabilitation also demonstrated potential (Worthington, Matthews, Melia, & Oddy, 2006). It is self-evident, therefore, that the organisation of rehabilitation services should involve greater attention to the process of reintegrating clients into the community from the hospital to address these potential secondary problems that might affect their engagement.

With regard to vocational rehabilitation Tyerman (2011) reports on the recommendations by the British Society for Rehabilitation Medicine (2010), calling for greater collaboration between neuro-rehabilitation services and vocational services, but rightly points out that "most vocational programmes are not geared to the complex needs of people with long-term neurological conditions" (p. 7). Furthermore, the British Society for Rehabilitation Medicine's report is limited to spinal cord injury, epilepsy, multiple sclerosis, and cerebral palsy, which, although providing exemplars for the four main clusters identified in the NSF (i.e., sudden onset, intermittent and unpredictable, progressive and stable conditions with unchanging needs), they do not encompass the particular difficulties encountered by clients with ABI, who often present with mainly cognitive (and particularly executive) difficulties.

It is our experience that vocational agencies and employers often have poor awareness of executive impairments in particular, and are less sympathetic to such problems as interpersonal impairments, unreliability of attendance and performance, impaired awareness, and poor monitoring and evaluation of performance. Thus, many people with ABI are unable to manage reintegration within the work setting because of pre-vocational impairments (e.g., time keeping, attendance, spotting and reporting mistakes, following instructions, appropriate help-seeking, managing changes in routines, distractibility, inappropriate social interactions, etc.). There is, therefore, a need to develop sheltered and protected vocational opportunities where these problems can be addressed prior to referral to more mainstream vocational rehabilitation programmes. Equally, rather than seeing vocational activities as the endpoint of rehabilitation, they are really an invaluable setting for further neuropsychological rehabilitation. Work environments are often very dynamic environments that bring the residual problem-solving difficulties suffered by many clients with a severe ABI into sharp relief and are an excellent context to explore abilities and difficulties.

The NSF for LTNC does not delineate the exact nature of residential resources for a graded approach for rehabilitation towards community re-entry. However, we suggest that a network of relatively small residential facilities is needed for an important proportion of persons with ABI. These would provide graded residential pathways with defined levels of support and structure. Indeed, the evolution of TRU has been to develop such residential options (ranging from post acute services, intensive neuro-behavioural programmes through community re-entry residential programmes and supported community houses, both individual and shared, to direct home support and rehabilitation). Each of these facilities provides different levels of support, intensity of clinical professionals' input, social milieus, community integration, and demands on the client with an ABI. Within each of these programmes, the client is seen not in isolation, but as part of a social milieu faced with the demands of interpersonal, mutual support, and personal responsibilities towards their environment and the welfare of others. In these settings, management of emotional behaviour, social interaction skills, empathy and mutual support, domestic responsibilities, recreational activities, planning and organisation, and social problem solving become core elements affected not only by rehabilitation staff, but also by peers.

These social environments should deviate markedly from traditional hospital or nursing/care home settings. In particular, there needs to be a blurring of the divide between the resident and the staff, although still with clear (and explicit) recognition of professional boundaries. Success and accomplishments should be focused on, and failures and impairments should be avoided. Residents should be encouraged to develop personal responsibilities and also social responsibilities in living with others. The role of the individual as a "cared-for person" or a client should be challenged. The social environment should encourage self-determination and the emergence of personal and social roles that will encourage the reconstruction of self-esteem and a valued personal and social identity. Under these circumstances, individuals are more likely to be willing to address the challenges caused by their brain injury without ever having to relinquish their denial or develop their insight.

Concluding remarks

Community neuro-rehabilitation exists in many formats and can be found in a wide range of settings. To some extent, this reflects the extreme variation in presentation in persons with ABI, some needing specialist residential input, while, at the other end of the continuum, some never access any rehabilitation services. It also often reflects the limited availability of funding, and, as a result, development of, at times, less than ideal services in some areas. In our own model described here, we posited that community-based neuro-rehabilitation is a complex and individualised process of adapting evidence-based approaches in an integrative, flexible, and systemic manner with individuals and their core supporters in ecologically valid settings. In this chapter, as the astute reader would have noticed, we drew upon a wide range of theoretical work, in particular that of Luria (1973), to suggest and advocate that, at an operational clinical level, it is these individuals who are most likely to be delivering the "real world" rehabilitation techniques and approaches that can make a meaningful difference for the individual with ABI.

In this specific context, clinical professionals have a fundamental role (and responsibility) in ensuring assessment and intervention approaches take into account the complex individual, interpersonal, and systemic factors and challenge traditional models of office-based therapy in isolation. Furthermore, we consider professionals to have a vital role in challenging the gulf that sometimes exists between theory and practice at both a clinical and social policy level in ensuring that clients with ABI have access to effective, real-world interventions, with trained and specialist support staff to support individuals to reach their potential, achieve their goals, and live an enriching and meaningful life. This is not an idealistic picture, but a core standard that should be expected. That said, there is clearly a need for service design, funding systems, and professional approaches to be better integrated and more robustly underpinned by this and other appropriate theoretical models to guide clinical practice. This continues to be a challenge, but one to be embraced by clinicians, academics, and specialist acquired brain injury services.

Note

1. Editors' note. An underlying theme of this book suggests successful engagement with the complex challenges of ABI demands that the therapist develops some understanding of the world of the ABI client and how their injury affects their whole way of being. Howard Jackson and Gemma Hague's comprehensive chapter shows why it is important to have both a philosophical and practical grasp of how executive dysfunction creates so many social difficulties for clients and can impede rehabilitation. While they present a particular holistic "total rehabilitation model", and there are others, we feel their explanation of the "TRU" approach will have implications for whatever approach you use.

References

Ben-Yishay, Y., Silver, S., Piasetsky, E., & Rattok, J. (1987). Relationship between employability and vocational outcome after intensive holistic cognitive rehabilitation. *Journal of Head Trauma Rehabilitation*, 2(1): 35–48.

British Society for Rehabilitation Medicine (2010). *Vocational Assessment and Rehabilitation for People with Long-Term Neurological Conditions: Recommendations for Best Practice*. London: BSRM.

Brooks, N. (Ed.) (1984). *Closed Head Injury: Psychological, Social, and Family Consequences*. New York: Oxford University Press.

Brooks, N., Campsie, L., Symington, C., Beattie, A., & McKinlay, W. (1986). The five year outcome of severe blunt head injury: a relative's view. *Journal of Neurology, Neurosurgery and Psychiatry*, 49: 764–770.

Carnevale, G. J., Anselmi, V., Busichio, K., & Mills, S. R. (2002). Changes in ratings of caregiver burden following a community-based behaviour management program for persons with traumatic brain injury. *Journal of Head Trauma Rehabilitation*, 17: 83–95.

Carnevale, G. J., Anselmi, V., Johnston, M. V., Busichio, K., & Walsh, V. (2006). A natural setting behavior management program for persons with acquired brain injury: a randomized controlled trial. *Archives of Physical Medicine and Rehabilitation*, 87: 1289–1297.

Department of Health (2005). *The National Service Framework for Long-term Conditions*. London: The Stationery Office.

Fleminger, S. (2010). Neuropsychiatric effects of traumatic brain injury: secondary symptoms that you need to watch for. *Psychiatric Times*, 27(3): 40–45.

Fleminger, S., Oliver, D. L., & Lovestone, S. (2003). Head injury as a risk factor for Alzheimer's disease: the evidence 10 years on; a partial replication. *Journal of Neurology, Neurosurgery and Psychiatry*, 74: 857–862.

Gracey, F., Palmer, S., Rous, B., Psaila, K., Shaw, K., O'Dell, J., Cope, J., & Mohamed, S. (2008). Feeling part of things: personal construction of self after brain injury. *Neuropsychological Rehabilitation*, 18(5–6): 627–650.

High, W. M., Sander, A. M., Struchen, M. A., & Hart, K. A. (2005). *Rehabilitation for Traumatic Brain Injury*. New York: Oxford University Press.

Jackson, H. F. (1988). Brain, cognition and grief: affective responses following brain injury. *Aphasiology*, 2: 89–92.

Jackson, H. F., & Bentall, R. P. (1991). Operant conditioning in amnesic subjects: response patterning & sensitivity to schedule changes. *Neuropsychology*, 5: 89–105.

Jackson, H. F., & Manchester, D. (2001). Towards the development of brain injury specialists. *Neurorehabilitation*, 16: 27–40.

Jackson, H. F., Hopewell, C. A., Glass, C., Ghadiali, E., & Warburg, R. (1992). The Katz social adjustment scale: modification for traumatically injured victims. *Brain Injury*, 6: 109–27.

Jackson, R., & Moffat, N. (1987). Impaired emotional perception following closed head injury. *Cortex, 1987*: 293–300.

Kreutzer, J. S., Marwitz, J. H., Hsu, N., Williams, K., & Riddick, A. (2007). Marital stability after brain injury: an investigation and analysis. *NeuroRehabilitation*, 22(1): 53–59.

Lezak, M. D. (1982). The problem of assessing executive functions. *International Journal of Psychology*, 17: 281–297.

Lezak, M. D. (1983). *Neuropsychological Assessment* (2nd edn). New York: Oxford University Press.

Luria, A. R. (1973). *The Working Brain*. New York: Basic Books.

Malec, J. F., & Basford, J. S. (1996). Postacute brain injury rehabilitation. *Archives of Physical Medicine & Rehabilitation*, 77(2): 198–207.
Manchester, D., Priestly, N., & Jackson, H. (2004). The assessment of executive functions: coming out of the office. *Brain Injury*, 18: 1067–1081.
Markus, H. (1983). Self-knowledge: an expanded view. *Journal of Personality*, 51: 543–65.
McDonald, S., & Flanagan, S. (2004). Social perception deficits after traumatic brain injury: the interaction between emotion recognition, mentalising ability and social communication. *Neuropsychology*, 18: 572–579.
Megginson, L. C. (1963). Lessons from Europe for American business. *Southwestern Social Science Quarterly*, 44(1): 3–13.
Miller, L. (1993). Family therapy of brain injuries: syndromes, strategies and solutions. *American Journal of Family Therapy*, 21: 111–121.
Onsworth, T., & McKenna, K. (2004). Investigation of factors related to employment outcome following traumatic brain injury: a critical review and conceptual model. *Disability and Rehabilitation*, 26(13): 765–784.
Panting, A., & Merry, P. (1972). The long-term rehabilitation of severe head injuries with particular reference to the need for social and medical support for the patient's family. *Rehabilitation*, 38: 33–37.
Prigatano, G. P. (1986). Psychotherapy after brain-injury. In: G. P. Prigatano (Ed.), *Neuropsychological Rehabilitation after Brain-Injury* (pp. 67–95). Baltimore, MD: Johns Hopkins University Press.
Roth, R. M., Isquith, P. K., & Gioia, G. A. (2005). *Behavior Rating Inventory of Executive Function—Adult Version*. Odessa, FL: Psychological Assessment Resources.
Royal College of Physicians and British Society of Rehabilitation Medicine (2003). L. Turner-Stokes (Ed.). *Rehabilitation following Acquired Brain Injury: National Clinical Guidelines*. London: Royal College of Physicians, British Society of Rehabilitation Medicine.
Sastre, M., Richardson, J. C., Gentleman, S. M., & Brooks, D. J. (2011). Inflammatory risk factors and pathologies associated with Alzheimer's disease. *Current Alzheimer's Research*, 8(2): 132–141.
Sohlberg, M. M., & Mateer, C. A. (1989). Theory and remediation of attention disorders. In: M. M. Sohlberg & C. A. Mateer (Eds.), *Introduction to Cognitive Rehabilitation* (pp. 110–135). New York: Guildford Press.
Soo, C., & Tate, R. (2007). Psychological treatment for anxiety in people with traumatic brain injury. *Cochrane Database of Systematic Reviews*, 3: CD005239.

Tajfel, H. (1982). *Social Identity and Intergroup Relations*. Cambridge: Cambridge University Press.

Tiersky, L. A., Anselmi, M. V., Johnston, Kurtyka, J., Roosen, E., Schwartz, T., & DeLuca, J. (2005). A trial of neuropsychologic rehabilitation in mid-spectrum traumatic brain injury. *Archives of Physical Medicine and Rehabilitation, 86*(8): 1565–1574.

Tyerman, A. (2011). Recommendations for best practice in vocational assessment and rehabilitation. *Division of Neuropsychology Newsletter, 10*(1): 6–7.

US General Accounting Office (1998). *Traumatic Brain Injury Programs Supporting Long-term Services in Selected States* (Publication No. GAO/HEHS-98–55).

Vogenthaler, D. (1987). An overview of head injury. Its consequences and rehabilitation. *Brain Injury, 1*: 113–127.

Williams, W. H., & Evans, J. J. (2003). Brain injury and emotion: an overview to a special issue on biopsychosocial approaches in neurorehabilitation. *Neuropsychological Rehabilitation, 13*(1/2):1–11.

Wilson, B. A., Gracey, F., Evans, J. J., & Bateman, A. (2009). *Neuropsychological Rehabilitation: Theory, Models, Therapy and Outcome*. Cambridge: Cambridge University Press.

Wolters, G., Stapert, S., Brands, I., & Van Heugten, C. (2011). Coping following acquired brain injury: predictors and correlates. *Journal of Head Trauma Rehabilitation, 26*: 150–157.

Wood R. L., & Yurdakul, L. K. (1997). Change in relationship status following traumatic brain injury. *Brain Injury, 11*(7): 491–502.

Worthington, A. D., Matthews, S., Melia, Y., & Oddy, M. (2006). Cost-benefits associated with social outcome from neurobehavioural rehabilitation. *Brain Injury, 20*: 947–957.

Yates, P. J., Williams, W. H., Harris, A., Round, A., & Jenkins, R. (2006). An epidemiological study of head injuries in a UK population attending an emergency department. *Journal of Neurology Neurosurgery and Psychiatry, 77*: 699–701.

PART II

BEING IN PRACTICE: WORKING WITH THE ISSUES FACED BY REAL CLIENTS WITH ACQUIRED BRAIN INJURIES LIVING IN THE REAL WORLD

ASSESSMENT IN SPECIFIC CONTEXTS

CHAPTER FIVE

Low awareness conditions: their assessment and treatment

Crawford Thomas

This chapter will focus on defining the terminology of low awareness conditions, assessment and rehabilitation techniques for those people who have sustained profound or severe brain injuries. Techniques covered include: the Coma Recovery Scale-Revised (CRS-R) (Giacino, Kalmar, & Whyte, 2004), the Western Neuro Sensory Stimulation Profile (WNSSP) (Ansell & Keenan, 1989) and the Sensory Modality Assessment and Rehabilitation Technique (SMART) (Gill-Thwaites, 1997; Gill-Thwaites & Munday, 1999). It is perhaps more important to understand the general principles involved in this kind of work. In this sense, this chapter is clearly not a training manual (go and get trained if you want that. No, seriously, it will do you a lot of good). So, to the purist, well-drilled, SMART-trained individual, it could be viewed as too impressionistic. I hope what it does is give an overview, with enough depth, maybe, for someone to become excited (as I am about this area of work) to actually go and be trained or, at the very least, think about some of the fundamental issues that work like this can raise. One little teeny tiny one being: what is consciousness? In order to have a better understanding of these principles, it will be necessary, to begin with, to examine what we currently understand to be profound and severe brain injury.

What is very severe or profound brain injury?

One of the difficulties in this area for the newly qualified clinician is the range of potentially confusing labels and other terminologies that sometimes appear quite distinct in what they are describing and, at other times, seem to blur between one type of presentation and another. This becomes even more strange when you are busy feeling out of your depth in your first interdisciplinary team meeting and you suddenly realise that medical person opposite is talking about the same patient, but is using terminology that you thought meant something else. To be balanced, though, we should not assume that other colleagues always have an in-depth knowledge of what we often talk about, and vice versa. Historically, much of the work on profound or severe brain injury began being sharpened at the same time as advances in medical knowledge made these conditions more common. Thus, our ability to enable patients to survive profound or severe brain injury took significant leaps forward in the late 1960s and 1970s, in both the UK and the USA. Partly as a result of this, one of the seminal papers was initially presented by Jennet and Plum in 1972, within which they coined the term "persistent vegetative state" (PVS) to describe people who, although still in coma, had progressed to a level of some wakefulness but without any signs of marked awareness.

Over a decade later in America, a presidential commission in 1983 for the study of ethical problems in medicine, biomedical and behavioural research accepted Jennett and Plum's definition. In particular, with regard to consciousness, and, more specifically, the patient's inability to experience his or her immediate environment. However, they were keen to make clear that PVS is only one of a number of forms of permanent unconsciousness. Others include the end stage in forms of dementia and untreatable mass lesions, for example. Subsequent to this, various position papers and working parties and committees have been formed to refine our understanding not only of PVS, but also other related conditions. Perhaps the most well known was the multi-society taskforce on PVS established in 1991. Rather like Jennet and Plum's 1972 paper, this multi-taskforce paper represented a watershed moment in our understanding of low awareness conditions. A quick reference guide for the main conditions is presented in Table 5.1 (adapted from Monti, Laureys, & Owen, 2010).

Table 5.1. Differential diagnosis in low awareness conditions.

Condition	Definition	Main clinical characteristics
Coma	Unarousable state of unresponsiveness	No eye opening (even after intense painful stimulation) No evidence of awareness of the self or environment In same condition for more than one hour
Vegetative state	Wakefulness but no sign of awareness	Eye opening and closing No reproducible purposeful behaviour including (a) no response to sensory stimulation; (b) no awareness of the self or the environment; (c) no language ability (comprehension or expression)
Minimally conscious state response	Wakefulness but some inconsistent and reproducible signs of awareness	Displays eye opening and closing Some inconsistent but reproducible purposeful behaviour including (any of) (a) non-reflexive response to sensory stimulation; (b) awareness of the self or the environment; (c) language comprehension or expression Lack of functional communication or object usage
Locked-in syndrome	Significant problems with voluntary motor behaviour	Discernible eye-coded communication Some awareness Significant impairments in motor behaviour

One of the key definitions with regard to PVS is that:

> the vegetative state is a clinical condition of complete unawareness of the self and the environment, accompanied by sleep–wake cycles with either a complete or partial preservation of hypothalamic and brainstem autonomic functions. (Multi-Society Task Force on PVS, 1996, p. 1499)

The paper then goes on to state the seven main criteria for diagnosing the vegetative state. This is a very important point for clinical practice.

A number of clinicians still use the terms PVS and vegetative states in a casual manner, leading to disharmony among family members and an inability to understand the prognosis properly.

Some use the term "minimally conscious", others "low level neurological states", and still others use the more global term "altered states of consciousness". For the purposes of this chapter, I will refer to those people who have some level of awareness of their environment but who have had a severe and profound injury as being in a low awareness condition. It is important to distinguish patients in minimally conscious states (MCS) from those in coma and PVS, because preliminary findings suggest that there are meaningful differences in outcome. These are outlined below.

Low awareness condition captures more of the sub-conditions under discussion in a more positive way. In my view, it is a more global term, and no one has to revert to the exceptionally frightening (for nearly all families I have worked with) term *vegetative*. In any case, I think this particular word will become lost over time; the main reason for this is the apparent clear (and repeatable) demonstration, using sophisticated PET and *f*MRI equipment, of consciousness in patients who had previously been termed vegetative (Cruse & Owen, 2010). However, currently, at its worst, this word connotes concretely adjacent words to this, such as vegetables. At best, while it is clinically accurate, it is just that, perceived as too extremely clinical a description for the human being they have known and loved now lying before them. Put another way, you might more easily move from discussion and clinical support using low awareness condition as your initial verbal anchor. This might eventually become a discussion and support based around a phrase including the word vegetative. For families, there is nowhere to go from there, but if you start the conversation with this terminology, where do you go, as the treating clinician?

Factors affecting the outcome

Another source of confusion to the new recruit to a neuro-rehabilitation unit is that there is no "gold standard" measure of severity of a brain injury. What one has to do is take a number of different measures and combine these into an overall assessment, so there is some room for more flexible interpretation of findings, using clinical judgement to integrate from different sources. A few examples of some commonly used measures are briefly described below.

One such measure is the Glasgow Coma Scale Score (GCS) (Teasdale & Jennet, 1974). This is a measure that aims to give a reliable and somewhat objective way of recording the level of conscious state for initial as well as subsequent assessment of a person after a head injury. There are three sub-components that make up this final figure. These are: best eye, verbal, and motor responses. Each is considered separately as well as their overall total being evaluated. Each one, at its base, runs from no response through eyes opening spontaneously, or orientated, or obeys commands. The lowest possible GCS (the sum) is three, which can mean a deep coma or, indeed, death. The highest overall score is fifteen, which means that the person is fully awake. While very widely used, there are some limitations with generating accurate scores. Examples include when patients are sedated and intubated at the scene of an accident before a rating is performed, or if extensive facial injuries prevent an accurate overall rating.

Another useful tool to understanding severity of brain injury is the length of time someone is in a coma. Although this does not usually apply to the low awareness patient, it is another useful rule-of-thumb (for the dangers of this approach, see below) for those less profoundly injured. Nevertheless, there is some evidence that length of coma does capture severity, and, perhaps more importantly, has an association with subsequent outcome. However, this is by no means a perfect association. One of the main difficulties here is that total time in coma is a problematic measure, as a number of hours, days, or even weeks might pass while the person is in an artificially induced coma, contaminating the judgement of the overall length of time of coma.

The final measure, often described as the best, is that of post-trauma amnesia (PTA). A person's orientation to themselves, where they are currently, and at what time should ideally be assessed on a continuous basis from the point at which they are deemed to have emerged from a coma. Most hospitals in the UK simply do not have the resources to do this. An understanding of PTA can be estimated by calculating the interval between the date the person emerged from coma and the point at which they began to lay down day-to-day memories for ordinary events, such as what they had for lunch today, and whether they know what month we are currently in, and what building they are in at the moment. There is evidence that length of

PTA is associated with subsequent psycho-social outcome (e.g., Kosch, Browne, King, Fitzgerald, & Cameron, 2010).

A standard definition of severity has been discussed by a number of authors (see, for example, Tate, Pfaff, & Jurjevic, 2000). The grading for estimating severity of brain injury is provided in Table 5.2. In my experience, most brain-injured clients who are deemed suitable for neuro-rehabilitation are in the extremely severe category.

A common dilemma for many clinicians is that they often have to rate the severity of injury of their clients retrospectively. Malec and colleagues (2007) provide a model for providing a clinical tool for retrospectively determining the severity of traumatic brain injury. In the Mayo Traumatic Brain Injury Severity Classification System (Malec et al., 2007) data from different sources are used in an attempt to overcome some of the above-mentioned difficulties that clinicians might encounter when faced with missing clinical data. For example, there may be no GCS score on file, or, indeed, PTA or reports or findings from neuro-imaging. Combining the available data, including GCS scores, period of PTA, loss of consciousness, and findings from neuro-imaging, traumatic brain injury in this model is classified as moderate–severe (definite), mild (probable) or symptomatic (possible). A potential advantage of this model is that it appears to correctly classify more cases of traumatic brain injury, as opposed to when a single indicator of potential severity, for example, neuro-imaging, is used.

In the acute and immediate post-acute phase of a brain injured client's recovery, mortality has been strongly linked to lowered post-resuscitation GCS scores (e.g., Marshall et al. (1991) found that there was a mortality rate of 76% for patients with a GCS of three measured after resuscitation, compared with 18% for those with a GCS score of

Table 5.2. Post-trauma amnesia (PTA) and severity of brain injury.

Severity	KPTA
Very mild	< 5 minutes
Mild	5–60 minutes
Moderate	1–24 hours
Severe	1–7 days
Very severe	1–4 weeks
Extremely severe	> 4 weeks

6–8). Brain stem injury, in particular, was one of the main types of injury associated with a higher mortality.

Apart from the above detour into severity, probably the main factor that affects outcome in the low awareness patient is the presence or absence of other medical problems. Common medical difficulties found to increase mortality are hypotension, hypoxia, post-trauma seizures, hypopituitarism (the latter can develop much later than originally thought, so another top tip: endocrine functions is a good thing to ask medical colleagues about if you think this could help to explain a person's presentation), and, finally, a greater amount of time where higher intracranial pressure is apparent. Pre-morbid substance misuse and age are other factors that will affect outcome (e.g., the extremes, under two years of age and over sixty-five years of age).

Of most obvious importance in the longer term is simply being relatively still and mainly bed-bound (humans need to move around for optimal health). The kind of complications that can occur here are: pressure sores, contractures, pneumonia and other infections, and deep vein thrombosis. Of all of those mentioned, in practice, the most common problem I have found in treating people who have sustained a profound brain injury is recurrent chest infections. This latter problem can be helped considerably by having a good physiotherapy and medical team who diagnose early and who also put in place measures to prevent (as far as is possible) these occurring in the first place (e.g., regular chest physiotherapy).

Before you undertake the assessment, ensure (as far as is possible—good phrase this, it might come up again) that you have spoken to your medical colleagues and found out whether any basic neurological examination has been attempted, such as I–XII cranial nerve assessment, deep tendon reflexes, and motor function testing, among other areas. This might not be possible, but it is good to talk to these people, since they might have done something that could provide you with clues about your own assessment. Finally, before assessment begins, the clinician should ensure (as far as is possible) that there is no significant sedating or cognitive dampening medication prescribed that could have an impact on the arousal systems of the patient. Patients should also be in a good nutritional state.

A short note on arousal (yes, that old chestnut). Arousal is both a psychological and physiological state. It implies wakefulness and an ability to react to external and internal stimuli. It involves three main sub-systems, the reticular activating system (RAS), the endocrine system (remember that stuff about hypopituitarism?), and the autonomic nervous system. If it is not working properly, then our ability to attend to anything is also not going to work properly; one is, in many respects, the bedrock of the other. Not only this, but it works optimally when we are upright and moving around. This is partly why positioning the patient is important (see below).

Basic principles of sensory assessment

One of the fundamental problems in psychology, and, indeed, its errant parent, philosophy, is how we determine what is inside someone else's head. We have to conclude that other people are conscious, through, in effect, a series of assumptions in our daily life. Unfortunately, this is not something we can do as a clinician presented with a person who has sustained a profound brain injury. We have to rely on finely grained observation and serial testing of targeted senses to ascertain behavioural outputs or responses as meaningful or not. Assessments, here, are attempts at making things slightly less subjective. However, the somewhat brutal truth is that there is a large degree of art and skill to these assessments. Ultimately, you are deciding whether a particular response is contingent on the quality of an external stimulus that you introduced at that particular moment. However, you then need to make collections, or sums, of particular moments in order to arrive at a meaningful whole.

If it is not clear from the above, one of the cardinal features of this area of work is that there are few absolutely agreed areas of diagnosis or assessment. The best tools we have devised all rely on systematic serial neuro–behavioural assessment. Moreover, the cardinal feature of this assessment is its very fine-grained attention to small nuances in an individual's presentation, so that you can begin to pick out evidence for awareness as opposed to the often reported clutter, or white noise, that the person displays. Developing astute observational skills is of paramount importance to the clinician working in this very complex area. There are some very important approaches to facilitating these types of assessments, outlined below (for a more complete explanation, see, for example, Majerus, Gill-Thwaites, Andrews, & Laureys, 2005).

Position

After re-checking that the client is essentially medically stable and able to take part in this kind of assessment, where possible she should be in some form of supported seating. This might not be possible, but clearly the results obtained will not be as robust (see earlier note on arousal).

Capturing the best presentation

Prior to any formal neuro–behavioural sensory assessment, careful examination of the person's best and worst times of day should have been made.

Stimulation management

There should be an uncluttered and reduced level of environmental stimulation in the examination room. Most people who have sustained a severe brain injury do not function optimally when overburdened by too much stimuli. By this, I mean anything. For example, too much visual information, too much general noise, too much talking, too many things happening around them. Treat everything in their room as a potential source of over-stimulation and find a way of "turning it off", or at least down. Thus, neuro–behavioural sensory assessments done on a general medical ward are almost doomed to failure before they have begun. Remember the two fundamental systems that you are trying to switch on for the purposes of the assessment are arousal and attention.

Understanding what you do and the effects you have

To begin with, it can be very useful to have a companion who silently observes your own behaviour in the room with the person being assessed. They need to silently analyse your micro-behavioural repertoire. It is remarkable how we are not aware of the amount of throat clearing, coughing, humming, and general flapping around we do when we are in a quiet environment. After you have sorted out the environment (see above), you are the biggest potential confounding variable present in the room with the person who needs assessment.

Control yourself and become more aware of those everyday things you do that might inhibit clarity of response from the person being assessed. One glaring example pointed out to me, in a very quiet room, was how loudly I was chewing gum (after yet another attempt at stopping smoking!). Remember also that you are observing without judging: in effect, what this means is that data are paramount; interpretation and, thus, judgement occurs after you have gleaned enough naturally occurring information that the patient himself has displayed. It is all too easy to decide upon the meaning of something before you know what it might mean for that particular individual at that particular time.

Baseline

After the above considerations have been taken into account, a systematic approach is necessary to observing what the patient does without anything actually being done at first. In other words, once the patient has accommodated to you being in the room (after you have introduced yourself), simply observe what they do for a distinct period for a certain number of sessions, for example, ten sessions of ten minutes' duration. Make scrupulous notes of what they did. For example, a number of profoundly brain-injured patients moan, grind their teeth, grimace, and sometimes twitch. All of these and anything else they do should be noted as these are part of the oft-reported clutter, or white noise, spoken about earlier. Incidentally, they are also the most commonly reported behaviours suggested as meaningful by inexperienced clinicians or family members in the early days of a person's recovery. Observing these baseline behaviours is a crucial first step in understanding whether someone is responding contingently later on in your assessment. In other words, you are beginning to filter out things that are extraneous to the heart of what you are attempting to find out.

The family and significant others

Having said that family members can over-interpret some behaviour, it is important to pay attention to what they have to say in a more general sense. They are uniquely qualified to show a deeper understanding of the person before the brain injury, which might influence final outcome. Remember, on the whole they know the person exceptionally well and they spend a larger amount of time with them than you may do. In this respect, relatives are very likely to have some useful information to impart. If nothing else, it behoves the clinician to involve them in the process, especially the treatment phase. This is undoubtedly a very important strategy for the long-term management of the client and their family.

A team approach

Although from the account thus far it may appear that the neuropsychologist is the key part of the team in this context, they are not. Historically, the groundwork in sensory stimulation approaches was undertaken by neuropsychologists (prominently, Sarah Wilson in the UK). Subsequently, occupational therapists pulled together a lot of this literature and produced standardised training for these assessments (importantly, Helen Gill-Thwaites in the UK). This work further progressed our knowledge and skills in this continually evolving area of clinical practice.

More recently, the clinical and training opportunities have further opened up to include more professionals who want to train and work in these methods. Moreover, as I have already stated, without medical and nursing colleagues, medical stability and optimal physical functioning will not be gained. Interestingly, the one profession that has been quietly fundamental to these approaches is physiotherapy. Without the expertise of physiotherapists with regard to positioning, seating, aids, and adaptations, many of these assessments could not even begin. In other words, done well, these assessments offer the opportunity to truly work together as a whole team.

Assessment

Above the obvious necessity of brainstem function (e.g., for breathing, temperature control, etc.), you need to find clues for something else. In effect, during your screening phase, you need to find something that suggests cortical functions are apparent or nascent after the injury (e.g., eye tracking to sound or vision, etc). The CRS-R, WNSSP, and the SMART appear to try to do at least three things. First, they attempt to differentiate levels of presentation that may fit with sub-categories of diagnostic classification. Second, they attempt to gauge how aware someone in a low awareness condition is. Third, they attempt to gain some leverage on their functional and communicative abilities.

All these assessments focus on stimulating vision, hearing, touch, taste, and smell. A couple of examples follow. The CRS-R examines in a systematic way the visual functions, and then notes what level the patient responded at consistently, from no response, visual startle, fixation, pursuit, object localisation, through to object recognition. The WNSSP consists of thirty-two items that assess clients' arousal and attention, expressive communication, and response to auditory, visual, tactile, and olfactory stimulation.

Other assessments include the SMART (Gill-Thwaites, 1997; Gill-Thwaites & Munday, 1999). The SMART utilises a methodology that is used across all the sensory modalities examined. This involves a five-point hierarchical scale, ranging from no response (level 1), reflexive (level 2), withdrawal (level 3), localising (level 4), to discriminating (level 5). Level 5 is the key here, as, if it can be demonstrated the client consistently operates at this level, then it can be more safely concluded that these behaviours are meaningful.

An example of this is through standardised graded exposure in the auditory modality. Auditory stimuli are presented, from quiet or whispered speech through shouting on the left, then on the right, side of the patient. Certain auditory–verbal instructions are provided which bring together information from the behavioural baseline and the information from staff and family members, such as he nods or moves his eyes to the right when he means yes. During this process, some contingent (meaningful?) understanding of responses may be gleaned. If the client responds in a particular way (e.g., put crudely, the person consistently localises to a clap made by the hands on the left side, at head height), this can be differentiated from other, perhaps artefactual, responses through comparison with the careful behavioural baseline observations made earlier in the assessment procedure.

All of the information gleaned from the assessment described above is then re-examined to ensure, as far as is possible, that the assessor actually understands something "real" as opposed to the "ordinary" random behaviours displayed without stimulation. This again highlights how vital it is to obtain an uncontaminated baseline of behavioural observations against which to interpret subsequent findings from the assessment, as described earlier.

Having been involved in a number of these kinds of assessments, I would suggest that, although great emphasis is placed in the manual and during training of SMART accredited assessors on standardisation, it takes an especially sensitive and intuitive (based partly on a deep understanding of the effects of brain injury) clinician to do this process well. Indeed, having been able to follow individual clients occasionally from initial SMART assessment through other assessments, with and without treatment being delivered, it is true to say that there is variation in results that appear in large measure to do with who assessed, rather than any other distinct difference.

In this sense, it might well have been that the assessor did not fully own themselves on that day (see earlier, but also see the next time you have a "bad day at the office"). It comes back to a central notion, in that, while almost any very bright person can be trained to administer and score a test, it is the interpretation of the results that is of paramount importance. With this in mind, SMART training works very hard at ironing out the differences between individual assessors to increase the validity of the tests and the final results. To a large extent, this works; for example, there is a high interrater reliability displayed. However, ultimately, this assessment is delivered, interpreted, and reported by human beings about other human beings, with all the in-built limitations that come with such an approach.

The interpretation of clinical findings in this area is no different from many other areas of assessment or medical investigations used in hospitals. For example, take radiology. Indeed, much medical research has been expended on whether there are clinically significant differences between newly qualified and senior radiologists. The answer is that there are differences, some of which are significant, but, as scanning and computer interpretation have advanced, fewer potentially clinically catastrophic scan interpretation results are being made.

It is here that I would make one of my brief asides. The best neuropsychologists I have had the pleasure of working with combine a good deal of expertise, understanding the effects of medication on cognition and behaviour, functional neuroanatomy, cognitive testing, neuropsychological, psychological, and social functioning, together with the ability to tap-dance. All right, that last bit might not apply, but you get my drift. Conversely, the worst clinicians test without properly bothering to understand any internal or external context, or fail to integrate different sources of data obtained to come to an overall interpretation.

Feedback

One of the cornerstones of the assessment should be about recommendations for the level of stimulation allowable in the environment (including the "dosage" of family and therapeutic input). See, for example, *The Multi-Society Task Force on Persistent Vegetative State* (1996), Royal College of Physicians (1996), Giacino and colleagues (2002), and, in particular, Gill-Thwaites (1997), and Gill-Thwaites and Munday (1999).

Treatment

After attempting to sort the wheat from the chaff, the assessor then might go on, if it is clinically appropriate, to start treating the client. In effect, this means stimulating in a systematic way either one or more senses that have shown the most promise for gains during the assessment phase. The phrase "uni- or multi-modal treatments" is often bandied about at this juncture. In essence, are you going to concentrate on one sensory modality, or more than one? After a set period (maximum eight weeks) a full re-assessment occurs. During this process, any increase in responses are noted to see whether there have been treatment effects.

Once these data have been collected and collated, the key is whether it can be accepted that the person has demonstrated contingent responses, and not simply an increase in those artefactual ones discussed earlier. This is almost never an easy question to answer with complete confidence. At the most fundamental level, this question is about outcome, or if the input provided to the patient had a clinically detectable effect.

Does it work?

Before I try to answer this question, I think it important to note that the CSR-R, WNSSP, and the SMART are, in essence, assessment tools. They are, thus, best suited for differentiating someone diagnostically from a vegetative state through minimally conscious and other forms of low awareness condition. It is, in some respects, unfair that they should be criticised for not delivering startling treatment results clinically, since they were never intended to be used for that purpose.

While it is not explicitly discussed in detail with family members, we should know, as neuropsychologists, something of the vast literature on memory research and, in this context, the work undertaken on emotion and memory functioning. There is a real basis for all those hackneyed images of the person in a coma, being played favourite music, for instance. Of course, in this regard, it is a legitimate question as to whether the person is aroused, able to attend, and subsequently process a memory (see, for example, McGaugh, 2003). Moreover, it is also true to say that even though this, and similar, literature demonstrates the power of emotion and memory, results of neuro–behavioural sensory treatments are less encouraging. Indeed, Giacino, Katz, and Schiff (2007) are among a number of clinicians who downplay the significance of sensory stimulation programmes as potentially useful for staff and family members, but, as yet, there is not enough evidence to promote them as a standard treatment recommendation.

Moreover, there is no meaningful and, at present, adequate evidence that sensory programmes of any kind improve clinical outcomes in those patients in low awareness conditions. In a recent review, they found no Class I studies,[1] and only one Class II study was found, which reported only one change in a single chemical marker at six days post injury. Of the remaining studies, some showed some improvements. Given this, the authors urge caution in providing definitive conclusions for this type of intervention. Moreover, they assert: "... it is incumbent upon clinicians to clearly elucidate to family members, the high degree of clinical uncertainty associated with this form of treatment" (Giacino, Katz, & Schiff, 2007, p. 431). Having said this, sensory-based treatments are the best hope, at present, for effecting any change.

In my experience, most do not produce the results the family and staff are hoping for, but extremely rarely they appear to do so. It is the latter instances that propel us; in any case, they have been demonstrated to cause no harm. At this point, it is also fair to point out that as there are no Class I studies available, it might well be that there is a treatment effect or effects, but, as yet, these have not been found owing to the paucity of really robust research. From the studies that have been undertaken, the conclusion appears to be that hospital stays are generally shorter for those that have been treated, more of those treated tended to return home, and that there appears to be a dose response benefit to treatment using sensory stimulation techniques in terms of some increase in functional gains (Giacino, Katz, & Schiff, 2007). However, all of this, it must be noted, is merely suggestive and not conclusive.

These kinds of treatments remain as options, not recommendations, in our current clinical repertoire. Of perhaps more significance are the small number of studies that appear to show sensory stimulation evoked clear neuro–behavioural responses on the one hand, but (and this is absolutely crucial) no apparent awareness (e.g., Giacino & Malone, 2008) on the other. In other, more clinically technical words, work over the past ten years seems to show (counter to their neuro–behavioural assessment results) that some patients deemed vegetative are aware and some patients deemed to have low awareness have none at all and are, thus, technically vegetative (Giacino et al., 2009). On the one hand, this might imply that the initial diagnosis was incorrect, or, alternatively, that for some patients, under some circumstances, these treatments have a valuable effect. Clearly, further research is needed in this emerging area of clinical work to clarify many of the remaining uncertainties.

Prognosis

Rather bizarrely, given the title of this sub-section, I am not going to unpack this much further. Remember, key factors previously discussed include age at injury, severity of insult, and pituitary function, among others. In this section, I want to discuss one of my many hobby-horses: specifically, time. Emergence from very profound low awareness conditions (vegetative states) depends, apart from what has previously been discussed, on the span of time subsequent to the point of injury. Two really important things should be noted here about this time: first, the greater the amount of time that has passed since injury the less likely emergence from this deeply impaired state becomes. This is a clinical fact and runs wholly counter to the often irresponsibly reported dramatic emergence stories in the media (see, for example, Giacino et al., 2007; Zasler, Kreutzer, & Taylor, 1991).

Second, and, once again, this is crucial, even if the person has emerged, the longer they have taken to do so the greater is the likelihood of a poorer outcome functionally. Conversely, the best outcomes happen when emergence occurs within the first few days or weeks, and concomitantly these produce the best functional outcomes. Typically, those people who emerge after a year has passed have permanent and highly severe functional deficits. As a general rule of thumb, severe hypoxic injuries result in worse disability than typical traumatic brain injuries (unless there has been a significant secondary insult with the latter injury). Of course, it is at the point when you are pontificating in your most self-important style with a family member that one of these thumbs pokes you in the eye. Yes, it is that old individual case stuff breaking down the general rule again.

Gradually, over the years, I have found it better to not get drawn into debates about larger stuff and prognostications *per se*. I think it is best to hope and plan for small incremental improvements in discrete "What we as a team are going to be concentrating on next is ..." terms. This helps oneself, the team, and the family to stay grounded. And, during profound uncertainty, as is the case when considering the prognosis of these patients, being grounded, while at the same remaining open to possible change, must be more productive than believing what is essentially impossible to predict with any degree of reliable accuracy.

Grief

What happens to significant others during this whole process is fantastically varied. The way some family members clearly manacle themselves to a rock of absolute denial of the prospect of decline, stasis, or, indeed, virtually anything negative can be astonishing. This usually occurs while other members of the family are progressing at a very different pace with their own emotional journey. The term mobile mourning has been coined by Muir and Haffey (1984) to describe the recurring and extended process of grieving for a loved one who has sustained a brain injury. I use it to guide my own thinking for those members of a family who are grieving. An important component is the impact of an uncertain prognosis. Moreover, at its heart is the recognition that even after it is apparently over, it might return in some unexpected way and that it is heavily influenced by medical setbacks or changes to the initial diagnosis (hmmm, you might need to re-read this chapter at this juncture).

Conclusion

If nothing else has occurred for you while reading this chapter than a better understanding of what neuro–behavioural sensory stimulation is, then I have achieved what I had intended in the first instance. Further than this, if, after reading the chapter, an excitement has developed to explore our understanding of consciousness, then I am all the more blessed. However, for me, of most importance is that I have discussed something about the importance of diagnosis to an audience of neuropsychologists. Of the many sage things he wrote, Wittgenstein (1958) once said, "A 'picture' held us captive. And we could not get outside it, for it lay in our language and language seemed to repeat it to us inexorably" (p. 115).

Put more simply, it is our own language that traps us. The words, phrases, and sentences, or ways of talking, we use have profound effects on how we make sense of the injured person—indeed, how we assess them. Our ways of talking have profound effects on how we understand our colleagues. Finally, our ways of talking have profound effects on how we support and affect a family member through the whole process of dealing with a loved one who has sustained a severe or profound brain injury.

Note

1. The generally accepted format for meta-analytic studies of other studies, is that a Class I study is a randomised, blind controlled clinical trial. A Class II study is a non-randomised control trial. A Class III study is an observational study with controls. Finally, a Class IV study is an observational study without controls. For a more complete explanation, see for example, French and Gronseth (2008).

References

Ansell, B. J., & Keenan, J. E. (1989). The Western Neuro Sensory Stimulation Profile: a tool for assessing slow-to-recover head-injured patients. *Archives of Physical & Medical Rehabilitation, 70*: 104–108.

Cruse, D., & Owen, A. M. (2010). Consciousness revealed: new insights into the vegetative and minimally conscious states. *Current Opinion in Neurology*, 23(6): 656–660.

French, J., & Gronseth, G. (2008). Lost in a jungle of evidence: we need a compass. *Neurology*, 71: 1634–1638.

Giacino, J. T., & Malone, R. (2008). The vegetative and minimally conscious states. *Handbook of Clinical Neurology*, 90: 99–111.

Giacino, J. T., Ashwal, S., Childs, N., Cranford, R., Jennett, B., Katz, D., Kelly, J., Rosenberg, J., Whyte, J., Zafonte, R., & Zasler, N. (2002). The minimally conscious state: definition and diagnostic criteria. *Neurology*, 58: 349–353.

Giacino, J. T., Kalmar, K., & Whyte, J. (2004). The JFK Coma Recovery Scale-Revised: measurement characteristics and diagnostic utility. *Archives of Physical & Medical Rehabilitation*, 85: 2020–2029.

Giacino, J. T., Katz, D. I., & Schiff, N. (2007). Assessment and rehabilitative management of individuals with disorders of consciousness. In: N. D. Zasler, D. I. Katz, & R. D. Zafonte (Eds.), *Brain Injury Medicine: Principles and Practice* (pp. 397–413). New York: Demos Medical.

Giacino, J. T., Schnakers, C., Rodriguez-Moreno, D., Kalmar, K., Schiff, N., & Hirsch, J. (2009). Behavioral assessment in patients with disorders of consciousness: gold standard or fool's gold? *Progress in Brain Research*, 177: 33–48.

Gill-Thwaites, H. (1997). The Sensory Modality Assessment and Rehabilitation Technique—a tool for the assessment and treatment of patients with severe brain injury in a vegetative state. *Brain Injury*, 11: 723–734.

Gill-Thwaites, H., & Munday, R. (1999). The Sensory Modality Assessment and Rehabilitation Technique (SMART): a comprehensive and integrated assessment and treatment protocol of the vegetative state and minimally responsive patient. *Neuropsychological Rehabilitation*, 9: 305–320.

Jennet, B., & Plum, F. (1972). Persistent vegetative state after brain damage; a syndrome in search of a name. *Lancet*, April 1: 734–737.

Kosch, Y., Browne, S., King, C., Fitzgerald, J., & Cameron, I. (2010). Post-traumatic amnesia and its relationship to the functional outcome of people with severe traumatic brain injury. *Brain Injury*, 24(3): 479–485.

Majerus, S., Gill-Thwaites, G., Andrews, K., & Laureys, S. (2005). Behavioral evaluation of consciousness in severe brain damage. In: S. Laureys (Ed.), *Progress in Brain Research* (pp. 397–413). Philadelphia, PA: Elsevier.

Malec, J. F., Brown, A. W., Leibson, C. L., Flaada, J. T., Mandrekar, J. N., Diehl, N. N., & Perkins, P. K. (2007). The Mayo classification system for traumatic brain injury severity. *Journal of Neurotrauma, 24*: 1417–1424.

Marshall, L. F., Gautille, T., Klauber, M. R., Eisenberg, H. M., Luerssen, T. G., Marmarou, A., & Foulkes, M. A., (1991). The outcome of severe closed head injury. *Journal of Neurosurgery, Special Supplements, 75*(1): S28–S36.

McGaugh, J. L. (2003). *Memory and Emotion: The Making of Lasting Memories*. London: Weidenfeld & Nicolson.

Monti, M. M., Laureys, S., & Owen, A. M. (2010). The vegetative state. *British Medical Journal, 341*: 292–296.

Multi-Society Task Force on PVS (1996). Medical aspects of the persistent vegetative state. *New England Journal of Medicine, 330*:1499–1508.

Muir, C. A., & Haffey, W. J. (1984). Psychological and neuropsychological interventions in the mobile mourning process. In: B. A. Edelstein & E. T. Couture (Eds.), *Behavioral Assessment and Rehabilitation of the Traumatically Brain-damaged* (pp. 247–272). New York: Plenum Press.

President's Commission for the Study of Ethical Problems in Medicine and Biomedical and Behavioral Research (1983). *Deciding to Forego Life-Sustaining Treatment*. Washington, DC: US Government Printing Office. March 171–192.

Royal College of Physicians Working Group (1996). The permanent vegetative state. *Journal of the Royal College of Physicians of London, 30*: 119–121.

Tate, R. L., Pfaff, A., & Jurjevic, L. (2000). Resolution of disorientation and amnesia during post-traumatic amnesia. *Journal of Neurology, Neurosurgery & Psychiatry, 68*: 178–185.

Teasdale, G., & Jennett, B. (1974). Assessment of coma and impaired consciousness. A practical scale. *Lancet, 2*: 81–84.

Wittgenstein, L. (1958). *Philosophical Investigations*. Oxford: Basil Blackwell

Zasler, N. D., Kreutzer, J. S., & Taylor, D. (1991). Coma recovery with coma stimulation: a critical review. *NeuroRehabilitation, 1*: 33–40.

CHAPTER SIX

Assessment of mental capacity

Helen Newby and Tracey Ryan-Morgan

Introduction

As discussed in Chapter Two, neuropsychological assessment can be used for many purposes. Here, we specifically discuss the assessment of mental capacity. Although many clinicians will have already been conducting such assessments prior to its arrival on the scene, the statute (*Mental Capacity Act* (MCA), 2005) has brought to the forefront such assessments. When assessing capacity it is essential that the clinician is familiar with the current legal situation for the particular capacity question you are assessing. We highlight in particular that the MCA does not replace existing common law tests but sits alongside them. In testamentary cases, for example, the MCA sits alongside the well-known case of Banks *vs*. Goodfellow (1870), which provides the leading common law test of testamentary capacity.

As a starting premise, the MCA enshrines in law five essential principles. These are listed below, and have been drawn directly from the *MCA 2005 Code of Practice* (Department of Constitutional Affairs, 2007).

1. *A person must be assumed to have capacity unless it is established that he lacks capacity.*
   Therefore, the burden of proof is upon the assessor to demonstrate that the person being assessed does not have capacity. That opinion is based on the civil standard of a "balance of probabilities". That is, is it more likely than not that the person does or does not have capacity? This can be extremely helpful in cases when the clinician might feel less certain about their clinical opinion than normal.
2. *A person is not to be treated as unable to make a decision unless all practicable steps to help him to do so have been taken without success.*
   This taps well into the skills of a neuropsychologist interested in rehabilitation and can also be augmented by the skills of speech and language therapists.
3. *A person is not to be treated as unable to make a decision merely because they make an unwise decision.*
   Here, the law is enshrining the importance of neuropsychological process rather than outcome. The focus, therefore, is on how the person makes the decision, not the decision itself. You, as the assessor, are therefore required to demonstrate whether the person's thinking process is impaired in some way. Often, of course, the reason a capacity assessment is requested is because the person appears to others to be making an "unwise" decision. However, this is merely the start of the assessment process.
4. *An act done, or decision made, under this Act for or on behalf of a person who lacks capacity must be done, or made, in their best interests.*
   Section 4 of the MCA devotes itself to what is meant by the term "best interests" and how this might be determined. Essentially, for those of us with psychological training, it encourages us to go "back to basics" and adopt a psychologically enquiring approach with formulation at its centre. You might want to ask questions such as, who is the individual in front of us (socially, cognitively, emotionally, physically), where did they come from, what are their values and beliefs and how do these sit with their historical values and beliefs, what is their current context, what was their past context?
5. *Before the act is done, or the decision is made, regard must be had to whether the purpose for which it is needed can be as effectively achieved in a way that is less restrictive of the person's rights and freedom of action.*

This principle reminds clinicians that the decision they are making in someone's "best interests" is not to be taken lightly, as it could affect the individual's human rights.

The Act goes on to stipulate how the assessment of mental capacity must relate to a specific decision at a particular point in time.

In the opinion of the authors of this chapter, the skills and expertise of neuropsychologists fit extremely well with the five principles of the MCA (2005). Our own, shared, philosophy is that mental capacity assessments should be conducted in a formulation-focused manner. It is a psychologically holistic process, with the individual and the specific capacity question at a particular point in time held at its core. This process is, therefore, familiar to clinical psychologists, as the roots of the approach are firmly entrenched in their training. It demands that the clinician gather and synthesise information from various sources, including clients, people in their surrounding system, including family, friends, and professionals, cognitive testing, and clinical notes.

The Act sets out how the capacity assessment is conducted in two steps, seeking to determine the answers to the following questions.

1. Does the individual have an impairment of, or a disturbance in, the functioning of the mind or brain (whether permanent or temporary). If so,
2. Does the impairment or disturbance cause the person to be unable to make a specific decision at the time it needs to be made?

Helpfully for the assessor, the Act goes further, specifically stating that the person is considered to be unable to make a decision if they are unable to do any one of the following:

- understand the information relevant to the decision;
- retain that information;
- use or weigh that information as part of the process of making the decision;
- communicate his decision (whether by talking, sign language, or other means).

This chapter will now focus on four questions in capacity assessment of particular relevance to the clinician working in rehabilitation settings.

1. What issues should be considered before and during the assessment process?
2. How is mental capacity assessed?
3. What is the role of neuropsychological testing in assessing capacity?
4. What issues may be pertinent after the capacity assessment?

What issues should be considered before and during the assessment process?

There is a raft of questions that you could ask yourself before embarking on a capacity assessment. The *Audit Tool for Mental Capacity Assessments*, published by the British Psychological Society in 2010, provides a practical and useful set of questions to be asked. These questions are helpfully grouped under different components of the assessment process (before starting the assessment, the assessment itself, enhancing capacity, conclusion, outcome, and recommendations). Some of the questions from the *Audit Tool for Mental Capacity Assessments* are listed below to provide an indication to the reader of some of the issues worth thinking about.

- Are the circumstances and rationale for the assessment clear?
- Do any of the exclusions apply to the person (e.g., is the person under eighteen years of age; are they subject to the Mental Health Act; has a valid and relevant Advance Refusal been made)?
- Do any of the exclusions apply to the decision (e.g., the capacities to make intimate relationships; vote; adopt or make decisions on matters affecting the person's child; or consent to care or treatment authorised under the Mental Health Act)?
- Is the question to be answered stated clearly and specifically?
- Does insight have an impact on the person's ability to understand the information relevant to the decision and of foreseeable consequences of the decision?
- What evidence is there of attempts to compensate for cognitive/communication/emotional disabilities or use support tools?
- Was there evidence of suggestibility/social influence in their responses?
- Were there any checks for consistency of responses?

Additional issues briefly discussed in the BPS document worthy of particular mention are: the potential skills and competencies assessors should have, standards for audit (in relation to factors you could consider in the assessment) and client consent. There are few studies to date exploring such matters and so, although legislation is likely to vary between England and Wales, and the countries of origin of the studies referred to below, both HN and TRM consider the results to be of interest and relevance to readers of this chapter. Mullaly and colleagues (2007), in their study of Australian neuropsychologists, explore some of the issues briefly discussed in the BPS document referred to above. In relation to the first issue, Mullaly and collaborators (2007) describe that around two-thirds of their sample had more than five years' experience in conducting capacity assessments at least once or twice a month. Sixty-two per cent of the sample felt confident about their conclusions, reflecting a reasonable degree of belief in their competence. In relation to the assessment process, respondents reported that the most commonly asked capacity questions surrounded (in order of frequency) lifestyle decisions and then financial decision-making. The issue of client consent was identified as one of the most problematic aspects of the process.

Another practical consideration of major importance is "How much time do I have to carry out the overall assessment?" The amount of time you have available might influence the reliability and/or validity of the assessment (as indicated in the *Audit Tool*, 2010). Mullaly and colleagues (2007) found that 39% of respondents took 6–8 hours to complete a capacity assessment and 31% 8–10 hours. Only 28% took less than six hours. It is not stated what this assessment includes but the implication is that this would include clinical interview/s, neuropsychological tests, gathering background information (for example, through past reports and clinical notes) and then a written report. Whyte, Wilson, Hamilton, Primrose, and Summers (2003) found that on an acute older adult ward, the average time spent by a neuropsychologist at the bedside in assessing capacity (under the auspices of the Adults with Incapacity Scotland Act 2000) was approximately eighty-three minutes (range 45–115 minutes). From our own practice, we would estimate our community-based assessments take a similar length of time to that indicated by Mullaly and colleagues (2007). This has potentially significant implications for service provision if capacity assessments are set to become an increasing area of work for neuropsychologists.

Finally, within this section, we would like to re-emphasise the formulation-driven philosophy underlying our approach to capacity assessment. The BPS's *Interim Guidance for Psychologists*, published in 2006, discusses a "functional approach" to capacity assessment. This appears to have much in common with our formulation-driven approach. The individual is considered within their unique situation and history. The capacity opinions are made in relation to specific capacity questions at specific points in time. As yet, there is no published model or framework that has been developed specifically for use with people who have an acquired brain injury.

The BPS guidance document referred to previously provides a visual representation of factors affecting capacity. This covers a wide range of factors, including psycho-social functioning, external factors, internal intrapsychic factors, and neuropsychological factors. In addition, the American Bar Association Commission on Law and Aging and the American Psychological Association published in 2008 a document titled *Assessment of Older Adults with Diminished Capacity: A Handbook for Psychologists* (ABA & APA, 2008). This presents a useful conceptual framework involving nine elements that can be used by clinicians when considering capacity questions with older adults. The nine elements are: legal standard, psychiatric and emotional factors, cognitive underpinnings, diagnosis, functional elements, values and preferences, risk considerations, steps to enhance capacity, and clinical judgement. We have found this to be a useful framework when conducting assessments with adults with an acquired brain injury, as the nine elements express concisely the complex array of factors commonly found to be relevant in cases we have dealt with.

How is mental capacity assessed?

A key component of our practice is a tailored clinical interview with the client whose capacity is being assessed. Newberry and Pachet (2008) suggest the essential characteristics of a clinical interview are "sensitivity and skill". Ideally, the client making the decision should be interviewed (alone). Any significant other(s), such as family and professionals involved in their care, should also be given the opportunity to provide relevant information to the assessment process.

Collateral information is particularly important in instances where the client (who is the focus of the assessment) might lack full awareness of their cognitive limitations or deficits.

It is well recognised that each practitioner may, through the process of acquiring experience, develop their own sets of interview questions pertinent to the decision in question (Newby, Anderson, & Todd, 2011). Such protocols subsequently become honed by experience and further professional development. However, to guide those who may feel relatively inexperienced in this area we would endorse Newberry and Pachet's (2008) "psychosocial" interview framework. A prompt sheet is attached to their journal paper and encompasses the following areas.

- Introduction to assessment (for example, discuss reason and purpose for interview, confidentiality and release of information, assuring ability to communicate in native tongue).
- Medico–legal issues (for example, is there an advanced directive in place? is there an existing Enduring Power of Attorney (EPA)? Is there a guardian or trustee? Any previous capacity assessment?).
- Establish the current living situation. For example, what are the relevant medical/post-injury issues, particularly in terms of activities of daily living (ADL)? Does the client live alone?).
- Social and family history (for example, education; occupation; work skills; genogram; who currently makes decisions? History of decision-making? Are there family conflicts that have relevance? What is the family view of the issue under assessment?).
- Social supports (for example, what supports are in place? Where is the client in the family life cycle? What are the client's perceptions of dependence/independence? What support is currently offered? By whom? On what basis? How frequently? How is it viewed?).
- Coping (for example, what coping styles/techniques does the individual use and apply day to day? Is there a history of not coping well?).
- Relevance of any religious or cultural factors (for example, current religious practice and its possible influence on decision).
- Risk factors (for example, what is the nature of any concerns? Is the client considered to be vulnerable to exploitation or abuse by others? What degree of self-protection can the client exert?).

As mentioned in our introduction, the MCA (2005) does not replace common law tests, but exists alongside them. The assessor, therefore, also needs to be familiar with such common law tests when thinking about question sets as well as the requirements of the MCA (2005). The British Medical Association and the Law Society (2010) have provided a clear breakdown of the legal aspects of different tests of capacity. This is invaluable in formulating structured interviews for clients. The case examples in the BPS's *Interim Guidance for Psychologists* (2006) also have questions you can incorporate into your interview schedule. On a final point, the circumstances of the particular individual you have in front of you will play a large part in forming the structure, content, and format of the interview questions. We have both found that having formatted semi-structured interview question sets for a range of capacity questions, it is often necessary to tailor them more precisely to the individuals we have referred to us.

What is the role of neuropsychological testing in assessing capacity?

The administration of neuropsychological tests might serve two purposes when considering capacity assessment. First, performance on neuropsychological tests could provide considerable objective assistance in establishing or confirming that stage one of the two-stage process enshrined in the Act is met. That is, that there is an impairment of, or disturbance in, the functioning of mind or brain, whether temporary or permanent. Second, neuropsychological testing might provide guidance as to whether this impairment means that the person has lost the capacity to make the particular decision being considered: that is, does the person fail step two of the test of capacity?

In the clinical practice of most neuropsychologists working in rehabilitation settings, the existence of any impairment in the functioning of the brain is often already well established. For example, it is typically already known that your client has an acquired brain injury. Therefore, the primary function of the neuropsychological tests in many cases might be to guide the capacity assessor in considering what perhaps could be argued to be the more complex question as to what impact this impairment might have on the person's decision-making abilities. It is essential to be clear in your mind about the precise function that neuropsychological testing is going to serve in the capacity assessment before you. This will ensure that your testing is relevant for that particular person at that particular point in time, in relation to a particular capacity question.

Caution must be exercised on the part of the neuropsychologist not to fall into the trap of believing that the more test data one can gather, the more certain one can be about an individual's capacity. Newby, Anderson, and Todd (2011) refer to neuropsychologists best occupying a position of safe uncertainty (Mason, 1993) in the same way that Kapp and Mossman (1996) previously warned against the "construction of a capacimeter". For the clinician, this simply means do not hide behind neuropsychological tests and consider them as the only or ultimate decider of the capacity question you are working on. We would implore you not to test in a formulaic and unthinking fashion and to consider instead using a range of sources.

To our knowledge, there are as yet no clear empirical relationships established between neuropsychological test findings, cognitive functions, and the ability to successfully make specific decisions. Perhaps this is an impossible task? For example, due to the nature of the task, we are dealing with specific decisions for a particular person at a particular point in time. Therefore, it will be intrinsically difficult to build up an appropriate sample. There are also the ergonomic limitations of tests to take into account. Although the tests you choose will, we hope, tap into the cognitive skills thought to be important to undertake the particular capacitous decision under question, those tests are intrinsically paper and pencil tasks that do not feel or look like the functional sequences the person must do in order to undertake the decision in the real world. This dislocation between the tests used and how the decision is actually carried out in the real world can lead to statistical noise and limited explained variance in the test data collected. The difficulties in relating test data to real world functions in meaningful ways has been discussed in related areas, such as fitness to drive after a brain injury (see Gavin Newby's chapter on driving). A useful way forward at this stage might be to build up the number of case studies in the published research literature.

Although we recognise that there are limitations to the predictive value of psychometric tests in determining a client's capacity, like Newby, Anderson, and Todd (2011), we recognise that they have a very important place in the capacity assessment process. A useful approach might be to focus on assessing those areas of cognitive functioning that appear to have face validity. Table 6.1 outlines the four criteria the MCA (2005) has laid out as requiring consideration when assessing capacity. As discussed in our introduction, if the client "fails", on the balance of probabilities, one of these tests, they are deemed to lack the capacity to make to decision in question.

Table 6.1. The four criteria of the MCA (2005), associated cognitive functions, and suggested neuropsychological tests.

MCA 2005 criteria	Associated cognitive function	Suggested neuropsychological tests*
Understanding the relevant information	Comprehension (orally provided) (written information) Visual perception (of pictures, objects)	Frenchay Aphasia Screening Test (FAST Comprehension subtest from the Wechsler Adult Intelligence Scale 4th edn (WAIS-IV) Figure copy subtest from the Repeatable Battery Assessment of Neuropsychological Status (R-BANS) Rey Figure Copy test
Retaining the information	Autobiographical memory Auditory and visual attention Working memory Verbal memory (immediate and delayed)	Autobiographical relevant Memory Interview Digit Span subtest from the WAIS-IV and/or R-BANS Coding subtest from the R-BANS Verbal memory tasks from the 4th edn of the Wechsler Memory Scale (WMS-IV), R-BANS; BIRT Memory and Information Processing Battery (BMIPB)

(continued)

Table 6.1. (*continued*)

MCA 2005 criteria	Associated cognitive function	Suggested neuropsychological tests*
Using or weighing up relevant information	Executive skills such as deductive reasoning, integrating feedback from another to inform your reasoning, cognitive flexibility, impulse inhibition, abstract reasoning and perspective taking	Various tests from the Delis–Kaplan Executive Function System (DKEFS), particularly Word Context Test, 20 Questions Test, Trail Making Test Hayling and Brixton Tests Similarities subtest from the WAIS-IV Kaplan Baycrest Neuropsychological Assessment Problem-solving subtests Matrix Reasoning subtest of 2nd edn of the Wechsler Abbreviated Scale of Intelligence (WASI-II) Social Moral Awareness Test
Communicating the decision by any means possible	Verbal expression	Frenchay Aphasia Screening Test (FAST) Graded Naming Test Picture Naming subtest from the R-BANS Verbal Fluency test (Controlled Oral Word Association Test; DKEFS; R-BANS)

*See pp. 205–206 for full test references.

Alongside each of the criteria are associated cognitive functions, with the suggested neuropsychological tests that could be used to assess these functions. It is also important that we practitioners do not forget, however, that our clinical judgement also plays a part in the contextual and dynamic nature of capacitous decision-making (Moye & Marson, 2007).

From our experience, the emphasis given to each area of cognitive functioning may vary depending on the specific capacity question being asked or the complexity of the capacity question. For example, the client required to make an investment decision involving large sums of money (such as might result from a personal injury claim settlement) would need to have more developed abstract reasoning skills than someone making decisions about how to spend their weekly allowance of £50.00. These considerations can then inform the test selection process in terms of cognitive functions being assessed and the level of difficulty of the test selected.

The time you have available to conduct the assessment might also contribute to your test choice, or whether you test at all. Anecdotally, in common with many other neuropsychologists we have spoken to, it might be possible to create some rules of thumb to help you if time is short. Generally, if your client has been neuropsychologically tested reasonably recently (e.g., in the past year or two), the last testing indicates that progress has plateaued, and there is no obvious evidence of a change in cognitive or real world functioning, the original test results could be used to inform the current capacity assessment. If you feel a particular issue has not been addressed from previous testing (e.g., reasoning ability) but the other important cognitive aspects of capacity have, then you might be able to undertake a very focused and specific battery. In this case, make sure when you write your final report that the tests reported, upon which you have based your opinion, were not undertaken by yourself.

We hope, therefore, that it is clear from this section that a diagnostic approach is unsuitable to address capacity questions. In other words, having neuropsychological deficits or impairment does not mean a person lacks capacity *per se*. The results from neuropsychological tests inform which cognitive functions might be impaired or compromised, and this is further corroborated by clinical interview of the client and a reliable collateral informant (as discussed above).

Case examples

We now present some case examples, which demonstrate the formulation-driven philosophy we have adopted in capacity assessments. We have focused on the four areas that have been the most commonly asked capacity questions in our clinical practice: living circumstances, managing finances, testamentary capacity, and capacity to undertake litigation on one's own behalf.

Capacity to decide about living circumstances

The paper by Mackenzie, Lincoln, and Newby (2008) provides suggestions for a semi-structured interview designed for use with patients who had suffered a stroke in an acute hospital setting. This can be easily adapted for use with clients who have suffered an ABI in community settings. With experience, we have come to realise that this particular assessment centres round the assessor having a full understanding of the main risks and advantages involved. For example, if the person wants to live alone, can they: remember if they have eaten or drunk anything recently; safely prepare food and drinks; take their medication correctly; wash and dress sufficiently well; get confused about whether it is day or night; have the opportunity (if they wish and have the ability) to socialise with others; deal with paying the bills for the house; sort out house repairs?

If you are lucky enough to have occupational therapy and physiotherapy colleagues involved, they will be able to provide you with a useful overview as to whether the person is able to carry out such activities. You can then collate a list of the potential risk areas for your client. It is then essential to think about what the advantages for the person would be if they returned home alone. The client and his family might provide particularly relevant and useful information here.

Case example: Wanting to go home alone when the team think a residential care environment is needed

> Terry is forty-six years old and suffered a head injury in a road traffic accident a year ago. At the time of his accident he had been working as a manager in a jewellery shop and had high standards about his physical appearance. He had been living alone in a flat and spent his spare time gardening and socialising with friends. His friends reported he had always tended to be "a bit of a worrier".
>
> He is currently in a temporary placement in a residential home. He has no physical problems and can eat and drink independently. Currently, carers

provide his medication and meals, prompt him regarding when to wash, and lay out clothes for him to then put on independently. He has sometimes left the home without saying where he was going and then been found disorientated and upset several hours later by concerned staff. He says he wants to live at home when asked directly, but does not ever ask to go home independently. He seems to be happy and content in the residential home, according to reports from staff and a friend. Any changes to his routine are anxiety-provoking, and he has been known to refuse to attend medical appointments because of this. He has formed good relationships with other residents and staff. The team were concerned that if he returned home alone, he would quickly start to neglect himself due to his poor memory.

Neuropsychological testing indicated severe attention, memory, and executive functioning impairments. His reading skills were in the normal range. No emotional disturbance was identified. The semi-structured interview with Terry initially focused on whether he understood what he needed to do if he lived alone and if he recognised the potential risks highlighted by the team. He was unable to provide a comprehensive account of what he would have to do if he went home and continually stated "I'll be all right" when potentially risky situations, such as him getting lost while trying to shop, were discussed with him. The assessor (HN) then discussed with the rest of the team how to test out some of the possible risks for the client in returning home alone. First, we gave him the chance to administer his own medication, using a blister pack. Second, we gave him the opportunity to practise preparing and cooking some simple meals with the occupational therapist. He was only able to use the blister pack if reminded. He had significant difficulties sequencing any kitchen tasks and was easily distracted from the task. A home visit was planned and Terry was due to be accompanied there by a familiar member of staff. He refused to attend the visit on the day and three attempts to rearrange it were met with excuses.

Consideration was then given to taking "all reasonable steps" to enhance Terry's capacity. HN compiled a list of the risks and advantages of staying where he was versus going back home alone. A sheet of A4 paper was used for each option, one headed "going home" and the other "staying here". Each sheet was divided into two columns, one entitled "advantages" and the other "risks". On discussing the results of the functional trials, Terry was unable to recall his difficulties freely during the session. However, he was able to see that there were more items on the "risks" side of the "going home" chart and more items on the "advantages" side of the "staying here" chart. He then said that he thought it might be better if he stayed where he was. This process was repeated on two more occasions and no marked changes in his cognitive processing were observed.

From the above, the evidence pointed to Terry lacking the capacity to make an *informed* decision regarding where he should live. This was on the basis that he was unable to understand what the requirements of living by himself were, that he could not retain the information for long enough, and that he was unable to weigh up the relevant information to make an informed decision. His stated desire to return home when specifically asked might have reflected a desire to feel "at home", rather than wishing to return to the "bricks and mortar" of his physical home. The settled nature of his behaviour in the home and his friend's report all supported this. Perhaps there was also an element of him saying what he thought the assessor (HN) wanted to hear, that is, he was giving what he perceived to be a socially desirable response when asked about where he wanted to live.

We hope that this case example shows how drawing on the legal standard, functional elements, diagnosis, cognitive underpinnings, psychiatric and emotional factors, risk considerations, and steps to enhance capacity of the American Bar Association and American Psychological Association (2008) framework can help in reaching a clinical judgement. The remaining element of "values and preferences" significantly informed the process of determining what was in his "best interests". The element of "values and preferences is discussed in our section "What are some of the issues that may come into play after the capacity assessment?"

Capacity to manage finances

This area of capacity assessment is usually referred to in legal circles as the capacity to manage "property and affairs". This is used interchangeably in the literature, but, for consistency purposes, we have used the term "finances".

Moye and Marson (2007), in their paper relating to the assessment of older adults, present a conceptual model of financial capacity, including:

- declarative knowledge (the ability to describe facts, concepts, and events related to financial activities, such as knowledge of currencies, loans and interest rates, and personal financial data);

- procedural knowledge (the ability to carry out learnt motor-based skills, such as withdrawing from a cashpoint (ATM), writing a cheque, obtaining change);
- judgement (the ability to make financial decisions consistent with self-interest in everyday and novel or ambiguous situations). This information, when collated and combined, provides a global view as to financial capacity.

Suto, Clare, and Holland (2007), in their work with people with learning disabilities, also provide some interesting ideas. These include an explanation as to when, developmentally, various financial concepts are developed. They then suggest how these concepts can be assessed and provide extremely practical tools to assist with this. For example, they provide five hypothetical stories that become progressively more difficult. Each story has pictures that develop the story and are shown one at a time in a given sequence. The pictures require adapting to make them more relevant for people other than those with learning disabilities, but this is easily done.

The approaches by Moye and Marson (2007) and Suto, Clare, and Holland (2007) discourage the assessor from thinking about capacity to manage finances as a black and white concept, where a client either has capacity to manage all of their finances or they entirely do not. Instead, they suggest it is more helpful to consider how a client might have capacity to manage certain aspects (perhaps the simpler ones) of their finances, but not others (maybe the more complex). This, in our view, reflects a central concept within the MCA. That is, capacity is complex and multi-factorial, and it is perfectly possible for a client to exercise reasonable capacity in part(s) of such a decision even if they might not be able to in more complex parts. This detailed way of assessing capacity questions could be considered the "gold standard" approach in capacity assessment and something to strive for. Practically, reporting such results can prove to be complicated. The Court of Protection forms provide little physical space (the boxes are really small) to facilitate clinicians presenting their information beyond a "yes they do have capacity" or "no they don't" format. This militates against the psychological formulation philosophy we adopt. In our view, the appointed financial deputy (if the person lacks some sort of financial capacity) is often left to judge for themselves how much autonomy to allow or not allow their client.

What follows is a list of useful questions, which could be included in a semi-structured interview (Table 6.2).

Table 6.2. Examples of interview questions regarding capacity for managing finances.

Managing money
How much money do you have at the moment?
Do you have bank account(s)?
If so, does anyone else have access to these?
What do you need money for?
Where do you get money from?
What financial decisions do you make now? (e.g., Do you manage direct debits? Do you budget for bills?)
What other kinds of decisions do you make now? (e.g., Do you choose what you wear each day? Do you choose how you spend your time? Do you choose your meals?)
How much money do you get each week and how do you spend it?
Do you have access to any other money such as savings?
How would you go about arranging a loan if you needed one?
Would you know what questions to ask the lender?
Do you know what "interest" is and how it is calculated?
Do you know what a mortgage is?
Would you know how to arrange a mortgage if you needed one?
Who would you ask to help you?
What questions do you think you might need to ask before signing any documents?
Would you write a cheque to buy a stamp?
How much is a pint of milk?
How much is a loaf of bread?
How much is a pint of beer?
How much is a daily newspaper?
How much is a litre of petrol?
How much is a cinema ticket?
What would you do if you had more money each week?
What would you do if you received a large cheque in the post?
In the future, would you like to change how your money is managed/handled?
Is there anyone you would trust to help you to look after your money?
How well do you think that you have managed your money in the past?
Have you got into money difficulties in the past?

Case example: Assessment regarding capacity to manage settlement monies

Jack was being seen for long-term community-based neuropsychological rehabilitation following a traumatic acquired brain injury (ABI) four years earlier. He had general cognitive impairment, communication difficulties, memory impairment, had marked visual difficulties (for which he was registered blind), and a history of turbulent and failed intimate relationships since his ABI. His medico–legal claim was about to settle, for a seven-figure sum, and he was adamant that he wished to manage his own finances. His solicitor had concerns about his vulnerability to financial exploitation. His ex-wife had claimed for gratuitous care compensation, which Jack's family felt was groundless. Jack wanted to pay her whatever it took to make her leave him alone, despite legal advice to the contrary. The neuropsychologist (TRM) was asked to complete a Court of Protection 3 (CoP3) form and provide an opinion that could guide the Court in its deliberations.

Neuropsychological assessments were already lodged with the Court as part of the medico–legal claim process (and which were recent enough to be considered relevant). Therefore, no further testing was undertaken. TRM used a structured and open-ended clinical interview, using the questions above (Table 6.2), as a basis to test out the four elements of stage two of the legal test enshrined within the MCA detailed at the beginning of this chapter. TRM had already been working with the client for over a year and was familiar with the pertinent and complex issues involved and had the trust of the client.

As a result of the interview and several hours of discussion, TRM was able to establish that Jack did not have the capacity to manage his settlement monies. What marked out this particular case was the manner in which the assessment was completed. By the end of the process, the client was able to acknowledge that he was vulnerable to financial exploitation, that his memory was unreliable, and that he could be easily confused if someone wished to do this. He was then able to agree that it was better for him to have the safety net of the Court of Protection until such time as it could be demonstrated that this was no longer needed. This was achieved through the assessor affording value to the client's wishes and taking time to ensure he grasped the complex issues at play. This then facilitated the long-term relationship between Jack and his appointed financial deputy.

Testamentary capacity

As mentioned above, the commonly accepted legal test for testamentary capacity is set out in the case Banks *vs.* Goodfellow (1870). The criteria for testamentary capacity laid out by the Lord Chief Justice in this case is archaic and perhaps somewhat impenetrable in its wording. However, there are four elements in this case requiring consideration.

1. Understanding the nature of the act of making a will.
2. Understanding the effects of making a will.
3. Understanding the extent of the property being disposed of.
4. Comprehending and appreciating the claims to which a person making a will ought to give effect.

Chapter Six within the British Medical Association and the Law Society's joint text (2010) provides a very helpful checklist of what the assessor could consider when assessing a person's testamentary capacity with regard to the four elements listed above. This checklist provides a useful starting point for the questions you could develop for a semi-structured interview.

Subsumed under the second element, "effects of making a will", some solicitors request the assessor to address specifically whether the person has the mental capacity to "create an orderly plan of disposition". This phrase has been taken directly from instruction letters sent to HN by various firms of solicitors. In simple terms, this means assessing whether the person can tell you how they would divide their estate among their beneficiaries. For example, you could assess the person's understanding of mathematical concepts such as fractions and percentages. The person's understanding of the relative relationships between different fractions and percentages is also important to establish.

We mentioned previously that such common law tests sit alongside the MCA statute (2005). Therefore, the requirements and principles of the MCA (2005) need equal consideration. The principle of "taking all practicable steps" to maximise a person's capacity can open up the possibility of enabling someone to make their own Will. However, the *extent* to which clients can be effectively assisted to make decisions by another person is unclear. The BMA and Law Society text (2010) discusses how certain elements can be explained and the person can be reminded of facts. However, they must be able to form the actual will themselves. Thus, they must be able to satisfy that they have, without assistance, created an orderly plan of disposition and been able to explain their choices.

Case study: Assessment of testamentary capacity

> Mary is a twenty-one-year-old who suffered from an acquired brain injury aged two, having fallen from a first-floor window. Her mother and father have been divorced since she was five years old. She lives with her mother and younger brother and sister. She has very little contact with her father and last saw him around a year ago. Her five maternal aunts and uncles live close to her and she sees them and her seven cousins at least weekly. She has a support worker to assist her with cooking, shopping, and various activities such as going to the gym. She has demonstrated an ability to learn new skills, such as cooking spaghetti bolognaise from scratch. At times, she struggled to ascertain how much money she needed to provide to purchase an item and also to calculate the change owing.
>
> On neuropsychological testing, she scored in the Extremely Low range on the Attention, Language and Visuospatial indices on the Repeatable Battery Assessment of Neuropsychological Status. She scored in the Extremely Low to Borderline ranges on the Immediate Memory Index. On the Delayed Memory Index she scored in the Extremely Low to Low Average ranges at the 4th percentile. The assessor (HN) used the Twenty Questions Test from the Delis–Kaplan Executive Function System to tap into Mary's ability to problem solve using abstract thinking and to incorporate feedback in formulating more effective questions. On this test, all her scores fell within the Severely Impaired to Borderline ranges.
>
> Every test does, of course, have its limitations, but the Twenty Questions Test can be particularly useful when assessing people who have acquired their brain injury early on in life and might be vulnerable to falling foul of floor effects on other tests. For example, the Word Context Test (also from the DKEFS-UK) appears to rely on knowledge of how a word's meaning can be gleaned from its context in a sentence. This sort of knowledge is often acquired through formal education. If someone has acquired their brain injury early in childhood, they might have been unable, or limited in their ability, to acquire such knowledge. Her mood on formal assessment, using the Hospital Anxiety and Depression Scale and based on her self-report and clinical impression, was normal.
>
> Regarding her Will, Mary appeared to understand the nature of a Will once various features of a Will were described to her. She was able to adequately summarise these descriptions provided to her. For example, she had been informed about the role of an executor and was able to tell HN it was to "sort out the will when you die"; they "gives the money out to people". She was able to provide a comprehensive description of her family tree. Although she understood her father might expect to be a

beneficiary, she was able to provide a logical and thought-through reason for not including him. HN therefore concluded Mary had the capacity to understand who would have a reasonable claim to benefit from her estate. She also appeared to understand the extent of her property, knowing it was made up of her property and some investments. She was not able to acknowledge the value of this, but this is not required in the capacity test.

Mary had extreme difficulty in expressing her wishes about an orderly plan of disposition. She wanted to include her mother, siblings, and also all her aunts and uncles and cousins individually in her will. She was unable to conceptualise beyond the concrete level regarding her assets. For example, she was unable to conceptualise that her property (90% of her assets) could be sold and then divided up. When discussing the potential distribution of the remaining 10%, she was easily influenced to change her mind. HN formulated that, due to her limited capacity to weigh up and consider information independently from such an early age, she had become highly dependent on other people's suggestions about many matters and was, therefore, vulnerable to being unduly influenced.

HN concluded Mary did not have testamentary capacity as she was unable to express her wishes clearly and consistently in an orderly plan of disposition and also to understand the effects of making a Will in the form she was proposing. If she had decided on a simpler format for the distribution of her estate, she might have had testamentary capacity. This case highlights how higher levels of cognitive functioning are required for more complex decisions and are substantively different from small-scale everyday choices (e.g., testamentary capacity versus deciding between beverages when a drink is wanted). Also, this case highlights the different cognitive demands of deciding simple and complex versions of the same category of decision. For example, a simpler Will (with one form of asset and one beneficiary) will require a lower level of mental capacity than a complex will (with multiple assets and beneficiaries).

Capacity to undertake litigation

This is a complex area of law with significant authorities referred to in established case law. It is agreed that the question of capacity has to be considered on an issue of specific basis, and the Courts have approved a three-stage formulation, as follows.

- First, the individual litigants must have the insight and understanding of the fact that they have a problem in respect of which they need advice.
- Second, having identified the problem, it will be necessary for the individual litigants to seek an appropriate adviser and to instruct them with sufficient clarity to enable them to understand the problem and advise them appropriately.
- Finally, the individual litigants need sufficient mental capacity to understand and to make decisions based upon, or otherwise give effect to, such advice as they may receive.

It is also important that individual litigants have capacity to understand, absorb, and retain sufficient information, including advice relevant to the matters in question, sufficiently to enable them to make decisions based upon such information.

Table 6.3 gives examples of questions to ask with a view to instructing a solicitor.

Table 6.3. Examples of interview questions for instructing a solicitor.

1.	Do you know what has happened to you?
2.	How has this affected you/changed you?
3.	Do you think that you need advice on how to deal with these matters?
4.	Who is the best professional to give you advice? Why do you think that?
5.	Do you know what a solicitor is?
6.	Who is *your* solicitor and what is their job?
7.	What do you think that you have asked your solicitor to do for you?
8.	What are the issues in the case?
9.	Who else is involved in this case?
10.	What are their jobs/roles?
11.	Who represents you?
12.	What can the Court do? (Expect reference to: trial/hearings; uncertainty of proceedings and outcome; potential for loss.)
13.	Who is the Court supposed to listen to?
14.	Who makes the decision at the end?

*Case example: Adult with TBI wishing to enter into
family law proceedings*

Keith had previously undertaken a lengthy programme of neuropsychological rehabilitation with one of the authors (TRM), but had not been seen for two years since discharge. Keith's solicitor asked TRM to now establish whether or not he retained the capacity to litigate on his own behalf or whether a litigation friend (appointed by the Official Solicitor) might need to be appointed to represent his interests.

At the time of assessment, he was five years post-injury. A complicating factor was that he was a "problem drinker" and had been so since before his injury. However, since his post-injury divorce, his alcohol intake had become such that he had spent time (unsuccessfully) in alcohol detoxification services and had been diagnosed with type II diabetes.

Keith has a support worker (Bradley) for forty hours per week. TRM interviewed Bradley to ascertain any key changes since he had been discharged and to establish the nature and level of the support currently required and provided.

Bradley confirmed that although Keith was still drinking at "problem" levels, he was drinking less alcohol than for several years and had also managed to sustain this reduction over several months. His motivation for this reduction was unclear.

TRM also interviewed Keith, using a structured interview approach (see Table 6.3, above). His responses indicated that he had a clear understanding of his role in evidence, the nature of court proceedings, and the potential course of events. He was clear about the roles of the Officers of the Court, as well as the advice of his solicitor in the context of his instruction to him or her.

Neuropsychological testing was subsequently undertaken to obtain data that could inform whether Keith's capacity to understand, recall, formulate, and communicate the elements of decision making was retained or under threat. The Wechsler Abbreviated Scale of Intellligence (WASI), Brixton, Spatial Anticipation Test, BIRT Memory and Information Processing Battery (BIMPB) Information Processing, Kaplan–Baycrest Neuropsychological Assessment Problem-Solving, Colour Trails and Repeatable Battery Assessment of Neuropsychological Status (R-BANS) tests were employed. Clinical observations made during the assessment were triangulated with the information obtained from formal interviewing and testing.

Keith had particular difficulties with processing speed, mental flexibility, and working memory. In formulating an opinion for the court, TRN particularly considered how Keith's problem drinking and insulin-managed Type II diabetes might well lead to his capacity fluctuating. TRM advised the court that there was clinical evidence to suggest he retained capacity to litigate, but would require specific assistance to ensure optimal access to proceedings.

What issues might be pertinent after the capacity assessment?

In clinical training, clinical psychologists are taught the importance of reflection and hypothesis testing in the development of formulations. In our view, this is of particular importance when conducting capacity assessments. There are some issues worthy of consideration across all capacity assessments.

We assess for the existence of factors that could cause fluctuating capacity and, also, factors that might be amenable to therapy or treatment. Knowing about such factors could lead to recommendations about the circumstances under which someone might have the capacity to make the decision. Some of these factors have already been drawn out in our case examples (e.g., current alcohol consumption). Others include mood problems, such as anxiety and depression, drug abuse, and the influence of another on decision making. If there is a concern about undue influence being exerted by others, it could prove useful to administer the Gudjonsson Suggestibility Scales (GSS) (Gudjonsson, 1984). Although not designed specifically for capacity assessment, it can give an objective psychometric indication of the susceptibility to alter one's position under pressure from others.

It is critical is that there is a benchmark for "reasonableness" (or the principle of parsimony) in the assessment. In pursuit of thoroughness, the clinician must guard against raising the assessment bar higher than it should be. For example, in the instance of testamentary capacity, it is important to establish that the person making the Will understands that this will be implemented after their demise. Clearly, they need to understand the concept of "death". The average person might describe death in terms of the person being "no longer here", or "no longer breathing". The assessor must take care not to expect more than this of the person being assessed, regardless of their cognitive deficits or disabilities. Suto, Clare, and Holland (2007) also emphasise the importance of this in relation to financial capacity, highlighting that to do so "would be discriminatory and unacceptable" (p. 15).

The concept of effort testing has been raised in the Assessment chapter of this book. The document *Assessment of Effort in Clinical Testing of Cognitive Functioning for Adults* (British Psychological Society, 2009) provides a useful overview on this thought-provoking and somewhat controversial topic. As the process of assessing capacity involves cognitive testing, the issue of effort testing within the field of capacity assessment necessitates consideration.

There are also issues specific to particular capacity assessments. For example, assessments of capacity to manage finances can occur in cases where large compensation claims (often into the millions) are at issue. This can complicate matters as, for example, many people without an impairment in the functioning of the mind/brain could have difficulty in managing such sums. In such cases, it is essential to be wary of concluding that someone lacks capacity because they could be making an "unwise" decision. For example, it is common for people receiving a large compensation sum to see it as a "lottery win", and wanting to "blow" part of it is a normal reaction.

The assessment process requires the assessor to set up the situation well. This will include discussing in depth the client's understanding as to what the money is expected to cover (both now and in the future). For example, issues such as the likely rehabilitation they will require for the rest of their lives across all domains (e.g., speech and language therapy, physiotherapy, occupational therapy, medical monitoring and intervention, support workers, carers, nursing), changes to life expectancy, and changes in dependency level across the life span. There are also issues specific to people who receive large lump sums (e.g., reactions of others, wanting to treat others, wanting to treat themselves, and wanting to change themselves).

The remaining point centres round maintaining the individual's "best interests". The person's values and preferences will particularly inform this process. Taking the example of capacity regarding living arrangements, it is, of course, essential to consider issues such as what sort of place would suit the person, how much personal space they require, and the other people that might be there. However, we also think it is essential to discuss what is in the individual's best interests regarding the following points.

- Who is going to discuss with the individual that a decision is going to be made in their "best interests"? Their next of kin, a professional they have got to know well, the professional with clinical responsibility? For each person, the decision will be different.
- When should the person be told? Way ahead so they can get used to the idea? The day before they are due to go? The moment they are due to go to their new home? Again, for each person, the decision will be different.

Theresa Joyce's excellent guidance booklet on helping professionals make best interests decisions (Joyce, 2007) is well worth consulting and, for example, includes suggestions on how to convene and manage a best interests meeting.

Conclusion

To conclude, we have summarised the fundamental principles of the Mental Capacity Act (2005) and the two steps required in the assessment of capacity. The importance of adopting a formulation-based philosophy to capacity assessment has been emphasised. This requires an emphasis on idiosyncratically developed interviews informed by the MCA and other relevant legislation, including case law. Neuropsychological testing has its place, an important one, but it is not *the* tool; it is *part* of the process. There are a considerable number of issues surrounding capacity assessments requiring thought and consideration, which have been discussed. We hope you now feel confident to approach capacity questions with renewed vigour and inspiration.

Useful resources

For a short introduction to the Mental Capacity Act (2005), please see www.bps.org.uk/sites/default/files/documents/mental_capacity_act_2005_-_short_reference_guide_for_psychologists_and_psychiatrists.pdf

For guidelines (including useful case studies) on conducting assessments of various capacity issues including: consent to health and social care, legal areas, sexual relations, and finances, please see

British Psychological Society (2006). *Assessment of Capacity in Adults: Interim Guidance for Psychologists, Professional Practice Board and Assessment of Capacity Guidelines Group*. Leicester: BPS.

British Medical Association and Law Society (2010). *Assessment of Mental Capacity: A Practical Guide for Doctors and Lawyers*. London: BMA.

Suto, I., Clare, I. and Holland, A. (2007). *Financial Decision-Making: Guidance for Supporting Financial Decision-making by People with Learning Disabilities*. Kidderminster: BILD.

Test references

Baddeley, A., Emslie, H., & Nimmo-Smith, I. (1992). *The Speed and Capacity of Language Processing Test*. London: Pearson Assessment, The Psychological Corporation.

Coughlan, A. K., Oddy, M., & Crawford, J. R. (2007). *BIRT Memory and Information Processing Battery*. Horsham: The Brain Injury Rehabilitation Trust.

Delis, D. C., Kaplan, E., & Kramer, J. H. (2001). *The Delis–Kaplan Executive Function System*. San Antonio, TX: Harcourt Assessment, The Psychological Corporation.

Dodd, K., Marlow, L., Jones, K., & Livesey, A. (2010). *Social–Moral Awareness Test (SMAT)*. Epsom: Surrey & Borders Partnership NHS Trust.

Enderby, P., Wood, V., & Wade, D. (2006). *The Frenchay Aphasia Screening Test* (2nd edn). London: Wiley-Blackwell.

Kopelman, M., Wilson, B., & Baddely, A. (1990). *Autobiographical Memory Interview*. London: Pearson Assessment, The Psychological Corporation.

Randolph, C. (1998). *Repeatable Battery for the Assessment of Neuropsychological Status (RBANS™)*. London: Pearson Assessment, The Psychological Corporation.

Richards, B., Rewilak, D., Proulx ,G. B., & Leach,L. (2000). *Kaplan–Baycrest Neurocognitive Assessment (KBNA UK)*. London: Pearson Assessment, The Psychological Corporation.

Robertson, I. H., Ward, T., Ridgeway, V., & Nimmo-Smith, I. (1994). *The Test of Everyday Attention – Manual*. London: Pearson Assessment, The Psychological Corporation.

Shallice, T. (1997). *The Hayling and Brixton Tests*. London: Pearson Assessment, The Psychological Corporation.

Snaith, R. P., & Zigmond, A. S. (1994). *The Hospital Anxiety and Depression Scale*. London: G. L. Assessment.

Wechsler, D. (2010). *Wechsler Adult Intelligence Scale – Fourth U.K. Edition*. London: Pearson Assessment, The Psychological Corporation.

Wechsler, D. (2010). *Wechsler Memory Scale (4th UK edn)*. London: Pearson Assessment, The Psychological Corporation.

Wechsler, D. (2011). *Wechsler Abbreviated Scale of Intelligence* (2nd edn). London: Pearson Assessment, The Psychological Corporation.

Wilson, B. A., Alderman, N., Burgess, P. W., Emslie, H., & Evans J. J. (1996). B*ehavioural Assessment of the Dysexecutive Syndrome*. London: Pearson Assessment, The Psychological Corporation.

References

American Bar Association and American Psychological Association (2008). *Assessment of Older Adults with Diminished Capacity: A Handbook for Psychologists*. Washington, DC: American Bar Association and American Psychological Association.

Banks *vs*. Goodfellow [1870]. 5 LR QB 549.

British Medical Association & the Law Society (2010). *Assessment of Mental Capacity: A Practical Guide for Doctors and Lawyers* (3rd edn). London: BMA.

British Psychological Society (2006). *Assessment of Capacity in Adults: Interim Guidance for Psychologists, Professional Practice Board and Assessment of Capacity Guidelines Group*. Leicester: BPS

British Psychological Society (2009). *Assessment of Effort in Clinical Testing of Cognitive Functioning in Adults*. Leicester: BPS.

British Psychological Society (2010). A*udit Tool for Mental Capacity Assessments, Professional Practice Board and Social Care Institute for Excellence*. Leicester: BPS.

Department for Constitutional Affairs (2007). *Mental Capacity Act 2005 Code of Practice*. London: The Stationery Office.

Gudjonsson, G. H. (1984). A new scale of interrogative suggestibility. *Personality and Individual Differences*, 5(3): 303–314.

Joyce, T. (2007). *Best Interests Guidance on Determining the Best Interests of Adults Who Lack the Capacity to Make a Decision (or Decisions) for Themselves [England and Wales]: A Report Published by the Professional Practice Board of the British Psychological Society*. Leicester: BPS.

Kapp, M. B., & Mossman, D. (1996). Measuring decisional capacity: cautions on the construction of a "capacimeter". *Psychology, Public Policy & Law*, 2(1): 73–95.

Mackenzie, J. A., Lincoln, N. B., & Newby, G. J. (2008). Capacity to make a decision about discharge destination after stroke: a pilot study. *Clinical Rehabilitation, 22*: 1116–1126.

Mason, B. (1993). Towards positions of safe uncertainty. *Human Systems: The Journal of Systemic Consultation & Management, 4*:193–200.

Mental Capacity Act (2005) (c.9). London: The Stationery Office. Electronic version: www.legislation.gov.uk/ukpga/2005/9/contents. Accessed 23 May 2012.

Moye, J., & Marson, D. C. (2007). Assessment of decision-making capacity in older adults: an emerging area of practice and research. *Journal of Gerontology: Psychological Sciences, 62B*(1): 3–11.

Mullaly, E., Kinsella, G., Berberovic, N., Cohen, Y., Dedda, K., Froud, B., Leach, K., & Neath, J. (2007). Assessment of decision-making capacity: exploration of common practices among neuropsychologists. *Australian Psychologist, 42*(3): 178–186.

Newberry, A. M., & Pachet, A. K. (2008). An innovative framework for psychosocial assessment in complex mental capacity evaluations. *Psychology, Health & Medicine, 13*(4): 438–449.

Newby, G., Anderson, C., & Todd, D. (2011). It takes time, practice and thought: reflections of a neuropsychologist's experience in implementing the Mental Capacity Act 2005. *Clinical Psychology Forum, 218*:16–20.

Suto, I., Clare, I., & Holland, A. (2007). *Financial Decision-Making: Guidance for supporting Financial Decision-making by People with Learning Disabilities*. Worcestershire: BILD.

Whyte, M., Wilson, M., Hamilton, J., Primrose, W., & Summers, F. (2003). Adults with incapacity (Scotland) Act 2000: implications for clinical psychology. *Clinical Psychology, 31*: 5–8.

CHAPTER SEVEN

Driving after acquired brain injury: rehabilitation and therapy

Gavin Newby

Throughout this book, we have discussed how the pernicious mix of cognitive deficits, emotional difficulties, behavioural and personality changes can wreak devastating changes on the lives of brain-injured people and their families. At face value, it would seem obvious that this combination of difficulties should affect a person's ability to drive safely.

The driving task requires the driver to be attentive, to concentrate, make judgements quickly in rapidly changing circumstances, and to be able to cope when the situation is demanding (Christie et al., 2001). However, currently, the research evidence about whether people who have experienced an acquired brain injury and have returned to driving are at increased risk of having an accident or are more likely to commit traffic offences is extremely equivocal. For example, both Lundqvist, Alinder, and Ronnberg (2008) (in a mixed traumatically acquired brain injured (TBI) and stroke group) and Bivona and colleagues (2012) (in a severely TBI group of thirty) found significantly more drivers reported accidents compared to controls post injury. Indeed, Bivona and colleagues' (2012) post-injury driver group report an increased accident rate that is over twice their reported pre-injury rate. However, Schultheis, Matheis, Nead, and DeLuca (2002), among others, found no evidence of an increased accident rate. There is also much debate about which aspects of cognitive functioning are important in the driving task, and still more debate about which aspects are linked to safe driving.

This situation has meant that there is no standard, validated protocol for assessing fitness to drive after acquired brain injury in the UK. Not surprisingly, as a result, current assessment practices are extremely variable. Many professional groups are extremely uncertain about the relevance and validity of the clinical data they collect to inform an opinion regarding their clients' driving. Indeed, when members of the then Special Group in Clinical Neuropsychology of the British Psychology Society were surveyed, of the ninety-two respondents, 23% did not know their clients' legal duties in relation to reporting the brain injury, of the 77% who said they did know, only 61% mentioned informing the DVLA and gave an opinion on fitness to drive based on the neuropsychological tests they routinely gave. Interestingly, only those who had been in practice for over five years and had given advice to large numbers of people regarding driving had any significant levels of confidence. Very few services had consistent operational policies (Christie, Savill, Buttress, Newby, & Tyerman, 2001). Although these studies are quite old now, the author's anecdotal discussions with colleagues do not suggest that the professional situation in neuropsychology is markedly or consistently different today. The cost of making the wrong judgement about an individual's fitness to drive is potentially high. If individuals are judged fit to drive when they are not, then their safety and that of other road users could be in jeopardy. If judged unfit to drive when they are fit, the loss of driving might mean unemployment, loss of independence, and social isolation.

In this chapter, I set out some of the key issues clinicians should consider when facing the issues surrounding returning to driving after brain injury and some suggestions about how to take their own practice forward.

Why is the return to driving such an important and thorny topic?

Driving is considered by most adults to be an "essential" activity of daily living (Fox, Bashford, & Caust, 1992) and a route to increased freedom and social standing within society for young people (Brooks & Hawley, 2005). In Western culture, driving is intimately associated with independence, a sense of self-worth, work, social, and leisure contexts, maintaining family roles, and undertaking personal business such as shopping and holidays. Thus, returning to driving after a brain injury is a key milestone for many clients and their families in rehabilitation and can be an important "gold standard" symbol of regaining both independence and a sense of "normality" (Brooks & Hawley, 2005; Newby, 1996). Returning to driving also has a strong association with increased life satisfaction (Novack et al., 2010).

Not surprisingly, clients are highly motivated to return to driving, with return rates for those with moderate to severe brain injuries tending to range between 40% and 60% (e.g., Brooks & Hawley, 2005; Novack et al., 2010).

With such highly charged importance attached to driving, this perhaps goes some way to explain why questioning clients as to whether they have returned to driving, or are continuing to drive, can be extremely difficult and challenging. Additionally, there is also consistent evidence from the social psychological literature that many drivers would tend to perceive their skills as above average (Groeger & Brown, 1989) and that they are below-average risk takers (Delhomme, 1991).

The lack of clear, consistent links between cognitive deficits and driving

Ironically, many people with brain injury who later turn out to have significant difficulties with managing the whole driving task are able to physically manipulate and control a car (e.g., undertaking manoeuvres such as steering, operating the pedals, and so on) because they are able to retain the blueprints for carrying out the motor sequences of the movements required (McKenna, 1998). Indeed, Lezak, Howieson, and Loring (2004) remind us that clients suffering from significant frontal lobe or dysexecutive difficulties can raise their levels of performance during assessment as a result of this retained ability. This can mean that on a one-off assessment, even people who show significant attention and concentration difficulties over longer periods can perform at near normal levels during stimulating short-term assessments.

Many of the clients we speak to also raise the issue of what is safe driving. Many so-called "normal" drivers exhibit a range of occasionally unsafe behaviours, such as pulling out in front of another car or driving too fast, but their driving is not questioned. However, many clients worry that their driving is being questioned solely because they happen to have a brain injury.

Not surprisingly, there have been at least three decades of research endeavour looking at the role of psychometrics in validating and reliably picking up on cognitive difficulties that lead to poor on-the-road driving (e.g., see British Psychological Society, 2001, Brouwer & Withaar, 1997; Classen et al., 2009; Christie et al., 2001; Van Zomeren, Brouwer, Rothengatter, & Snoek, 1988, and Novack et al., 2010 for reviews). However, the research has not been conclusive about which neuropsychological deficits predict driving performance, due, in part, to a range of conceptual and methodological problems. Among these difficulties have been poor study designs: for example, trying to develop a general neuropsychological tool with small numbers of participants (which tries to take into account a wide variety of deficits after brain injury), taking a "test everything" theoretical approach, and over-reliance on test procedures which bear little resemblance to the actual driving task (Christie et al., 2001). A number of researchers have attempted to validate their neuropsychological batteries on a structured, closed driving course. However, this is unlikely to be representative of the twists, turns, and chance events of real traffic. Indeed, the spontaneity of real road assessment makes it difficult to replicate or reliably include particular driving challenges, for example, reacting to a car pulling out in front of you. Further, as driving assessors acknowledge, they have to make on-road assessments difficult in that they do not give directional cues to actions that can help maximise performance, such as "turn left ahead", "stop over there". Interestingly, the findings of a Swedish study by Lundqvist, Alinder, and Ronnberg (2008) suggest that on-road assessment is a poor predictor of driving status ten years later. The authors tentatively suggest this might be due to on-road assessments being relatively insensitive to brain injury-related residual symptoms which have progressively greater influence on driving status over time.

Of course, traditional psychometric assessment is not the only way of assessing possible relevant deficits. Indeed, they are, by their very nature, rather static tools that theoretically assess underpinning relevant neurobiological systems considered relevant for driving. They do not pick up the dynamics of the visual experience of driving, for example. Until relatively recently, the use of computer-based assessments have been restricted by the limited sophistication of the visual experience. Put most simply, such simulations did not look or feel like driving and led in some circumstances to subjects experiencing vestibular disturbance such as nausea and dizziness. However, recent advances have made this much more acceptable. A good recent example is that of a French study carried out by Milleville-Pennel, Pothier, Hoc, and Mathe (2010) using the useful field of view (UFOV) paradigm. In brief, a driver's UFOV is the range/circumference of visual stimuli that a driver can attend and react to when scanning their visual environment. It incorporates visual sensory functioning, visual processing speed, and visual attention (Novack et al., 2006). Better driving is associated with a broader UFOV and poorer driving with a narrower UFOV. While by no means conclusive, the UFOV paradigm holds promise as a useful diagnostic adjunct.

The legal context: the role of the UK Driver, Vehicle and Licensing Agency (DVLA)

It is fair to say that the typical enduring deficits experienced by many severely brain-injured people raise intuitive concerns about driving. Chief among these in any written review are likely to be attention and concentration, planning and judgement, reaction times, and any visuo-perceptual deficit (Rapport, Hanks, & Coleman Bryer, 2006). Additionally, epilepsy, which is found at higher than general population levels after severe ABI, is a very real risk to safe driving and is a proscribed medical condition for driving in the UK if it is uncontrolled (DVLA, 2012). By statute (the Road Traffic Act, Department of Transport, 1988), licence-holders have to notify the DVLA as soon as they become aware of any health condition that might influence their ability to drive safely. Once notified, the DVLA requires licence-holders to complete and return medical information forms. The DVLA Medical Branch has the responsibility of reviewing these forms and deciding on how they will undertake a "medical investigation". This might include requesting further information from a GP or consultant, obtaining an independent medical opinion, or referral for a specialist clinical assessment. The licence-holder may occasionally be required to re-take the standard driving test or, more likely, be referred to a specialist driving assessment centre. Despite it being a legal requirement to inform the DVLA, a survey of clients who had rehabilitation after a severe head injury (post-trauma amnesia three weeks) indicated that 70% had resumed driving but most had done so without any specialist assessment or advice (Newby & Tyerman, 1999). Only 50% had actually notified the DVLA. Indeed, many clients point out that the section on the driving licence that asks you to inform the DVLA about any medical condition is innocuous. Although these findings are relatively old now, and it might be that informing rates have changed to some extent with the introduction of online notification, it is my clinical experience that a substantial number of clients are both surprised that they need to notify the DVLA and can be reluctant to do so for the reasons discussed above. However, when a client declines to accept advice to notify the DVLA and continues to drive, clinicians are faced with trying to persuade their client or with dealing directly with the DVLA (Brooks & Hawley, 2005). DVLA procedures allow for others, such as clinicians and GPs, to inform the DVLA of a medical condition likely to affect safe driving (British Psychological Society, 2001). The UK's General Medical Council (the professional body of medical doctors) has produced an excellent guidance document which gives some suggestions on how to resolve the ethical dilemma of how to persuade compliance with DVLA procedures and how to go about informing the DVLA if required (e.g., persuade to contact DVLA, do not drive until the DVLA has made a determination, and suggest a second opinion) (General Medical Council, 2009). In the event that the DVLA is contacted, they will write to the licence-holder seeking permission to obtain further medical information, and if the patient fails to comply within three weeks, then the driving licence will be revoked for non-compliance. That questionnaire is then passed on to a relevant clinician before a request is made for a more detailed medical report that will be received by the DVLA (Brooks & Hawley, 2005).

The Specialist Driving Assessment Centres previously referred to are a regional collection of centres run under the auspices of the Forum organisation. For a list of Forum-accredited centres, please see Forum of Mobility Centres (2012). Of course, many clients might be concerned about the costs of any assessment, and such concerns can contribute to non-compliance. Costs are incurred if a client seeks an assessment outwith the DVLA medical investigation process. However, the DVLA can mandate a Forum-accredited assessment (which is free) if the medical adviser handling the case feels that such an assessment is required to clarify a client's driving fitness. Clinicians might wish to discuss this possibility with the responsible driving adviser as required. The possibility of reducing costs could be another positive reason for suggesting DVLA compliance to clients. While the exact nature of the assessments undertaken by such centres varies to some extent, each centre will ask clients to come for roughly a half-day assessment during which they will have an initial interview to delineate their current difficulties, and possibly undertake a visual field assessment and/or test of reactions. Forum-accredited centres are working towards the standard use of psychometric instruments such as the Rookwood Driving Battery (McKenna & Bell, 2007). The client is then invited to go out on the roads under observation. All assessments are undertaken in a dual-controlled car with a driving adviser. An initial assessment is usually made in the centre's car park to check on basic manoeuvring ability. Should the adviser feel it is safe to do so, the client is then asked to drive on local roads. The assessment will usually involve driving in a range of situations, such as dual-carriageways, country roads, approaching roundabouts, and driving in busy urban environments. Rating systems vary to some extent. Clients requiring in-car adaptations due to physical disabilities also have the opportunity to drive with the adaptations. Following the assessment, the driving adviser will make a recommendation about the client's driving fitness that is then sent to the DVLA Medical Branch. Currently, recommendations will usually range from fit to drive (i.e., return to driving), definitely unfit to drive (i.e., recommend licence is rescinded), or they might recommend a period of further driving tuition before being reassessed. The DVLA has recently introduced Provisional Disability Assessment Licences (PDALs) that can allow up to three months' worth of tuition under what is essentially a provisional driving licence. In my experience, the DVLA Medical Branch almost always follows the advice given by the assessment centres and can make a number of determinations on the driving licence. First, they might restrict categories—most likely to ordinary motor cars or, in the case of physical disability, to automatic and/or in-car adaptations. Second, they might restrict the length of the licence—typically initially to an annual, bi-annual, or tri-annual basis. At the end of each review period, the client will be asked to see a local GP who is employed specifically by the DVLA to check that there have been no significant changes to the client's medical condition. It is possible, following a number of successful reviews, that the DVLA may give a licence until the driver reaches seventy years of age.

The DVLA Medical Branch operates according to a number of medical/diagnostic rules contained in their *At a Glance Guide to the Current Medical Standards Regarding Fitness to Drive* (DVLA 2012). This guide is available online, is regularly updated, and outlines, for example, the suggested time off from driving following a neurological disorder (e.g., year off after an epileptic seizure, and six months off after intracranial aneurysm with surgical craniotomy and deficit). At the end of the "ban" period, the client can reapply for their licence and undertake an assessment.

It is also important to note that the DVLA may also reissue a licence, or assent to the client continuing to drive, pending the outcome of a further assessment or evidence that a person should not drive. In these circumstances, the client will receive a letter explaining this. Another route to returning to driving post-ABI can be via the opinion of a medical practitioner—often a client's GP.

From all of the above, while the enduring difficulties faced by many people who have an acquired brain injury might naturally raise concerns about driving, there are no consistent research findings to guide professionals on which deficits definitively lead to unsafe driving. Additionally, one must balance both the socio-psychological loading of the role of driving in many people's lives and recognise that we must not expect brain-injured drivers to be better drivers than ordinary drivers. However, we must recognise that the statutory notification process is dependent on clients understanding their responsibilities and having the insight to recognise that they are in difficulty. Not surprisingly, returning to driving is both a fraught and confusing matter for many professionals. Below, we have made a number of suggestions that may inform your practice.

Ensuring clinical service consistency

I would recommend that each service develop an auditable and governable clinical protocol about driving. This would normally include recognising the importance of driving and ensuring that driving is routinely discussed with clients, not only in initial assessment, but throughout your period of treatment with them. I would also recommend that you develop routine information-giving protocols through the collation of leaflets and/or pointing clients towards the DVLA website. We have included driving information for our clients on our original website. Our website was recently evaluated for ease of use by our clients in a research project (Newby & Groome, 2007, 2010).

Supporting clients throughout the driving assessment process

It can be helpful for clients to know you are someone to talk to about the re-licensing process. You can play a major role in reassuring clients, helping them to complete forms, and ensuring they understand what an assessment is likely to involve. It is also important at the end of the process in helping clients understand what the DVLA has actually decided.

Facilitating early disclosure

I would also recommend that services routinely encourage clients and their families to notify the DVLA Medical Branch about their difficulties as soon as it is practicable. This could include referring them to the DVLA website to download forms. Clinicians may, of course, wish to help clients do this and help to complete forms where appropriate. On occasion, I have sought consent from clients to inform the DVLA of their brain injury on their behalf. On an anecdotal level, we feel that this approach has certainly increased the notification rate of our client group.

Facilitating local co-operation and team working

Given the highly emotive nature of returning to driving after ABI, advising on driving can place great strain on therapeutic and clinical relationships. Nouri (1988) recognised that GPs can often find that their relationships with clients do not survive the returning to driving issue. As such, we find that one of the most important decisions to make is who within a client's care network is the right person to pursue the question of returning to driving and potentially be the bearer of bad news. Obviously, each situation will be unique, but it can be useful to raise such questions as:

- who has the right skills to assess driving-relevant skills?
- who is central to the client's future care?
- is there someone with the right skills and credibility who can specifically work on driving and then withdraw once the issue is resolved?

For example, I have regularly met clients and their families with their GPs at the surgery, completed any assessments there, and then fed back jointly with the GP.

Develop working relationships with the DVLA Medical Branch and local Forum-Accredited Driving Assessment Centres

In our experience, we would strongly recommend that practitioners contact the DVLA Medical Branch whenever clients present with driving-related issues that they are unsure of how to handle.

In my experience, I have been able to contact the DVLA to discuss anonymously the client's situation and request advice on how to proceed. On occasion, I have expressed concerns regarding the outcome of a Forum-Accredited Driving Assessment due to my long-standing knowledge of the consequences of a client's executive functioning difficulties. (See case example, below.)

Case example

> Jeff is a fifty-one-year-old former sales executive who developed a thrombosis of the left carotid artery following a serious road traffic accident. This led to extensive right-sided hemispheric infarction and post-stroke epilepsy. His MRI scans showed a site of dissection and that he was left with a right distal internal carotid irregularity but good vessel flow. Although Jeff had been left with relatively preserved intellectual functioning, he retained significant difficulties with attention and concentration, and extremely poor social cognition that consistently led to difficulties in exercising judgement about interpreting the intention of others and the nature of their interest in him. In everyday activities, Jeff was helped by a community support buddy, who assisted him to under-

take small and time-limited targeted amounts of voluntary work, but noted that he had had to continue to prompt Jeff when his attention wandered.

Around four years after the accident, Jeff's ongoing wish to return to driving began to increase, as he wished to access a sports club. Jeff asked my advice about returning to driving. I advised him that I felt that his difficulties with attention were so severe that I thought it was unlikely that he would be able to drive safely. Despite this, he remained extremely keen to return. I undertook a neuropsychological reassessment to help reinforce my advice. The assessment showed continued severe attention and concentration difficulties. I advised him accordingly that my advice about driving had not changed. However, he wished to reapply to the DVLA for his licence. I helped him complete the application forms and recommended in my report to the DVLA that he at least undertook an assessment at a Forum-Accredited Driving Assessment Centre. Jeff duly undertook the assessment and passed. I was immediately contacted by his wife, who was extremely worried about the prospect of her husband driving again. I then spoke to a DVLA Medical Branch Adviser and expressed my concerns, given my functional knowledge of Jeff's abilities. I had also previously contacted the Driving Assessment Centre who were also surprised that Jeff had passed. On considering my opinion, the Medical Branch disregarded the outcome of the driving assessment and determined that Jeff was now unsafe to drive.

Jeff was obviously extremely upset and more than a little angry with me. However, we have been able to work through his anger and he is now more settled in receiving his community mobility via his wife and support buddy.

We would also encourage practitioners to contact their local Driving Assessment Centre. You might benefit from seeing around the centre and, if possible, undertaking a driving assessment to get an idea of what is required. This can be invaluable in assuring clients of what will happen in a driving assessment.

Giving a circumspect opinion on driving

Although research to date does not give any clear guidance on developing specific assessment protocols, documents such as the British Psychological Society's *Assessment of Driving Fitness Following Acquired Brain Injury* (2001), as well as a number of research initiatives (such as those of Christie et al., 2001, and McKenna & Bell, 2007) suggest the primacy of executive functioning difficulties, such as attention, concentration, and information processing, as well as visuo-perceptual and psychomotor speed in determining clients who might have eventual difficulties in returning to drive safely. This is very consistent with the three-part hierarchy conceptualisation of driving (Michon, 1985), as listed below.

- Operational tasks: for example, braking speed, position control, steering, and gap judgement—requiring fast information processing speed.
- Tactical tasks: for example, adjusting speed and estimating distance when overtaking—requiring judgement and anticipation as well as awareness of other road users.
- Strategic tasks: for example, knowing whether you tend to feel comfortable driving in certain weather conditions or unfamiliar cities—requiring accurate knowledge of your own cognitive and driving abilities and their adequacy in certain situations (after Newby, 1996, and Lundqvist & Alinder, 2007)

Interestingly, Lundqvist and Alinder (2007) have found in their study that brain-injured drivers who failed an on-road assessment significantly overestimated their performance compared to those that passed.

As such, I am routinely asked by the DVLA for my neuropsychological assessment results and, where appropriate, I will often point out the existence and relevance of any executive functioning difficulties in any correspondence or discussion with the DVLA Medical Branch.

Supporting clients if the DVLA feels they are unsafe to drive

If the outcome of the whole process is to be "bad news", it is important that practitioners think sensitively about how the information is delivered to anxious and cognitively impaired people. Sensible guidelines might include:

- ensuring family/friends are present to help process the outcome and reasons for not returning to driving (provide concrete examples where possible);

- feed back in a safe and quiet environment;
- speak in a manner appropriate to the client, with opportunities for questions and summary;
- back up the feedback with a written explanation;
- offer additional opportunities to discuss the outcome again.

However, it is vital, if at all possible, not to leave your intervention at the stage of telling clients that they will never drive again. Many people with an ABI are relatively young, have families, and want to work—what are they going to do without a car? Professionals often neglect to address this with clients. As might be guessed from both your own clinical experience and the above review, many clients can be devastated if they are not allowed to drive. It can be important to work with clients and their families to help them look at alternative modes of transport, investigate whether they might be eligible for free bus passes, or whether their DLA could be converted into a Motability car for a relative or carer to drive, for example.

Conclusions

Returning to driving after an ABI is a highly charged and fraught issue. In Western culture, driving is hard-wired into the psyche of most of us as a right and a fundamental component of accessing and participating in society. Not surprisingly, after an ABI, the prospect of losing your driving licence can be devastating and regaining your driving licence is a gold standard symbol of recovery. While gross and profound cognitive deficits will probably mean that the practitioner can be reasonably certain in advising against a return to driving, the research to date does not lead to crystal-clear predictions about how less severe cognitive impairments affect safe driving. On top of this, the current relicensing process after ABI depends, in the main, on insightful self-disclosure. However, in this section, I have made some suggestions to help practitioners adopt consistent procedural and psycho-educational protocols, consider the likely crucial cognitive deficit domains to assess, and to make strong working relationships with local driving assessment centres as well as with the DVLA itself.

Useful resources

Driver and Vehicle Licensing Agency (2012). Driver information webpage: www.dft.gov.uk/dvla/drivers.aspx. Accessed 29 May 2012.

Forum of Mobility Centres (2012). Driving assessment webpage: www.mobility-centres.org.uk/services/drivingassessment.htm. Accessed 29 May 2012.

References

Bivona, U., D'Ippolito, M., Giustini, M., Vignally, P., Longo, E., Taggi, F., & Formisano, R. (2012). Return to driving after severe traumatic brain injury: increased risk of traffic accidents and personal responsibility. *Journal of Head Trauma Rehabilitation*, 27(3): 210–215.

British Psychological Society (2001). *Fitness to Drive and Cognition. A Document of the Multi-disciplinary Working Party on Acquired Neuropsychological Deficits and Fitness to Drive*. Leicester: BPS.

Brooks, N., & Hawley, C. A. (2005). Return to driving after traumatic brain injury: a British perspective. *Brain Injury*, 19(3): 165–175.

Brouwer, W. H., & Withaar, F. K. (1997). Fitness to drive after traumatic brain injury. *Neuropsychological Rehabilitation*, 7(3): 177–193.

Christie, N., Savill, T., Buttress, S., Newby, G. J., & Tyerman, A. D. (2001). Assessing fitness to drive after head injury. A survey of clinical psychologists. *Neuropsychological Rehabilitation*, 11(1): 45–55.

Christie, N., Savill, T., Grayson, G., Ellison, B., Newby, G., & Tyerman, A. (2001). *The Assessment of Fitness to Drive after Brain Injury or Illness*. Crawthorne: Transport Research Laboratory.

Classen, S., Levy, C., McCarthy, D., Mann, W. C., Lanford, D., Waid-Ebbs, J. K. (2009). Traumatic brain injury and driving assessment: an evidence-based literature review. *American Journal of Occupational Therapy*, 63(5): 580–591.

Delhomme, P. (1991). Comparing one's driving with others': assessment of abilities and frequency of offences. Evidence for a superior conformity or self bias? *Accident Analysis and Prevention*, 23: 493–508.

Department of Transport (1988). *The Road Traffic Act*. Electronic version: www.legislation.gov.uk/ukpga/1988/52/contents. Accessed 29 May 2012.

Driver and Vehicle Licensing Agency (2012). *For Medical Practitioners: At a Glance Guide to the Current Medical Standards of Fitness to Drive*. Issued by Drivers Medical Group. Swansea: DVLA. Electronic version: www.dft.gov.uk/dvla/medical/ataglance.aspx. Accessed 29 May 2012.

Fox, G. K., Bashford, G. M., Caust, S. L. (1992). Identifying safe versus unsafe drivers following brain impairment: the Coorabel Programme. *Disability Rehabilitation*, *14*(3): 140–145.

General Medical Council (2009). *Supplementary Advice: Confidentiality: Reporting Concerns about Patients to the DVLA or the DVA*. Electronic version: www.gmc-uk.org/static/documents/content/Confidentiality_reporting_concerns_DVLA_2009.pdf. Accessed 24 May 2012.

Groeger, J. A., & Brown, I. D. (1989). Assessing one's own and others' driving ability: influence of sex, age and experience. *Accident Analysis and Prevention*, *21*: 155–168.

Lezak, M. D., Howieson, D. B., & Loring, D. (2004). *Neuropsychological Assessment* (4th edn). New York: Oxford University Press.

Lundqvist, A., & Alinder, J. (2007). Driving after brain injury: self awareness and coping at the tactical level of control. *Brain Injury*, *21*(11): 1109–1117.

Lundqvist, A., Alinder, J., & Ronnberg, J. (2008). Factors influencing driving 10 years after brain injury. *Brain Injury*, *22*(4): 295–304.

McKenna, P. (1998). Fitness to drive: a neuropsychological perspective. *Journal of Mental Health*, *7*: 9–18.

McKenna, P., & Bell, V. (2007). Fitness to drive following cerebral pathology: the Rookwood Driving Battery as a tool for predicting on-road driving performance. *Journal of Neuropsychology*, *1*: 85–100.

Michon, J. A. (1985). A critical view of driver behaviour models. What do we know, what should we do? In: L. Evans & R. Scwing (Eds.), *Human Behaviour and Traffic Safety* (pp. 485–520). New York: Plenum Press.

Milleville-Pennel, I., Pothier, J., Hoc, J., & Mathe, J. (2010). Consequences of cognitive impairments following traumatic brain injury: pilot study on visual exploration while driving. *Brain Injury*, *24*(4): 678–691.

Newby, G. J. (1996). Following-up the head injured driver: self versus family assessment. Unpublished dissertation. Open University

Newby, G. J., & Groom, C. (2007). How accessible are website-based informational resources for disabled people? Electronic Letter to the Editor. *British Journal of Psychiatry*, *190*(1): 81a. Electronic version: www.bjp.rcpsych.org/cgi/eletters/190/1/81-a. Accessed 7 December 2011.

Newby, G. J., & Groom, C. (2010). Evaluating the usability of a single brain injury (ABI) rehabilitation service website: implications for research methodology and website design. *Neuropsychological Rehabilitation*, *20*(2): 264–288.

Newby, G. J., & Tyerman, A. D. (1999). Driving after a severe head injury: the need for assessment. *British Journal of General Practice, 49*: 301–302.

Nouri, F. (1988). Fitness to drive and the general practitioner. *International Disability Studies, 10*(3): 101–103.

Novack, T. A., Banos, J. H., Alderson, A. L., Schneider, J. J., Weed, W., Blankenship, J., & Salisbury, D. (2006). UFOV performance and driving ability following traumatic brain injury. *Brain Injury, 20*(5): 455–461.

Novack, T. A., Labbe, D., Grote, M., Carlson, N., Sherer, M., Arango-Lasprilla, J. C., Bushnik, T., Cifu, D., Powell, J. M., Ripley, D., & Seel, R. T. (2010). Return to driving within 5 years of moderate–severe traumatic brain injury. *Brain Injury, 24*(3): 464–471.

Rapport, L., Hanks, R., & Coleman Bryer, R. (2006). Barriers to driving and community integration after traumatic brain injury. *Journal of Head Trauma Rehabilitation, 21*(1): 34–44.

Schultheis, M. T., Matheis, R. J., Nead, R., & DeLuca, J. (2002). Driving behaviors following brain injury: self-report and motor vehicle records. *Journal of Head Trauma Rehabilitation, 17*(1): 38–47.

Van Zomeren, A. H., Brouwer, W. H., Rothengatter, J. A., & Snoek, J. W. (1988). Fitness to drive a car after recovery from severe head injury. *Archives of Physical Medicine and Rehabilitation, 69*: 90–96.

CHAPTER EIGHT

Vocational rehabilitation after acquired brain injury

Bernie Walsh

Introduction

Imagine not being in work ... sounds good at first, doesn't it? Many of the readers of this chapter will have extremely demanding and stressful jobs and the prospect of not working would be an enormous release of pressure and give you a feeling of freedom. But imagine being told you cannot work for a while by your partner, family, or your work manager. Imagine the idyllic few weeks away from the pressure turning into months and you feel that people seriously doubt your ability to return to work. You go on to reduced pay and money starts to get tight. However, some friends and work colleagues seem to have forgotten about you most of the time. When you do see them, they keep asking when are you coming back to work. Sometimes you have the distinct impression they think you are faking it a bit. At home, you start to feel a bit useless and not sure who you are. Not being in work suddenly does not sound so attractive, does it?

This chapter describes a community based vocational rehabilitation service for adults with an acquired brain injury (ABI). Much of the information will be more relevant for readers in the UK; however, readers from other countries should be able to take something from this chapter. For people with a serious disability after ABI, not working can become a huge and debilitating problem. On a personal level, it can have a huge impact on a person's self efficacy and self-confidence. At a sociological level, not working after ABI can fundamentally erode that person's sense of inclusion and participation in society.

Vocational rehabilitation: a philosophical, legislative, and organisational tour

Vocational rehabilitation (VR) is one approach that can facilitate inclusion and participation of disabled people in society, regardless of their disability. VR can take an active lead role in advocating the rights of disabled people by removing the physical and attitudinal barriers, and by promoting their abilities and the capacity they can offer in society.

Vocational rehabilitation: definitions and links with ABI

There is no single definition of VR in the UK (Department of Work & Pensions (DWP), 2004a). It is defined in different ways by the voluntary, private, and public sectors (DWP, 2004a), which results in a variation in the types of services provided within an individual's local area. There is a strong view that VR should be an integral part of the traditional rehabilitation process and not seen as an add-on (British Society of Rehabilitation Medicine (BRSM), 2000; BSRM & Royal College of Physicians (RCP), 2003). While national initiatives (DWP, 2003, 2006b; Job Centre Plus (JCP), 2006) are looking at addressing the work needs of disabled people, there is no specific focus on ABI. The UK's Department of Health has failed to act on recommendations to develop a service specifically for the needs of ABI (BSRM, 2000). Historically, this client group has been excluded, from both work initiatives and other services, because they do not meet the criteria of service provision, which tends to be categorised into learning disability, physical disability, and mental health. Often, due to the invisible nature and complexity of their deficits, some brain-injured clients become "lost" to health and social care (BSRM & RCP, 2003).

VR and the UK legislative and national context

The UK government's attempt to develop a national VR framework (DWP, 2004b) only served to highlight the huge variation in the provision of VR and did not translate into practical increases in resources or additional funding for service development (Beaumont, 2002). While the government has attempted to address the civil rights of disabled people by statute (*Disability Rights Act*, 1999, and subsequently *The Equalities Act*, 2010. See the Equality and Human Rights Commission website for current information, 2012), many of their policies are still based on the medical model (Drake, 2000). For example, disabled people are caught between having to "medically" prove their incapacity to work to enable them to claim financial benefits, thereby gaining some financial security, and yet, if they want to find paid employment, they have to prove their capacity to do the job with an emphasis on "medical fitness" (Howard, 2002). Despite this, there are governmental initiatives that do acknowledge the value of VR and demonstrate an increased awareness of the environmental and societal barriers that disabled people have to overcome to be able to achieve paid employment (Drake, 2000; DWP, 2003, 2006a,b; JCP, 2006). For example, the replacement of the sick note with a fit for work note reflects a change in the therapeutic value of work to promote recovery and rehabilitation (DWP, 2010).

The government's top-down approach has contributed to creating incentives for getting disabled people back to paid employment, but it does little to address the crucial role of the health service and rehabilitation in enabling disabled people to achieve this. Over the years, the "National Health Service (NHS) has largely lost the culture and skills to facilitate employment as a key element of effective health care" (BSRM, 2000). The emphasis is often more on discharge from hospital care and return to the home environment, rather than achieving optimal functional level of ability, which would encompass assisting people to return to their workplace or other alternative activity. This is largely due to lack of resources and time constraints imposed by management (Main & Haig, 2006). It is evident that there is a need for a bottom-up approach, for the health professionals to take the lead in recognising the value of work and their role in enabling people to return to work (Frank, 2002; Frank & Thurgood, 2006).

Not surprisingly, given the above, VR within the UK is poorly developed in comparison to the provision in America, Canada, Australia, and New Zealand. In each of those countries there are government funded vocational rehabilitation programmes and some health services have directives to focus on a return to work or social integration (Beaumont, 2002; BSRM & RCP, 2003; Disler & Pallant, 2001; Main & Haig, 2006). The number of UK studies is limited, and it could be argued that a review of the worldwide research does not provide robust evidence, since many of the studies use case study methodology. The major conclusion of a literature review by Brewin and Hazell (2004) was that there is no national standard for work practice in VR. Also, despite the strong evidence for the benefits of VR, the results are inconclusive in finding a direct link between employment outcome and the type of VR intervention (Blitz & Mechanic, 2006).

VR and the organisation of services

Unlike other disabilities, ABI can result in life-long effects that have an impact on an individual's ability to perform daily activities, and the additional serious neuropsychological constraints can make it difficult for a person to cope in a work environment (Kowalske, Plenger, Lusby, & Hayden, 2000) or be able to interact within social settings (see Chapter Four, by Jackson and Hague, in this volume). Consequently, the ABI client group can be low in volume with a high demand on resources due the complexity of their needs, which has a major implication for any service provision.

A typical community-based service could include any or all of the following professions:

- case manager;
- clinical neuropsychologist;
- clinical psychologist;
- occupational therapists;
- physiotherapists;
- rehabilitation assistants;
- speech and language therapists;
- vocational rehabilitation practitioner.

Community VR: a service example

Initial set up

In the North West of England, an ABI service was developed in 2001 to create an equitable community based service on a countywide basis, with collaborative commissioning. The service manager recognised the need for addressing the vocational needs of this ABI client group, who are predominantly males of working age, between the ages of eighteen and thirty-five years. An occupational therapist (OT) was selected for the VR practitioner role, due to the profession's capacity to explore the complex roles, to be able to understand the relationship between the medical condition, functional abilities, and psychosocial status (Davis & Rinaldi, 2004; Main & Haig, 2006; Stuckey, 1997).

Philosophy and conceptual frameworks

I would strongly argue that VR for ABI must encompass all the occupational aspects of an individual's life that have been affected by the ABI. It is important to understand what occupation (activity) means to the individual; the same occupation can have a different purpose and meaning for two people. Occupation is one factor that defines who a person is. The resultant effects from occupations, such as increased self-confidence, personal worth, structure to the day, and a sign of success, equate to the benefits of paid employment (Jahoda, 1979; Johansson & Tham, 2006; Kielhofner, 2002).

For occupation to be central within this VR service, the OT uses an occupational performance method. This approach promotes that the individual's optimal performance is achieved when the person, his environment, and his occupation fit harmoniously with each other (Kielhofner, 2002; Pratt & Jacobs, 1997; Strong et al., 1999). It embodies the principles of a client-centred practice and provides a framework for helping people with an ABI to successfully engage in personally meaningful activities (Fleming & Strong, 1997; Pratt & Jacobs, 1997). Within this framework, people with an ABI can be divided into three categories: those that wish to return to previous work, those who are vocationally ready and need assistance in vocational activities, and, finally, those for whom just engaging in meaningful activity is the primary goal.

It is essential that VR is an integral component of any community-based service for ABI. The principles, within this North West service, are based on client choice, initial and ongoing assessment, unlimited time frame, support for occupation and workplace activities. Also, in view of difficulties with sustainability and the risk of relapse, it is paramount that there is follow-up and ongoing monitoring (Brewin & Hazell, 2004; BSRM, 2000; Main & Haig, 2006).

Information gathering

The initial interview, which forms the foundations of the VR process, uses a narrative approach. This technique is chosen for its qualitative benefits, primarily allowing the individual to tell their story (Brewin & Hazell, 2004; Strong et al., 2004). The therapist gains an understanding of the individual's self-perception, how the individual views his disability and current level of function, and, more importantly, an understanding of the person the individual was before the ABI and who he or she is now. Formal information gathered ascertains the pre-morbid educational achievements, skills and employment history, current ability to self medicate, and any support needed to carry out everyday activities; these are all aspects that would impact current and future occupational performance.

Some typical things to ask initially are listed below.

- What difficulties do you experience?
- How has your life changed since your brain injury?
- What work have you done since leaving school?
- What did you like about work?
- Describe your daily routine.

It is a recognised skill of the therapist to use open-ended questions to identify the individual's level of self-efficacy, insight, and aspirations. Dependent on the individual's needs, this "interview" can be informal or formal, and take place over a number of sessions. This individualised approach is paramount to allow an opportunity for a rapport to develop between the individual and the therapist, progressing to a collaboration to set realistic and achievable goals (Frank & Thurgood, 2006; Innes, 1995).

Assessment

Assessment is a key component of VR, as well as being a continuation of the information gathering process (Kielhofner, 2002; Pratt & Jacobs, 1997). There are questions that need to be asked before using any assessments.

- What is the ultimate role and purpose of the assessment?
- What information is needed and what is the best method to gather that information?
- When and where is the appropriate time and place to conduct the assessment?

The assessment has a number of purposes within this VR provision: providing a baseline of an individual's level of ability, providing a basis for advice, and identifying areas of deficit and capacity. The assessment can be carried out using a structured or unstructured approach. Structured assessments are standardised tests that have a highly organised format with guidelines for administration, recording data, and scoring. They are guarded against bias and are specifically targeted to give detail on particular skills. To gain a baseline of an individual's general intellect, cognitive, behavioural, and emotional ability, the clinical neuropsychologist conducts a number of psychometric assessments (see Chapter Two, by Jones and co-authors, in this volume).

In contrast, unstructured assessments provide qualitative information on ability and can occur naturally, informally and spontaneously. It is an approach that is adaptable and flexible to the needs and ability of the individual. The main benefit of this approach is that it provides a measure of performance within a real-life context (Strong et al., 2004) and, hence, has robust ecological validity. To provide a level of reliability, the service has designed their own documentation to record behaviour and ability that is observed during these informal assessments. Although the results of unstructured assessments can complement the findings of standardised assessments, it can often be the case that an individual with ABI can perform contrary to the findings. An individual can do very well with pen and paper exercises that are highly structured and distraction free, but in a real-life context their overall performance is impaired (Kowalske, Plenger, Lusby, &

Hayden, 2000). In contrast, an individual can perform poorly in a test situation, but is able to function at a high level in everyday performance. This provides a strong argument for each client to be treated on an individual basis, and that there are benefits in using both approaches.

The selection and use of assessments is based on what contribution they can give to the VR process and clinical reasoning (Kielhofner, 2002). The OT uses a triangulation method of assessment with an emphasis on occupation. This includes the information gathered from the initial interview, the results of formal assessments, and observations of performance within environmental contexts. Standardised assessments selected for use have a functional basis, and unstructured assessments are observation of everyday skills within the individual's home environment and, more importantly, within their local community. For example, this can involve the individual's ability to cope within a coffee shop, which involves skills of orientation, selection process, decision making, calculation, and social skills.

Some standardised assessments are listed below.

- Chessington Occupational Therapy Neurological Assessment Battery (Tyerman, Tyerman, Howard, & Hadfield, 1987).
- Assessment of Motor and Process Skills (Fisher, 1995).
- Behavioural Assessment of Dysexecutive Syndrome (Wilson, Alderman, Burgess, & Evans, 1996).
- Test of Everyday Attention (Robertson, Ward, Ridgeway, & Nimmo-Smith, 1994).

The most significant element of any assessment is how the results are analysed, interpreted, and used within the VR process. On a formal basis, the results provide evidence of deficit and capacity, which can be used for a report whether that is for medical, insurance, or legal purposes. From an intervention perspective, it is the skill of the therapist to relay the outcome of any assessment in an understandable format for the individual and to relate this information to everyday function (Birkin & Meehan, 2004). This information can guide the discussion between the therapist and the individual, and be used to develop goals and a plan of action.

For a return to paid employment, the specific work-related assessment involves a job site evaluation and work analysis, to ascertain both workplace and job requirements. This can involve an ergonomic assessment and task analysis, looking at the actions and positioning required to carry out the job, such as equipment used, mobility, bending, carrying, pace, duration, and frequency of actions, cognitive skills, such as concentration, memory, decision making, and multi-tasking (Strong et al., 2004). These requirements are matched against the individual's level of ability and used to identify goals for the intervention programme which could be component based to improve a specific deficit, or to develop compensation strategies for areas of weakness (Royal College of Physicians, 2004). These can be progressed to functional or simulated tasks, or even job trials, to ascertain performance within a contextual environment. The overall aim is to retrain previous work skills, develop coping strategies, and build up work tolerance (Innes, 1995).

Examples of work requirements are:

- independent use of public transport;
- standing tolerance;
- ability to cope with variable shifts;
- recall of information;
- ability to make decisions
- judgement;
- ability to multi-task.

Vocational outcomes

Returning to work (RTW)

An RTW programme could commence with voluntary hours within the workplace or a voluntary work placement. The main advantage of this opportunity is to enable the individual to experience working in a more flexible manner without any work pressures. An RTW programme must include a planned, graded return with specified tasks, hours, and days, as well as planned reviews with both the individual and their employer to monitor and agree progress (Main & Haig, 2006). There is evidence to support the crucial role that this graded process has within the RTW programme, to ensure that it is managed and progressed according to the individual's level of ability (Main &

Haig, 2006). Also, job coaching is incorporated within this service to provide direct support within the work environment if it is required. It is invaluable to providing support for the individual within a real work environment and to maximise his/her vocational skills. A number of studies provide sound evidence of the benefits and effectiveness of such support within the workplace and to achieving successful employment outcomes (Bond, Becker, & Drake, 2001; Buffington & Malec, 1997; Davis & Rinaldi, 2004; Wall, Niemczura, & Rosenthal, 1998).

Education

Education is an important element of the RTW process; it enables the individual to gain insight into their difficulties, particularly in relation to their work environment. Also, it is essential for the individual's employer, manager, and colleagues to facilitate their understanding of the individual's disability and the need for any necessary adjustments within the workplace (Frank & Thurgood, 2006). This education, together with the timing of a return to work, is crucial to the overall process. If someone returns too soon, the individual can experience failure due to slow speed and fatigue. Also, the individual might not be able to sustain their initial level of ability due to the prolonged effect of being in work or cognitive overload (Powell, Heslin, & Greenwood, 2002). Consequently, any difficulties might not arise for months. Any lack of success can result in an impact on the overall VR process. Alternatively, a delay in addressing the work issue, time appropriate, can result in the individual experiencing anxiety or depression and developing the cycle of hopelessness.

The overall aim is to avoid any misperceptions of the individual's level of ability. Often an assumption is made that if a disability cannot be seen, it does not exist, and a prediction can be made that the person has made a good recovery. A cognitive impairment is not as visible, obvious, or as easily recognised as a physical or behavioural impairment. The positive consequence of this, for the individual, is that he or she is readily accepted; the negative effect is that there is a lack of understanding of why he or she behaves or responds in a certain way (Kielhofner, 2002). The fact that the difficulties of ABI are often hidden and the individual can look normal means that their disability is often not understood. Therefore, both the individual and their colleagues can have raised expectations of the individual's ability.

Collaborative working

Any return to paid employment usually involves collaborative working between a number of people. These include: the individual, therapist, employer, personnel, occupational health, and benefits agency. Communication is an important element of the therapist's role. You will need to negotiate with employers for modifications within the workplace and facilitate access to available resources. One example is Access to Work, which is a government scheme to provide help to people whose disability is affecting the way they are able to do their job. You are likely to need to liaise with the general practitioner or consultant to gain their support for the individual to return to the work environment. This can be a major hurdle to overcome, particularly in a culture where the medical profession is expected to continue to be the gatekeeper for sanctioning whether the individual can access services, including health, transport, and benefits. Also, more importantly, you might need to liaise with the benefits agency, within which the decision makers can often lack understanding of the needs of someone suffering from an ABI, or the cognitive and psychological deficits of ABI. This is an important area to ensure that the individual has financial security during the VR process.

Returning to alternative employment

For those not able to return to their previous employment, but who are assessed as capable to look at alternative employment, the therapist's role is to facilitate the individual in accessing services for career guidance or other vocational opportunities through Jobcentre Plus, for example, the Disabled Employment Adviser, or Looking for Work Schemes.

Meaningful occupation

There are a number of different reasons why an individual is not able to return to work; they might lack the capacity to work, their employment contract has terminated, or they are retired on ill health grounds. The national statistics and research studies identify that a proportion of people with ABI, due to their level of disability, will not be able to achieve paid employment, even with a change of role or work conditions (Brewin & Hazell, 2004; BSRM & RCP, 2003; Main & Haig, 2006).

For these, the emphasis of intervention is on occupation in the broader context and involves exploring other occupations and opportunities (RCP, 2004). This can be in the form of developing a structured routine at home, being able to have choices, gain some control over their life, have access to available community and leisure activities, educational opportunities, or voluntary work. This is an important aspect of VR for ABI. Following ABI, the individual experiences a number of losses and a wide range of long-term restrictions: in their ability to live independently, to drive or use public transport, to participate in leisure or social activities, possible changes to their family role or relationships, and loss of employment (BSRM & RCP, 2003; Coetzer, Hayes, & Du Toit, 2002).

Studies have indicated that the negative impact of these losses on the individual, and specifically not being in employment, can be loss of self-esteem, apathy, isolation, frustration, and can lead to depression and other emotional difficulties (Coetzer, Carroll, & Ruddle, 2011; Davis & Rinaldi, 2004; Jahoda, 1979; Thomas, 2004). This further reinforces the importance of the therapist's role in facilitating and empowering the individual to rebuild a purposeful satisfying life and to come to terms with his or her limitations. As recognised by studies (Barnes & Mercer, 2005), there is strong evidence of the cumulative effect of success in increasing an individual's self esteem, self-confidence, and self-belief to be able to achieve (Bandura, 1995). This provides a robust argument for the influence that social integration and participation, including vocationally, has on the individual's quality of life, which can lead to overall positive effects and reduce the life-long health needs.

Reintegration

Reintegration into previous lifestyle for the individual is an important goal of their rehabilitation and an indication of their recovery following their ABI (Brewin & Hazell, 2004; Davis & Rinaldi, 2004; Johansson & Bernspang, 2001; Kowalske, Plenger, Lusby, & Hayden, 2000; Main & Haig, 2006; Roberts, Coetzer, & Blackwell, 2004). However, this level of reintegration is complicated by the diverse range of cognitive, behavioural, emotional, physical, and social interaction difficulties (Brewin & Hazell, 2004). For the individual with an ABI, an RTW is seen as "tangible evidence of progress and achievement" (Japp, 2005) with high face validity. On a personal level, a number of clients have indicated that being able to resume previous activities, or level of ability, is a sign that life is returning to normal. From a service provider's perspective, the challenge for this VR provision is to be able to provide evidence that the service is achieving results, but the ultimate question to be asked is whether the outcome expected by the commissioning bodies is the same as that desired by the ABI clients.

Meaningful outcomes

Much of the research focuses on an RTW as an outcome measure without considering the changing role in what work means to the individual or the different levels of disability that can occur. There is a change in life priorities for the individual and a re-evaluation of work. The adjustments that have been made to the job can make it less enjoyable and too effortful for the rewards gained (Johansson & Tham, 2006). Although the research provides evidence that individuals with ABI achieve employment (Buffington & Malec, 1997; Coetzer, Hayes, & Du Toit, 2002; Johansson & Bernspang, 2001; Kowalske, Plenger, Lusby, & Hayden, 2000; Wall, Niemczura, & Rosenthal, 1998), the studies are limited to looking at sustainability following ABI (Brewin & Hazell, 2004; Powell, Heslin, & Greenwood, 2002). The study by Coetzer, Hayes, and Du Toit (2002), which looked at the long-term implications of employment, suggests that there are significant changes to be found in employment status after two years following ABI. It is my view that while an RTW can be a key factor in evaluating the effectiveness of achieving paid employment within the VR process, it is limited as an outcome measure because it eliminates the influence of environment on psychosocial and cognitive function, which has major implications for ABI (Kowalske, Plenger, Lusby, & Hayden, 2000). It is of interest to note that while the External Reference Group for the National Framework for Long-term Conditions does acknowledge the need to recommend outcome measures, none is identified (Department of Health, 2008).

A majority of the national public and private VR services provided within the UK are target led with a selection criterion and time limited constraints on the service provision. In many cases, a successful RTW is the outcome measure used by these services (Main & Haig, 2006). It is evident from the literature that with no clear indicators for selection of an appropriate tool there is an *ad hoc* use of measures. The development of an outcome measure, within a community based brain injury setting, would benefit not only clients, but also clinicians and service provision. A national implementation of a single measure would strengthen the ABI rehabilitation evidence base. For a community-based provision, such as this North West team, which provides a service for clients of all levels of ability and uses the individual's local community resources, it is more relevant to consider the level of achievement and engagement.

There is a need to take into account the different stages at which an individual recovers from his or her ABI, is able to engage with the process, and the impact of external influences. Due to the wide range of diverse deficits, which require a range of different types of interventions, there is no single outcome measure that could be expected to cover the full range of vocational restrictions or potential after brain injury (Tyerman, 1999, cited in RCP, 2004; Turner-Stokes, 2002). For such a client group, the service needs to be proactive as well as reactive (Tyerman, 1999, cited in RCP, 2004) to the needs of the clients. A prescriptive service would not be appropriate (Johansson & Bernspang, 2001). This is strongly supported by my experience of providing VR within this North West service. The client outcomes have demonstrated that the VR process needs to be highly individualised in intensity, duration, and forms of therapy to be able to meet the needs of the individual, reflecting the diversity of impairments and psychosocial problems (Powell, Heslin, & Greenwood, 2002).

It would be beneficial for this understaffed vocational rehabilitation service, which has established a strong network with the relevant agencies, and is working within the constraints of the current NHS reconfiguration, to use a number of outcome measures for the varying components of the service provision. The major drawback would be that it does not provide a robust quantitative evidence base and is not conducive to demonstrating the direct cost effectiveness of the overall service. However, the stronger argument for this approach would be that it addresses the individual's capacity, performance, and self-perception, and meets the needs of the individual in relation to his or her life: education, work, quality of life, housing, and transport.

Conclusions

A client with an ABI experiences a transition from their pre-injury "old self" to an emerging, different person who is a combination of their "old and new self" (McGrath, 2004). In the current political and economic climate, where there is increasing pressure for people of working age to return to work, survivors of a brain injury feel they are being judged by others, particularly the general public, due to the lack of understanding and the misconceptions that they often have about brain injury. This is often the result of the "invisible" nature of the complex impairments associated with ABI, resulting, for many persons, in significant disability.

In conclusion, the evaluation of the development and implementation of this VR provision, within a community based ABI service, has highlighted that the ultimate goal is to facilitate the individual's quality of life and level of engagement within his or her local community post-ABI, to maximise the level of recovery, minimise the adverse outcome of the brain injury, and to promote overall health with access to medical and non-medical services (Disler & Pallant, 2001; Frank & Thurgood, 2006; Langlois, Rutland-Brown, & Wald, 2006). While the individual's quality of life is, of course, the main focus, ultimately these VR initiatives also, by default, serve the wider function of reducing the burden on society.

Useful resources

Volunteer Bureaus (2012). I want to volunteer: Where do I start webpage: www.volunteering.org.uk/iwanttovolunteer/where-do-i-start?q=ch2. Accessed 29 May 2012.
Disabled Employment Adviser. Please contact your local Job Centre.
Learning Support at Further Education College.
Healthy Living Centres.
Libraries.
Directgov (2012). Access to work: Practical help at work webpage: www.direct.gov.uk/en/DisabledPeople/Employmentsupport/WorkSchemesAndProgrammes/DG_4000347. Accessed 29 May 2012.

References

Bandura, A. (1995). *Self-Efficacy in Changing Societies*. Cambridge: Cambridge University Press.

Barnes, C., & Mercer, G. (2005). Disability, work, and welfare: challenging the social exclusion of disabled people. *Work, Employment and Society*, 19(3): 527–545.

Beaumont, D. (2002). Rehabilitation and retention in the workplace. The interaction between GPs and occupational health professionals. A consensus statement. *Rehabilitation Network*, 64: 11–22.

Birkin, R., & Meehan, M. (2004). Talk, walk or drive with employment assessment? Thanks for the Obee–Snodgrass jump start. *Journal of Occupational Psychology, Employment and Disability*, 6(1): 3–6.

Blitz, L., & Mechanic, D. (2006). Facilitators and barriers to employment among individuals with psychiatric disabilities: a job coach perspective. *Work*, 26: 407–419.

Bond, G. R., Becker, D. R., & Drake, R. E. (2001). Implementing supported employment. *Psychiatric Services*, 52: 313–312.

Brewin, J., & Hazell, A. (2004). How successful are we at getting our clients back to work? The results of an audit. *British Journal of Occupational Therapy*, 67(4): 148–152.

British Society of Rehabilitation Medicine (2000). *Vocational Rehabilitation: The Way Forward. Executive Summary of a Working Party Report*. London: Lavenham Press.

British Society of Rehabilitation Medicine & Royal College of Physicians (2003). *Rehabilitation Following Acquired Brain Injury: National Clinical Guidelines*. London: Lavenham Press.

Buffington, A., & Malec, J. (1997). The vocational rehabilitation continuum: maximizing outcomes through bridging the gap from hospital to community-based services. *Journal of Head Trauma Rehabilitation*, 12(5): 1–13.

Coetzer, R., Carroll, E., & Ruddle, J. (2011). Depression, anxiety and employment status after traumatic brain injury. *Social Care & Neurodisability*, 2(4): 200–208.

Coetzer, R., Hayes, N., & Du Toit, P. (2002). Long-term employment outcomes in a rural area following traumatic brain injury. *Australian Journal of Rural Health*, 10(4): 229–232.

Davis, M., & Rinaldi, M. (2004). Using an evidence-based approach to enable people with mental health problems to gain and retain employment, education and voluntary work. *British Journal of Occupational Therapy*, 67(7): 319–322.

Department of Health (2008). *The National Service Framework for: Long-term Neurological Conditions: National Support for Local Implementation.* Electronic version: www.dh.gov.uk/prod_consum_dh/groups/dh_digitalassets/@dh/@en/documents/digitalasset/dh_084580.pdf. Accessed 29 May 2012.

Department of Work and Pensions (2003). *Pathways to Work: Helping People into Employment.* London: The Stationery Office.

Department of Work and Pensions (2004a). *Developing a Framework for Vocational Rehabilitation: A Discussion Paper.* London: The Stationery Office.

Department of Work and Pensions (2004b). *Building Capacity for Work: A UK Framework for Vocational Rehabilitation.* London: The Stationery Office.

Department of Work and Pensions (2006a). *A New Deal for Welfare: Empowering People to Work.* London: The Stationery Office.

Department of Work and Pensions (2006b). *Impacts of the Job Retention & Rehabilitation Pilot.* London: The Stationery Office.

Department of Work and Pensions (2010). *Statement of Fitness for Work, A Guide for General Practitioners and Other Doctor*s. London: The Stationery Office.

Disability Rights Commission (1999). *The Disability Rights Act.* London: The Stationery Office.

Disler, P., & Pallant, J. (2001). Vocational rehabilitation: everybody gains if injured workers are helped back into work. *British Medical Journal, 323*(7): 121–123.

Drake, R. (2000). Disabled people, New Labour, benefits and work. *Critical Social Policy, 20*(4): 421–439.

Equality and Human Rights Commission (2012). Homepage: www.equalityhumanrights.com. Accessed 29 May 2012.

Fisher, A. G. (1995). *Assessment of Motor and Process Skills.* Fort Collins, CO: Three Star Press.

Fleming, J. M., & Strong, J. (1997). The development of insight following severe traumatic brain injury: three case studies. *British Journal of Occupational Therapy, 60*(7): 295–300.

Frank, A. (2002). Vocational rehabilitation: helping those with illness or disability remain in, or enter work: a challenge for the NHS. *Rehabilitation Network, 64*: 11–22.

Frank, A., & Thurgood, J. (2006). Vocational rehabilitation in the UK: opportunities for health-care professionals. *International Journal of Therapy & Rehabilitation, 13*(3): 126–134.

Government Equalities Office (2010). *Equality Act*. London: Government Equalities Office.

Howard, M. (2002). An "interactionist" approach to disability. Processes and barriers that exclude disabled people from work. *Rehabilitation Network*, 64: 6–10.

Innes, E. (1995). Workplace-based occupational rehabilitation in New South Wales, Australia. *WORK: A Journal of Prevention, Assessment & Rehabilitation*, 5: 147–152.

Jahoda, M. (1979). The impact of unemployment in the 1930s and the 1970s. *Bulletin of the British Psychological Society*, 3: 309–314.

Japp, J. (2005). *Brain Injury and Returning to Employment: A Guide for Practitioners*. London: Jessica Kingsley.

Job Centre Plus (2006). Condition management web page: www.jobcentreplus.gov.uk. Accessed on 5th January 2011.

Johansson, U., & Bernspang, B. (2001). Predicting return to work after brain injury using occupational therapy assessments. *Disability & Rehabilitation*, 23(11): 474–480.

Johansson, U., & Tham, K. (2006). The meaning of work after acquired brain injury. *American Journal of Occupational Therapy*, 60(1): 60–69.

Kielhofner, G. (2002). *Model of Human Occupation*. Baltimore, MD: Lippincott Williams & Wilkins.

Kowalske, K., Plenger, P., Lusby, B., & Hayden, M. (2000). Vocational re-entry following TBI: an enablement model. *Journal of Head Trauma Rehabilitation*, 15(4): 989–999.

Langlois, J. A., Rutland-Brown, W., & Wald, M. M. (2006). The epidemiology and impact of traumatic brain injury. *Journal of Head Trauma Rehabilitation*, 21(5): 375–378.

Main, L., & Haig, J. (2006). Occupational therapy and vocational rehabilitation: an audit of an outpatient occupational therapy service. *British Journal of Occupational Therapy*, 69(6): 288–292.

McGrath, J. (2004). Beyond restoration to transformation: positive outcomes in the rehabilitation of acquired brain injury. *Clinical Rehabilitation*, 18: 767–775.

Powell, J., Heslin, J., & Greenwood, R. (2002). Community based rehabilitation after severe traumatic brain injury: a randomised controlled trial. *Journal of Neurology, Neurosurgery & Psychiatry*, 72: 193–202.

Pratt, J., & Jacobs, K. (1997). *Work Practice: International Perspectives*. Oxford: Butterworth-Heinemann.

Roberts, C., Coetzer, R., & Blackwell, H.C. (2004). Is performance on the Wechsler Abbreviated Scale of Intelligence associated with employment outcome following brain injury? *International Journal of Rehabilitation Research*, 27: 145–147.

Robertson, I. H., Ward, T., Ridgeway, V., & Nimmo-Smith, I. (1994). *The Test of Everyday Attention – Manual*. London: Pearson Assessment, The Psychological Corporation.

Royal College of Physicians (2004). *Vocational Assessment and Rehabilitation after Acquired Brain Injury: Inter-agency Guidelines*. London: Lavenham Press.

Strong, S., Baptiste, S., Cole, D., Clarke, J., Marcos, C., Shannon, H., Reardon, R., & Sinclair, S. (2004). Functional assessment of injured workers: a profile of assessor practices. *Canadian Journal of Occupational Therapy*, 71(1): 13–23.

Strong, S., Ridby, P., Stewart, D., Law, M., Letts, L., & Cooper, B. (1999). Application of the person–environment–occupation model: a practical tool. *Canadian Journal of Occupational Therapy*, 66(3): 122–133.

Stuckey, R. (1997). Enhancing work performance in industrial settings. *British Journal of Occupational Therapy*, 60(6): 277–278.

Thomas, M. (2004). The potential unlimited programme: an outdoor experiential education and group work approach that facilitates adjustment to brain injury. *Brain Injury*, 18(12): 1271–1286.

Turner-Stokes, L. (2002). Standardized outcome assessment in brain injury rehabilitation for younger adults. *Disability & Rehabilitation*, 24(7): 383–389.

Tyerman, R., Tyerman, A., Howard, P., & Hadfield, C. (1987). *The Chessington O.T. Neurological Assessment Battery*. Ashby de la Zouch: Nottingham Rehabilitation Supplies.

Wall, J., Niemczura, J., & Rosenthal, M. (1998). Community-based training & employment: an effective programme for persons with traumatic brain injury. *NeuroRehabilitation: An Interdisciplinary Journal*, 10: 39–49.

Wilson, B. A., Alderman, N., Burgess, P. W., Emslie, H., & Evans J. J. (1996). *Behavioural Assessment of the Dysexecutive Syndrome*. London: Pearson Assessment, The Psychological Corporation.

CHAPTER NINE

Opportunistic group work: service-based and community support group examples

Stephen Weatherhead, Bernie Walsh, Phillippa Calvert, and Gavin Newby

Group therapy can be useful in neuro-rehabilitation as a way to spread resources further, normalise experiences, develop support systems, and include systemic networks (Bowen, et al., 2009). It can also benefit other forms of clinical work, by providing a flexible environment in which to get to know clients, and be a privileged witness to their rich narratives, all of which can take place in a setting that is often more relaxed than formal neuro-rehabilitative environments.

Examples from residential brain injury services have provided evidence of the usefulness of group-based interventions in improving, among other things, family relationships (Kreutzer, Kolakowsky-Hayner, Demm, & Meade, 2002) and self-concept post-injury (Vickery, Gontkovsky, Wallace, & Jerome, 2006). Unfortunately, community-based brain injury services often face logistical challenges in facilitating such groups, as the services are often under-staffed and under-resourced. Attendance, participation, and functional gain from the groups can also be limited, due to individuals' cognitive and practical challenges (Bowen et al., 2009; Coetzer, 2007).

The Acquired Brain Injury Service based in Chester is a small community team consisting of a service manager, a specialist occupational therapist, a consultant clinical neuropsychologist, clinical psychologist, and a part-time administrator. Trainee clinical psychologists and volunteers also contribute to the service. The service regularly facilitates group therapeutic interventions, such as an epilepsy support group, informal group coffee mornings for service users and their families, a parenting group for fathers who have experienced an ABI (Weatherhead & Newby, 2008), and a narrative therapy group for men who have experienced an ABI (Weatherhead & Newby, 2011).

Two examples of successful groups are discussed below: the first is a group for the mothers of adult survivors of a brain injury, and the second is a support group for people with an ABI, which has now achieved charitable status. The consistent feature between them is that (in line with most groups at the original South Cheshire ABI service) they were developed in response to the needs of the service users at the time. Furthermore, both examples show that when group work is effective, it can provide camaraderie, social support, and help to build momentum in recovery by breaking down professional stereotypes and creating a space for clients with ABI to discover possibilities (rather than problems), and possibly more positive aspects about themselves, others, and their situation (Steffen, 1997).

Supporting mothers whose son/daughter has sustained a brain injury as an adult

Published literature has tended to focus on the experiences of parents in relation to children with an ABI. In contrast, the experiences of parents whose child sustained a brain injury as an older teenager or adult have largely been ignored. Yet, from clinical experience, the issues reported in the literature in relation to younger children with an ABI would appear to be highly relevant to an older cohort. Parents are said to experience an ongoing grieving process, as the object of their grief is still alive but changed, yet this is rarely acknowledged by society (Collings, 2008). This type of grief is often referred to as ambiguous loss (Boss, 1999), as the injured person is lost but still present, and so the grief, unlike bereavement, defies closure. This type of grief tends to have two components.

1. Loss for the child: this includes the change in the developmental projection for the child, such as hopes and dreams the parent held.
2. Loss for self: this focuses on the changes the child's ABI brings about for the parent, including less freedom and independence as well as a loss of mastery and control.

Research on how parents of disabled children (defined broadly and including physical and developmental disorders) cope suggests coping strategies fall into three groups: (1) problem orientated; (2) perception orientated, and (3) emotion orientated (see Benn & McColl, 2004 for a brief ABI-related review and Table 9.1 for details of the coping styles of parents who have an ABI child).

Benn and McColl (2004) reported that mothers have a tendency to have a larger repertoire of coping strategies that also tend to complement the fathers' strategies if the couple are still together. The process of coping for mothers involves adapting to their changed

Table 9.1. Coping styles of parents with an ABI child.

Type of coping	General examples of coping style	Specific examples of coping style statements reported by parents of children with ABI (from Benn & McColl, 2004)
Problem orientated	Try to change or eliminate causes of stress with new information and skills	Changing how things are done, redoubling efforts, coming up with a number of practical solutions
Perception orientated	Try to change how they think about the causes of stress	Thinking what's important in life, reminding self how much worse things could be, looking for silver linings, preparing for the worst
Emotion orientated	Try to manage the emotions that accompany the stressors	Expressing anger, letting feelings out, avoiding being with people

roles, needing to rebuild relationships, and receiving support from immediate family and specialist services (Clark, Stedmon, & Margison, 2008).

Our group for mothers was developed and facilitated by a trainee clinical psychologist (PC), and a clinical psychologist (SW). The mothers who attended either lived with their injured adult child and were their primary carer, or were heavily involved in the care. The group was particularly heterogeneous, as were the demographics of the injured children. The brain injury onset of the "index clients" ranged from 1–17 years from the start of the group. As they were not clients of the service, precise demographics were not collected, but the mothers' ages approximately ranged from 50–70 years and their known demographics are shown below.

Mother 1. Runs a small business, and lives with her son, who was in his early twenties at the time of the accident. Her son sustained an ABI approximately one year ago.
Mother 2. Describes self as a housewife, and lives with her daughter, who was in her mid-teens at the time of the accident. Her daughter sustained an ABI approximately three years ago.
Mother 3. Retired, and does not currently live with her son, who is in his early thirties. Her son sustained an ABI as an infant over twenty years ago.
Mother 4. A healthcare professional, who lives with her daughter, who was in her mid-teens at the time of the accident. Her daughter sustained an ABI approximately three years ago.
Mother 5. Retired, and lives with her son, who is in his early thirties. Her son sustained an ABI in his mid-teens.

The group had a narrative therapy orientation, and each session aimed to build on the previous session and identify the mother's narratives of their experiences of parenting an adult child with a brain injury, being a parent, and their reflections on their own experiences and stories. The later sessions aimed to help the mothers notice and develop an alternative narrative focusing on a more affirmative description of these three areas.

The group was facilitated over six sessions on a weekly basis, taking place in the evening to maximise attendance. A range of interactive approaches were used, including group and one-to-one discussions, art-based tasks, and home tasks aimed at reinforcing the session content, or preparing for the next session. Specific areas for exploration during the group included:

- understanding brain injury;
- hopes and expectations;
- who am I (as a person and as a parent);
- successes;
- life before and after the injury;
- looking after oneself;
- values, beliefs, attitudes, and experiences;
- the future.

Each group member completed three questionnaires at the beginning and end of the six sessions:

- Hospital Anxiety and Depression Scale (HADS) (Zigmond & Snaith, 1983)
- Family Head Injury Semantic Differential Scale (cited in Tyerman & King, 2004)
- Parenting Locus of Control (PLOC) (Campis, Lyman, & Prentice-Dunn, 1986)

These questionnaires aimed to assess the mothers' current levels of intrapersonal psychological distress and interpersonal experiences, as both an individual and as a parent.

As a whole, the questionnaire scores suggested a modest improvement in the group members' sense of wellbeing, both intra- and interpersonally. The total HADS scores for anxiety and depression, and individual semantic differential items, for all but one group member, indicated a modest reduction in psychological distress levels. The total PLOC scores were less consistent. Half of the group moved towards a more internal locus of control (LoC), and the other half's scores indicated a shift towards an external LoC. However, each score must be considered in the context of where they each initially saw the LoC as being situated. Overall, the scores suggested a tendency to have a more balanced locus of control after the group; that is, moving towards the midpoint between internal and external.

The participants themselves highlighted that these questionnaires were only "snapshots". During the initial session, all the mothers present stated that they were not seeking help for themselves. Instead, they reported that they were attending the group to either help other mothers by sharing their experiences, or to learn about how they could best support their child. However, interestingly, by the end of the group, all the mothers agreed that they had continued to attend because they themselves had gained from experience. They reported enjoying having a space to talk and explore their experiences, with the most important element being the opportunity to meet with other women who had been through similar experiences. They believed that the other members would immediately understand their perspectives without judging them. For many, it had been the first opportunity to talk about how having an adult child with an ABI had affected their lives. There was acknowledgement of the difficulty in reliving some of the experiences and the painful emotions associated with them, but that this had been worthwhile. Importantly, all the group members said that they would recommend the group to other mums.

Community support group

The ABI service was all too aware of the lack of a support group in the area that would provide a forum for people with ABI to be able to share experiences, improve their coping skills, not feel alone, and to make connections in a non-judgemental environment. As such, staff members of the service worked closely with service users, their families, and other organisations to facilitate the development of a support group for people with an ABI in Cheshire, and, in 2007, the support group Head Injured People in Cheshire (HIP in Cheshire) was established. The group's primary aim was to: "provide a means for the carers of, and survivors of, a brain injury who live in Cheshire to have social interaction and support" (HIP, 2012).

The Trust's board and the Committee consisted of both people with ABI and professionals who had an interest in promoting services to meet the needs of those living with a brain injury. A guiding principle of HIP was that the meetings were (and still are) intended to be a social event for people to meet and share experiences, rather than having an educative focus. This is reflected in its running; committee members are not required to have experience in management or related areas to be elected, although many do have relevant skills. The support group is a non-profit organisation that depends on monies from fundraising events or sponsorship from local companies. Monies are used to hire halls for events or to subsidise transport costs to events.

During the initial years after the group was formed, three or four annual regional events were held. These were primarily meetings in local centres or village halls and picnics in the park. The emphasis of these events was on provision of an opportunity for members and their families to meet others with an ABI in a relaxed, familiar environment using local areas of interest and community resources. Due to transport issues, these events took place at different locations around the county to enable different members to attend (consideration of accessibility, car parking, toilets, and cost were all important). However, due to the geographical and transport constraints of the Cheshire area, it was found that only a small number of people were able to attend these events.

Therefore, four local satellite groups were organised to run on a monthly basis in the main towns within the county. Meetings of these local groups were typically held in coffee shops, chosen primarily for their location and access. These local group meetings enabled members to get to know others from their area, the locations for the meetings were more familiar, and they provided opportunity for members to form friendships. In view of some members' memory difficulties, it was found that it was beneficial for members to receive a simple reminder about the group meeting either by telephone, text message, or email. Also, each local group meeting took place on a specific day each month (e.g., always the first Tuesday of each month). In addition to these local meetings, the county-wide HIP-Cheshire group continued with one annual regional meeting.

The Trustees and Committee members have been in post since the support group was established, which resulted in events being organised by the same small number of people. The Trustees and Committee were all too aware of the need for new people to be involved, at both the local and county levels, to share the load and to facilitate new ideas. One new development was to encourage members of the more local support groups to attend the HIP committee meetings as observers, with the opportunity to be supported to take on a designated role, such as chairperson, secretary, and treasurer. Also, a future progression for the support group is to develop the role of designated volunteers for the local groups to assist with organising other events, to provide additional support for members, and to help address transport issues. It is hoped that by developing the local groups, with progress, this will lead to further developments for the regional events.

Conclusions

These are just two examples of how groups for service users and their families have been developed within a busy community ABI service; we hope there may be other examples of such work occurring across other ABI services. Whether you wish to consider this approach to group working as organic, opportunistic, or responsive, it clearly demonstrates that it is possible for services to meet the changing needs of the people who access them if the service is willing to be responsive and flexible in how it works with clients. However, it can be difficult to offer such a dynamic approach, especially in small teams where resources are stretched, but well worth the effort, and is a good way to reach more people with a single intervention (a point not lost in an economically demanding environment).

Therapeutic groups such as these need to be flexible and client centred. Ownership of the group is a key feature in their success. Once the HIP group was running regularly, the ABI service staff were able to step back a little, attending occasionally, but still being available for support if required. Where groups such as these can be offered, there is the immediate impact of providing a support network, and some structure to what is often a disjointed, confusing life post-ABI. In the long term, as has been shown with HIP, such groups can become self-motivated and self-sustaining, particularly in the digital age of social networks, blogs, and emails.

Essentially, this form of working in ABI settings presents an opportunity for individuals to gain more control over their rehabilitation, feel understood by others, and, perhaps most importantly, increase their confidence and develop a more rounded perspective of their own and others' shared experiences.

References

Benn, K. M., & McColl, M. A. (2004). Parental coping following childhood acquired brain injury. *Brain Injury*, *18*(3): 239–255.

Boss, P. (1999). *Ambiguous Loss: Learning to Live with Unresolved Grief.* Boston, MA: Harvard University Press.

Bowen, C., Hall, T., Newby, G., Walsh, B., Weatherhead, S., & Yeates, G. (2009). The impact of brain injury on relationships across the lifespan and across school, family and work contexts. *Human Systems: The Journal of Therapy, Consultation and Training*, 20(1): 65–81.

Campis, L. K., Lyman, R. D., & Prentice-Dunn, S. (1986). The Parental Locus of Control Scale: development and validation. *Journal of Clinical Child Psychology*, 15(3): 260–267.

Clark, A., Stedmon, J., & Margison, S. (2008). An exploration of mothers whose children sustain traumatic brain injury (TBI) and their families. *Clinical Child Psychology and Psychiatry*, 13(4): 565–583.

Coetzer, R. (2007). Psychotherapy following traumatic brain injury: integrating theory and practice. *Journal of Head Trauma Rehabilitation*, 22(1): 39–47.

Collings, C. (2008). That's not my child anymore! Parental grief after acquired brain injury (ABI): incidence, nature and longevity. *British Journal of Social Work*, 38(8): 1499–1517.

Head Injured People in Cheshire (2012). Web homepage: https://sites.google.com/site/wwwhipincheshire/ Accessed 12 December 2012.

Kreutzer, J. S., Kolakowsky-Hayner, S. A., Demm, S. R., & Meade, M. A. (2002). A structured approach to family intervention after brain injury. *Journal of Head Trauma Rehabilitation*, 17(4): 349–367.

Steffen, V. (1997). Life stories and shared experience. *Social Sciences & Medicine*, 45(1): 99–111.

Tyerman, A., & King, N. S. (2004). Interventions for psychological problems after brain injury. In: L. H. Goldstein & I. E. McNeil (Eds.), *Clinical Neuropsychology: A Practical Guide to Assessment for Clinicians* (pp. 385–404). Chichester: John Wiley.

Vickery, C. D., Gontkovsky, S. T., Wallace, J. J., & Jerome, J. S. (2006). Group psychotherapy focusing on self-concept change following acquired brain injury: a pilot investigation. *Rehabilitation Psychology*, 51(1): 30–35.

Weatherhead, S., & Newby, G. (2008). Supporting dads: a parenting programme for fathers with an acquired brain injury. *Clinical Psychology Forum*, 182: 36–39.

Weatherhead, S. J., & Newby, G. J. (2011). The warehouse of responsibilities: a group for survivors of a brain injury. Institute of Narrative Therapy: Papers & Resources, Web-based article: www.theinstituteofnarrativetherapy.com/Papers%20and%20resources.html. Accessed 29 May 2012.

Zigmond, A. S., & Snaith, R. P. (1983). The Hospital Anxiety and Depression Scale. *Acta Psychiatrica Scandinavica*, 67: 361–370.

CHAPTER TEN

The use of emails and texts in psychological therapy after acquired brain injury*

Gavin Newby and Rudi Coetzer

Introduction

The huge explosion in the use of both email and SMS mobile phone texting over the past ten years has made electronic communication almost universally accessible. For young and old, rich and poor, electronic communication is a massive presence in almost all of our lives. It is a medium that allows for information transfer at any hour of the day, three hundred and sixty-five days a year. Excitingly, it is also a medium that can allow us to express ourselves in informal and personally meaningful ways and then reflect on what we have said and how we have said it. It also then follows that the receivers of our communication will do the same and, potentially, a whole process of construction and co-construction about meanings and thoughts is born. As such, emails and texts can offer clients, families, and the services that work with them

---

* This chapter is adapted from a conference presentation by Gavin Newby at the World Congress of Neuro-technology in October 2010.

opportunities to both maximise the understanding and retention of information and also provide ways in which very personally meaningful insights can be created and hard wired.

In recent times, social networking media, such as Facebook and Twitter, have also become important forms of electronic communication. Through the ability to create cohesive networks and a space to have opinions heard and valued, these media could have great potential in helping people with an ABI feel less isolated and increase their sense of self-belonging to a community. However, to date, this has been relatively unexplored within the ABI literature and is not considered in detail here. Of interest, a recent US online survey of ninety-six clients with an ABI, by Tsaousides, Matsuzawa, and Lebowitz (2011), reported that 60% regularly used Facebook. Seventy per cent of the non-users reported that they would use it if they were more knowledgeable. There is, of course, a literature describing the effectiveness of telephone-based psychotherapy (e.g., follow-up cognitive–behaviour therapy for clients with acquired brain injury (Bradbury et al., 2008) and multiple sclerosis (Beckner, Howard, Vella, & Mohr, 2010)) and, more recently, Skype[1] (e.g., Dobson, 2010, and *Therapy Today*, 2011, which describes a national network of UK-based professional counsellors who offer face-to-face counselling via Skype). Again, these therapeutic modes are not considered further in this chapter, although interested clinicians might want to consider their use.

In the following discussion, we hope the reader will feel reassured by research and service examples of the use of emails and texts in prompting and reminding our clients. We like to think of this as the "traditional" use of emails and texts. However, we also feel that there is an exciting, but, as yet, relatively unexplored role for emailing and texting in the process of psychotherapy. It is our contention that electronic messaging has huge potential not only to remind clients about what has happened in a therapeutic session, but also to allow therapists and clients to construct and reconstruct new and alternative meanings and insights. In particular, we suggest that electronic messaging can enhance each of the five stages of psychotherapy described by Orlinsky and Howard's generic model of psychotherapy (1986, 1995).

Electronic communication is normal and could be a communication standard

As stated above, electronic communication is present in all of our lives almost all of the time. One of the challenges for neuropsychological rehabilitation in the long term is not only to introduce clients to strategies that help, but also to introduce strategies that they are not embarrassed to use, can use regularly, and will continue to use. As many readers will know from their own experiences of working with people with ABI, it can be extremely difficult for them to accept rehabilitative strategies in the first place and, even if they do accept them, to maintain and regularly apply their use in the long term (Kennedy & Coelho, 2005). While there are many factors that contribute to whether a strategy is adopted and consistently used in the long term (such as the severity of the brain injury in itself, family support and insight), one factor that, in our experience, helps the adoption of a strategy is its cultural salience. By that, we mean whether a strategy looks normal, whether or not it makes you stand out, is easily used, and is easily a part of someone's life. In our opinion, two primary carriers of electronic communication—mobile phones and internet use—could not be more culturally salient. Indeed, many of our community based clients already have great experience of using texting to prompt attendance at appointments (for example, a partner who is at work might text their brain-injured loved one to remind them to attend their GP appointment).

In our opinion, facilitating electronic communication should be a service standard. Practically, this would most often mean services routinely asking clients and families for their email and mobile phone details and discussing their potential uses, such as in reminding about appointments, checking out information, confirming the points discussed in therapy, or (as discussed later in this chapter) as a medium to enhance the processes of psychotherapy. The eventual use of emails and texts would, of course, be a negotiated and consent-based discussion between clients, families, and services that should be regularly reviewed and could change over time.

Use of email and texts: a service example

The Cheshire & Wirral Acquired Brain Injury Service is a community based NHS outpatient service that works with clients with acquired brain injuries (ranging from traumatic brain injuries from assaults/accidents through to anoxia, cerebral poisonings, subarachnoid haemorrhage, and younger people who have had strokes) in a mixed urban and rural context. In our experience, we regularly use emails and texts as prompts to cue appointments, "finding" clients when they are not where they are supposed to be, reminding them of agreements, such as return to work meetings with employers, and to clarify any misunderstandings (South Cheshire Acquired Brain Injury Service, 2005).

We also know that clients with a range of disabilities and cognitive difficulties can use and access not only computers, but also web-based material (Newby & Groome, 2010). During our initial assessment process, email addresses and mobile phone numbers are gained with the consent of clients, who are also asked if they would be happy to communicate in this way if necessary. In our experience, this is almost universally accepted.

What does the empirical literature say about traditional uses of emails and texts?

By traditional, we mean the simple use of electronic messaging to prompt clients.

- *Prompting appointments*: There has been both governmental and media interest in increasing attendance at GP and other medical appointments (Newby, 2009). Practical examples include the development of software for text messaging dental surgery clients (e.g., the Dental Plus Appointment Software (2010)). Studies such as those by Koshy, Carr, and Majeed (2008) and by the iPlato Organisation (2011) report that text prompting led to 38% and 26–40% reductions in non-attendance at ophthalmic appointments and Camden GP surgeries, respectively.
- *Increasing information transfer*: Leadbeater (2005) described a nurse-led email service for breast cancer information, with the suggestion that it was a convenient and effective way of increasing patient understanding about their condition.
- *Health promotion*: Thomas and Shaikh (2007) suggested that email could be an excellent way of supporting and encouraging breastfeeding.

However, as Atherton, Huckvale, and Car (2010) admit, in common with many aspects of this area, there is a relative lack of systematic review and/or research-controlled trials in the UK.
- *Compensation for cognitive impairment*: Many readers will be familiar with the NeuroPage messaging system developed by Wilson and colleagues at the Oliver Zangwill Centre in Ely, Cambridgeshire. The system essentially works by clients/carers putting weekly information about the likely alerts required during the next week into a central communications hub. The alerts/cues to action typically involve reminders to attend appointments and to take medication, along with specific reminders/therapeutic suggestions related to ongoing therapy work (e.g., reminding clients about their anger triggers prior to going to a predictably anger-provoking situation). There are a number of studies confirming that this is an effective strategy (e.g. Wilson, Emslie, Quirk, & Evans, 2001). Of course, the eagle-eyed reader will have picked up that NeuroPage is a paging system rather than a mobile phone text service, but the brevity and syntax of the messages are relatively similar. In GN's experience, although the messaging system can be extremely helpful and effective, many clients can become irritated at the perceived "constant interruption" of the NeuroPage alarm and can also struggle to consistently recall that it was they themselves who chose the content of the message. In a more recent study, Pijnenborg and colleagues (2010) have shown that phone text messages have good effectiveness in prompting clients with schizophrenia-related cognitive impairments.
- *SMS texting, brain injury, and goal setting*: In a recent study, Culley and Evans (2010), using a single blind within-subjects trial, showed that text messaging can increase the recall of therapy goals in rehabilitation, thus leading to greater levels of compliance.
- *Email and brain injury*: While GN's service has a long history of using emails to communicate with clients in the fashions previously discussed, there is relatively little or no published work on using emails with brain-injured people. Interestingly, Daisley (2010) has talked about her long experience of communicating with child relatives of brain-injured people in Oxford. She particularly notes that emails are often constructed by the children and young people she works with early in the morning or late evening, and clearly are a way of formulating difficult questions that they

would find hard to ask on a one-to-one basis, or possibly be unable to ask without a forum in which to send messages at virtually any time of the day. Finally, GN has written about how we as professionals can use emails to construct, co-construct, and re-construct meanings about events during group work with people with a brain injury. (Newby, Bushell, Cotter, & Nangle, 2004).

The therapeutic potential of texts and emails

Dean (2008) makes an excellent case for considering electronic communication as an adjunct to the basic interactional requirements of a counselling relationship. Used well and sensitively, electronic communication can be acknowledging, confirming, educational, and revelatory. In Table 10.1, we have adapted the details of the therapeutic advantages of electronic communication described by Dean. We hope that the advantages of convenience, portability, accessibility, universality, and normalcy, being a reflective, co-constructive, and safe space, add up to a powerful argument for using emails and texts psychotherapeutically. However, as Dean (2008) does acknowledge, it is important to ensure such communication be sensitively and thoughtfully handled, particularly as messages can easily be misinterpreted because subtle meanings, such as sarcasm, can be lost without face-to-face contact and the communication can have a syntax that could exclude those who have not come across it before.

Making a case for emails and (even) texts in neuropsychotherapy

It is our contention that electronic communication can also act as much more than an analogue counselling media, and can also allow for development of neuropsychotherapeutic insight. Texts and emails in this context provide a brief, pertinent, and spare language, but can use familiar grammar and syntax (e.g., "thnk", "OMG", etc.) that can be extremely personally meaningful. The processes of reflection, review, and narrative co-construction can not only confirm feelings, but can also lead to new meanings. It is with this in mind that we feel strongly that electronic messaging can be a media for catharsis, the maintenance and extension of in-session meaning, and can promote out of session processing (in line with the therapy process work of

Table 10.1. Potential advantages of electronic communication used with brain-injured patients (adapted from Dean, 2008).

Potential advantage	Why this is important
Convenience	Mobile phones and internet access is often immediately accessible, easy to use and, therefore, more likely to be undertaken.
Portable	Mobile phones can be taken wherever you are and allows for further immediate response. The development of Smart phones also allows the creation of text messaging "on the hoof".
Accessible	Mobile and email use is highly accessible for a range of clients even with disabilities (e.g., Newby & Groome, 2010).
Universal and normal	It is not difficult to persuade clients to use their mobile phones as they may already be using them to prompt themselves; they do not make the client stand out.
Allows cognitive reflection	Means the act of typing out your thoughts allows you to further process what your thinking is, view it, and to think further about what you have written looks like.
Allows co-construction of narrative	You can express difficult and/or embarrassing issues. The interchange between therapist and client allows the creation of a shared story. The constant processes of cognitive reflection, reviewing and re-reviewing can help the client and therapist take on board each other's viewpoints. In GN's experience, therapists can find seeing long-held thoughts being written down and considered by another person as being extremely acknowledging and confirming.
You can express difficult and/or embarrassing issues	In GN's experience, this relative anonymity, divorced from the immediate face-to-face contact, can allow clients to talk about potentially difficult and/or embarrassing issues, such as sexual dysfunction, marital difficulties, loss of emotional feelings, etc. This can be true of family members and children of brain-injured people.

such as Hardy and Llewelyn, in press). Of note, the development of smartphone technology and the use of QWERTY keyboards within them allow for even more personal elaboration.

To act as a basic framework to hang our contention on, it seems natural to create links with Orlinsky and Howard's (1986, 1995) generic model of psychotherapy.

The second author (R2) has written extensively about how this model can be applied in neuropsychotherapy—that is, when working psychotherapeutically with people who have an acquired brain injury (e.g., Coetzer, 1997a,b, 2010). Detailed operational explanations of the five-part model are shown in Table 10.2.

Neuropsychotherapy using the Orlinksy and Howard model: a practical service example

Although the first author (GN) has worked with a number of brain-injured clients using electronic media over the past decade or so, the communication of seven recent clients are presented here. The seven clients include three males and four females who were injured in a range from one to fifteen years prior to therapy and ranged in age

Table 10.2. Orlinksy and Howard's generic model of psychotherapy (adapted from Coetzer, 2007).

Generic element	Explanation
Therapeutic contracting	The early and ongoing process of working out roles and practicalities of how the sessions will work.
Therapeutic operation	The collaborative process where the client presents information for evaluation and treatment decision by the therapist.
Self-relatedness	The intrapersonal process of becoming self-aware, and reflecting how people respond to themselves during their interactions.
In-session impact	The process of therapeutic realisation, which can include emotional relief, insight, and counter-transference.
Phases of treatment	This is a way of conceptualising all the events that happen during the sessions that give the sense of a journey of experience.

from thirty-four to fifty-two. Six out of the seven suffered a traumatic brain injury, with one having a cerebral tumour at the age of thirteen (she is now twenty-eight). Their Glasgow Outcome Scale-Extended scores (Teasdale, Pettigrew, Wilson, Murray, & Jennett, 1998; Wilson, Pettigrew, & Teasdale, 1998) are shown in Table 10.3.

Table 10.3. Glasgow Outcome-Extended Scores for seven users of a community ABI service.

Client	Glasgow Outcome Scale Rating
A (texter)	Lower moderate disability.
1	Lower good recovery.
2	Upper moderate disability.
3	Lower moderate disability.
4	Upper moderate disability.
5	Upper good recovery.
6	Lower moderate disability.

In Table 10.4, we give examples of where we feel a text or email interchange indicates each of the generic psychotherapeutic elements.

Table 10.4. Text and email examples of generic psychotherapeutic processes in action.

Generic psychotherapeutic processes	Text and email examples
Therapeutic contracting (where GN thought clients were negotiating their roles within therapy and the practicalities of the session.)	*Soz I can txt but u wont always ansa? U cumin evry other week. It's a chance 2 let off steam. Lik way u lisen & talk thru pros and cons* (Client A).
	Its very helpful to have your thoughts on email ... I'd say they fit ... with my own memories ... I don't think I would have been able to articulate them as clearly (Client 5)
	Getting the room and length of session right Agreed we'd have the lights off and limit the session to 45 mins, to minimise how tiring the session is (ought to practice what I preach) (GN to Client 6).

(continued)

Table 10.4. (continued).

Generic psychotherapeutic processes	Text and email examples
Therapeutic operations This is where GN felt the client was presenting information for his evaluation and treatment decision	*Im in the middle ov town sweating + shaking bcoz ive gon out of my house + can't wait 2 get home. This isnt normal* (Client A). Text response after phone call: *2 confirm. These r panic symptoms coz u not been out 4 a while. U def not mad. We gona look at strategies 2 get u in control* (Client A).
	GN email: You talked a lot about feeling "paranoid". I do not feel you are paranoid in any mental-health type of a way ... I think your worries stem from the fact that you don't have another grown-up at home to check things out with. *Thank you, I read it and it made me realise how I've been operating as a mum ... I need to find out ways of checking out* (Client 4).
Self-relatedness This is where GN felt the interchange showed the client being self-aware and reflecting how other people might respond to them in their everyday lives.	*... & if I stay my mums goin 2 lose the plot bcoz she cant handle my crazy thoughts + that not gona help my sister is it?* (Client A). *Your mention of the need to mark moving on has been a very positive thought ... It made me think ... planning for family events and to have the feeling that the event is special ... is something I can't just take for granted; that it is something to be glad to experience, something to appreciate.* (Client 5).
In-session impacts This is where GN felt therapeutic realisations were being made including countertransference and emotional relief.	*U made me think 2day* (after a session) *... im 2 easy 2 get in with + take advantage ov. Need 2 think abt who im talkin 2. If they make me feel bad then don't get in wiv them. Im better than that* (Client A). *(Email) supports the powerful thoughts from the session, boosts confidence, at the same time helping me to stand back and more measured way, perhaps making connections to other things* (Client 5).

(continued)

Table 10.4. (continued).

Generic psychotherapeutic processes	Text and email examples
Phases of treatment This is where GN felt the comments were suggesting they were beginning to piece together a journey of experience and how they had come to be where they are now.	*This is wot happens. I sort things out wiv my finances then wen it starts goin wrong I give up + spend a yr or 2 stoned. Well that's not happening again. In the time ive seen u Ive seen that cycle* (Client A). *I can look back now and see I wasn't coping . . . I was resistant to the work strategies because I've go this perfectionism thing. But you kept going with me. Now I feel I've got mastery of the strategies and can work better* (Client 1).

Comments from clients

GN asked each of the participants to give their overall reflections on the process in a relatively free and unstructured method to try to minimise his influence on the outcome.

Examples are shown below.

OK suppoz (Client A)

Supports very well your approach in sessions. In both you are focused on the person and thinking of them in their particular context . . . their positive tone, combined with warmth and understanding . . . (your comments about) . . . things that otherwise might seem unimportant . . . shows you are open to whatever is occupying their thoughts . . . The emails prompted me to mull over certain points in more detail, and prompted me to notice my reactions and feelings perhaps more than I would otherwise have done. (Client 5).

The clear structure of your emails was very helpful . . . (Client 5).

You are someone I felt drawn to trust on meeting you the first time and your emails have strengthened this (Client 5).

They also build to provide a useful history to reflect on progress made and themes that emerge (Client 3).

No downsides apparent . . . how are the records managed from your side to ensure confidentiality is maintained and data protection covered? (My response: Your emails are printed out and placed in your files and the originals deleted. The paper copies in the files are then kept according

to data protection rules regarding paper data). *A system that makes sense to me* (Client 3).
Confirmed what I had said had been understood and noted and interpreted (Client 2).

From this, what was clearly important was the structure of the emails, as well as supporting what had been discussed in the session. The clients clearly enjoyed the communication, warmth, and understanding, and the clear indication that the therapist had thought about and formulated a response to their difficulties. This is reminiscent of Bion's ideas of reverie in therapy (see Vaslamatzis, 1999 for a review). The participants felt the process was trustworthy and enjoyed the sense of testament and history. Interestingly, one participant was rightly interested in the governance of the emails, protection, and confidentiality. To confirm the response in the comments above, in our service emails are printed out and placed in files, the originals deleted, with the paper copies being kept according to data protection rules.

Some preliminary cautions

From our own experience, while the use of electronic communication is undoubtedly a positive addition to therapeutic work, the user must be reminded of a number of cautions.

As stated above, it is extremely important to ensure that correspondence is kept confidentially according to data protection rules. A service's solution to this has already been stated. Texts represent a challenge to note-keeping, but, given they are not easily printed out or retained electronically, and that a potentially large number of texts may be sent over a short period of time, our service's solution is to maintain regular updates in the notes, summarising the main themes and issues discussed. Given that also, particularly, emails are recorded in the notes on a verbatim basis, it is important to respect and understand the heartfelt meanings imparted by clients, but also that they can reflect different levels of literacy and readability. The most important issue is that they are meaningful for clients and the therapist should resist the temptation to "improve" grammar and spelling, remove swearwords, etc. Allied to respecting meaning, it is also important that therapists check out potential perceived meanings of texts and emails, particularly if they contain extensive comments, as relationships can be knocked sideways by unintended slurs or misinterpretation. While this cannot be totally avoided, it might be worth therapists asking a team colleague to read through the communication before sending it.

From a practical point of view, it is also worth noting that dealing with a series of involved and extensive emails can be fairly time consuming. The therapist should consider the practicalities involved in being able to provide extensive replies and reviews. GN is lucky to be able to count on administrative support within the team for producing extensive emails. Allied to this, long delays between sessions and replies can lead to loss of therapeutic momentum and, unless absolutely unavoidable, it is important to provide responses fairly quickly.

The need for more research . . .

Many readers will sigh at seeing this section at the end. However, we feel it is particularly warranted here. As stated previously, there is very little or no clinical work in this area and many of the practical comments are based on 20–30 clients in GN's practice over 10–15 years. There is clearly a need for research-controlled trials and more detailed outcome work. However, I feel that, albeit limited, work shown here suggests the real psychotherapeutic potential of electronic communication.

Conclusions

Electronic communication through texting and emailing is an almost universal and a highly accessible way in which professionals can interact with clients. Lay people have begun to recognise the practical potential of such communication in enhancing what clients understand and know about their condition, as well as simply prompting and cueing action. A burgeoning literature is beginning to develop around the use of text messaging in compensating for memory difficulties and in enhancing compliance with rehabilitation, for example. However, exploring the processes of interchange, review, and reflection also suggests electronic communication has great potential both in counselling and in enhancing and providing neuropsychotherapeutic insight and progress. Not only is electronic communication potentially a succinct but personally meaningful form of communication, but it is clearly a medium that supports and enhances many psychotherapeutic operations. Practical examples are shown in this chapter of just how clients' responses to not only emailing, but also texting, can fit within Orlinsky and Howard's generic psychotherapy model, and also show how clients value such communication. There is very little literature or empirical work in this area and there is a clear need to develop this if electronic neuropsychotherapy is to develop.

Note

1. A video-based Internet communication system.

References

Atherton, H., Huckvale, C., & Car, J. (2010). Communicating health promotion and disease prevention information to patients via email: a review. *Telemed Telecare*, 16: 172–175.

Beckner, V., Howard, I., Vella, L., & Mohr, D. C. (2010). Telephone-administered psychotherapy for depression in MS patients: moderating the role of social support. *Journal of Behavioural Medicine*, 33: 47–59.

Bradbury, C. L., Christensen, B. K., Lau, M. A., Ruttan, L. A, Arundine, A. L., & Green, R. E. (2008). The efficacy of cognitive behavior therapy in the treatment of emotional distress after acquired brain injury. *Archives of Physical Medicine and Rehabilitation*, 89(Supplement 12): S61–S68.

Coetzer, R. (2007a). Psychotherapy following traumatic brain injury: integrating theory and practice. *Journal of Head Trauma Rehabilitation*, 22(1): 39–47.

Coetzer, R. (2007b). *Traumatic Brain Injury Rehabilitation: A Psychotherapeutic Approach to Loss and Grief*. New York: Nova Science.

Coetzer, R. (2010). *Anxiety and Mood Disorders following Traumatic Brain Injury: Clinical Assessment and Psychotherapy*. London: Karnac.

Cully, C., & Evans, J. J. (2010). SMS text messaging as a means of increasing recall of therapy goals in brain injury rehabilitation: a single-blind within-subjects trial. *Neuropsychological Rehabilitation*, 20(1): 103–119.

Daisley, A. (2010). Working with children of people with brain injury, Head First conference presentation, 13 May, London

Dean, A. (2008). Communicating with patients using email and the internet. *Nursing Times*, 104(7): 29–30.

Dental Plus (2010). www.dentalplus.co.uk/dental-software. Accessed 24 May 2012.

Dobson, L. (2010). The net generation. *Therapy Today*, 21(4): 29–31.

Hardy, G. E., & Llewelyn, S. (2013). Psychotherapy process research. In: O. Gelo, A. Pritz, & B. Rieken (Eds.), *Psychotherapy Research: General Issues, Outcome and Process* (pp. 00–00). [[CITY]]: Springer, in press.

iPlato (2011). www.iplato.net/news-appointment-reminders-and-mobile-health-promotion/gp Accessed 29 May 2012.

Kennedy, M. R. T., & Coelho, C. (2005). Self-regulation after traumatic brain injury: a framework for intervention of memory and problem solving. Seminars in Speech and Language, 26(4): 242–255.

Koshy, E., Carr, J., & Majeed, A. (2008). Effectiveness of mobile phone short message service (SMS) reminders for ophthalmology outpatient appointments: an observational study. *BMC Ophthalmology*. Electronic version: www.biomedcentral.com/1471-2415/8/9. Accessed 29 May 2012.

Leadbeater, M. (2005). A nurse-led email service for breast cancer information. *Nursing Times*, 101(39): 38–40.

Newby, G. (2009). Programme contributor to *Your Call*, Radio Programme, BBC 5 Live, 12 August.

Newby, G. (2010). The use of emails and texts in psychological therapy after acquired brain injury. Paper presented to the World Congress of Neuro-technology, Rome, 12–14 October.

Newby, G., & Groome, C. (2010). Evaluating the usability of a single brain injury (ABI) rehabilitation service website: implications for research methodology and website design *Neuropsychological Rehabilitation*, 20(2): 264–288.

Newby, G. J., Bushell, S., Cotter, I., & Nangle, N. (2004). Therapist "hear thyself": using email and de-brief to acknowledge therapists stories in narrative group work. *Clinical Psychology*, 37: 27–34.

Orlinsky, D. E., & Howard, K. I. (1986). Process and outcome in psychotherapy. In: S. L. Garfield & A. E. Berglov (Eds.), *Handbook of Psychotherapy and Behaviour Change* (3rd edn) (pp. 311–383). New York: Wiley.

Orlinksy, D. E., & Howard, K. I. (1995). Unity and diversity among psychotherapies: a comparative perspective. In: B. Bongar & L. E. Beutler (Eds.), *Comprehensive Textbook of Psychotherapy* (pp. 00–00). Oxford: Oxford University Press.

Pijnenborg, G. H. M., Withaar, F. K., Timmerman, M. E., Brouwer, W. H., van den Bosch, R. J., & Evans, J. J. (2010). The efficacy of SMS text messages to compensate for the effects of cognitive impairments in schizophrenia. *British Journal of Clinical Psychology*, 49: 259–274.

South Cheshire Acquired Brain Injury Service (2005). Progress in the palm of your hand. Northwest NHS Innovation Award Winner.

Teasdale, G. M., Pettigrew, L. E., Wilson, J. T., Murray, G., Jennett, B. (1998). Analyzing outcome of treatment of severe head injury: a review and update on advancing the use of the Glasgow Outcome Scale. *Journal of Neurotrauma*, 15: 587–597.

Therapy Today (2011). Skype your therapist: Unaccredited opinion piece. *Therapy Today*, 22(7). Electronic version: www.therapytoday.net/article/show/2634/. Accessed 29 May 2012.

Thomas, J. R., & Shaikh, U. (2007). Electronic communication with patients for breast feeding support. *Journal of Human Lactation*, 23(3): 275–279.

Tsaousides, T., Matsuzawa,Y., & Lebowitz, M. (2011). Familiarity and prevalence of Facebook use for social networking among individuals with traumatic brain injury. *Brain Injury*, 25(12): 1155–1162.

Vaslamatzis, G. (1999). On the therapist's reverie and containing function. *Psychoanalytic Quarterly*, 68: 431–440.

Wilson, B. A., Emslie, H., Quirk, K., & Evans, J. (2001). Is NeuroPage effective in reducing everyday memory and planning problems? A randomised control crossover study. *Journal of Neurology, Neurosurgery and Psychiatry*, 70: 477–482.

Wilson, J. T., Pettigrew, L. E., & Teasdale, G. M. (1998). Structured interviews for the Glasgow Outcome Scale and the Extended Glasgow Outcome Scale: guidelines for their use. *Journal of Neurotrauma*, 15: 573–585.

CHAPTER ELEVEN

Working with relationships in standard neuro-rehabilitation practice

Giles Yeates and Audrey Daisley

Introduction and overview

Over recent years there can be said to have been a 'relational turn' in the neuro-rehabilitation and neuropsychological literature. That is, a move away from a narrow inward focus on the brain and mind of the individual client with a brain injury to considering the effect of the injury on the many different kinds of relationships that connect a client to significant others: family, lovers, friends, work colleagues, and community members. Considerations of this kind have involved the application of ideas from family and couples therapy, social neuroscience, social and community psychology, critical social theory, and other specialist areas (see Bowen, Yeates, & Palmer, 2010).

However, many of these specialisms have their own languages and concepts, often unfamiliar and inaccessible to clinicians working in brain injury services. Acquired brain injury (ABI) clinicians might also feel they lack specialist skills in applying some of these ideas, such as in family or couple work. Equally, many readers might be very "relational" in their everyday clinical practice, without realising it. This might be particularly so for those who work in community, vocational, or social services, who, out of necessity, have to, and are keen to, work with significant others during the course of their involvement with a client. However, those working in inpatient or residential services may also prioritise their liaison with those important to the client. This chapter aims to provide an accessible relational focus on the bread and butter of ABI clinical work. We hope to make explicit those everyday practices that are already inherently orientated towards relationships, and to also suggest some concepts and practice tips that might extend and sharpen practice to fully encompass all things relational. The authors work within acute and post-acute inpatient, outpatient (AD) and community (GY) service contexts, and, while there is much overlap in techniques and strategies used, particular suggestions for each service environment will be made accordingly.

Importantly, no assumption is made here of specialist expertise relevant to relationship/family work within an ABI service. For those readers who are interested in acquiring such specialist knowledge and expanding their service to offer family (including child relative work), couples, and vocational counselling, they are encouraged to read Bowen, Yeates, and Palmer (2010), Daisley and Webster (2008), and Tyerman and King (2008). This chapter will proceed by identifying relationships of relevance for the brain injury clinician, and then explore the various ways in which these relationships can be encountered and supported at all points of liaison across service contexts.

Why focus on relationships?

For most of us, having one or more close relationships is an essential and positive part of our lives. Relationships are typically associated with feeling secure, safe, and loved, and can breed a sense that you belong and are accepted by the networks that are important to you. A positive sense of self-worth often depends on these feelings. Pleasurable and meaningful interactions with other people—family, friends, and the wider community—are desired and valued by most. However, chiming with many clinicians' experiences, the literature consistently shows that ABI devastates relationships of all kinds. Strain and burden in marital relationships are noted, with some studies suggesting that divorce and separation are higher following injury (for a review, see Godwin, Kreutzer, Arango-Lasprilla, & Lehan, 2011).

Although it is often a very difficult conversation for both clients and partners to have with professionals, many of us will be familiar with hearing their heart-rending accounts of changed roles, altered communication, widening of previously shared interests, reduced ability to take part in activities together, sexual issues, and much more. It can feel very much like a living severance of a relationship. Many of these conversations are punctuated with comments such as "I just can't relate to her any more", "it's like living with a stranger", or "it's like having another child to look after but he's my husband", all of which attest to the huge relational shifts and impacts that can occur following ABI.

Other family relationships can suffer following adult injury, including those with aging parents (Minnes, Woodford, Carlson, Johnston, & McCall, 2010), siblings (Orsillo & McCaffrey, 1993), and child relatives (Pessar, Coad, Linn, & Willer, 1993; Uysal, Hibbard, Robillard, Pappadopulus, & Jaffe, 1998). In the workplace, a client with an ABI might remain competent in specific task-related job skills, might have minimal memory or perceptual cognitive difficulties, but interpersonal and executive difficulties might result in social *faux pas* during coffee breaks, relationships with work colleagues might break down, and demotion or job loss might result (Bowen, Yeates, & Palmer, 2010). Clients with an ABI often lose close friends and extended family might withdraw contact. As well as difficulties maintaining existing relationships, clients with an ABI can also experience problems in making new relationships and friendships (Elsass & Kinsella, 1987; Morton & Wehman, 1995); this can be particularly problematic for young people with disabilities who have little or no relationship history or experience to draw upon (Rintala et al., 1997).

For many people with ABI, the losses associated with changed roles and relationships are often of primary concern, but might not always be addressed by services. This can be for a variety of reasons; for example, Webster and Daisley (2007) surveyed rehabilitation professionals about the reasons they might not address child–parent relationship issues after ABI. They found that contextual factors (such as the service ethos, lack of support from managers), practical issues (time, limited child and family focused training), and personal views (attitudes and beliefs) explained why family focused services could have been slow to develop. For many ABI clinicians, a focus on relationships might be outside their own clinical "comfort zone", yet, if we fail to address these issues, clients with ABI might become lonely, isolated figures and those close to them might also become progressively social isolated over time (Bowen, Yeates, & Palmer, 2010). Mental health and wellbeing might suffer without the proximity of caring and fulfilling relationships, the very stuff so many of us rely on and value in life. Such interpersonal devastation can occur even when many cognitive and physical abilities remain unaffected by the injury.

Which relationships?

You are sitting in a consulting room with a client who suffered a brain injury, just the two of you. You ask about his or her story, their life before the injury, how things have changed since. Who do you start to hear about? Who is mentioned?

The first relationships that a client could reflect on might not be the one that immediately springs to mind for the clinician, and that is the many relationships a client has with himself. Noted originally by Tyerman and Humphrey (1984) and more recently explored in a special issue of *Neuropsychological Rehabilitation* on identity after brain injury (Gracey & Ownsworth, 2008), a client's adjustment and life post injury involves a constant dynamic relation of comparisons, judgements, and evaluations. These involve past (pre-injury) self, future or idealised self, and the present self, who is often experienced as lacking or insufficient in relation to those others. That is, "I am not as quick as I was before, my memory is not as reliable, I am not valued as the employed professional in the way I was pre-injury, so uncertain in my own self-ability now, or convinced everything will recover and work out if only I was given the chance by others", and so on. In an unpublished study, Edwards (2011) asked six parents with ABI to talk about the issues related to the parent–child relationship following injury. Among the themes that emerged were that of multiple losses, including loss of parental role and abilities, changes in the child and parent relationship, and loss of self-confidence as a parent (see also Chapter Twelve, by Rachel Skippon, in this volume). Similarly, clients might talk about comments they have received from significant others about their post-injury changes ("you're not the man you used to be") and this is then, in turn, integrated with, and confirms, their already diminished sense of self. As stated earlier, this is so often associated with emotional distress and negative self-evaluation for people with ABI.

Beyond the individual's own internal community of selves[1] (Mair, 1977), a story might be told of people once important to the client who have been lost, or who are distant, or even who have rejected and abandoned them. These could be lovers, friends, or family members. Others may be still in the client's life, but relationships might be tense or strained. The client's experience of this might be one of confusion, not clearly seeing their role in such strains, and, thereby, feeling passive and powerless in the face of negative reactions from others. Alternatively, the client might see their role in things clearly, and feel intensely self-critical, apathetic, and ashamed (psychological therapy work focusing on issues such as depression, social anxiety, and worry inevitably encounters the internalised perspectives and judgements of others). Some of these significant others might make attempts to contact the clinician themselves, to express their concern and exasperation regarding the impact of the injury. At all stages of recovery, families might attribute difficulties and problems to the injured individual. Sometimes, they correctly attribute problems to the cognitive and emotional consequences of the injury, but might, in situations where families have become overwhelmed, seek explanations for problems through perceived impairments within the injured person's motivations and intentions.

Help is usually asked to "fix" the problem (and the person). The message to the clinician is clear—they want their "old" relative returned to them. The challenges for the clinician are many: there is the need to contain the distress of those close to the client, to hear their concerns, while, at the same time, attempting to limit the damage of such accounts on the injured person, to consider how best to engage the family in working with you, and, crucially, how best to work with them towards a framing, understanding, and a description of the problems they are facing as being "relational" rather than "individual". This can be particularly challenging with those relatives who seem to wish to engage with us (at least initially) only as the "information providers", or advocates for their relative, as if positioning themselves slightly apart from the problem. Families seeing themselves in such a way might not always ask for help for themselves and might not offer themselves as part of any solution. We will address this later in the chapter.

Other relationships within a family network can be affected by ABI: child–parent relations can become strained and difficult. Uysal, Hibbard, Robillard, Pappadopulus, and Jaffe (1998) reported that parents with ABI described fewer feelings of love towards, and acceptance of, their children, which affected their relationships. Similarly, Pessar, Coad, Linn, and Willer (1993) reported that almost half of the families they studied described problems in the relationship between the injured parent and the child. Given the permanence of post-injury changes, this is a potentially chronic problem. Child difficulties might also be highlighted by other agencies at the same time, with insufficient awareness of the role of ABI. For example, child relatives might show their distress or struggles within the school context and attract less than helpful labels or responses.

Clients might also describe, and be concerned about, changes in working and professional relationships, either with colleagues, managers, or, indeed, their own clients, depending on the nature of their pre-injury employment. Vocational rehabilitation interventions will necessarily require liaison with pre-injury employers and colleagues, or, if job retention is not possible, the introduction of a whole new system of relationships. In both cases, successful job placement and long-term maintenance of a position will require that work colleagues engage with the reality of ABI over a sustained period of time and be supported by the clinical service to manage the more difficult aspects of this liaison. Often, one key contact in an enduring relationship with the client in the workplace is essential for placement success, the departure of which can lead to many new problems and challenges after often a long period of satisfactory work performance. These issues are addressed more fully by Bernie Walsh in Chapter Eight of this volume.

All of those just mentioned, the client and those around them, will also all have relationships with the brain injury itself. For this reason, it is important for us as clinicians to try to understand the beliefs, ideas, and assumptions that those close to the client hold about the ABI and its consequences in order to fully appreciate the relational impact. Family belief systems are also considered to be central to understanding family resilience, so it is important that we address this (Walsh, 2006). Furthermore, we will also hear stories from clients that reflect their relationships and daily encounters with the wider community, community resources and facilities, and with the public and negotiating public spaces such as shopping centres or supermarkets. These accounts are characterised by repeating stories of prejudice, misunderstanding, ignorance, and stigma. The hidden disability of brain injury is commonly responded to by unhelpful comments or suggestions by workers within employment or benefits agencies, and is frequently misrepresented in the media. At other times, unspoken negative judgements seem to surround the client during their daily interactions with others. For example, unfortunate encounters with the police might become a topic in therapy and could reflect misinformed police officer judgements of intoxication or antisocial behaviour in response to ataxia, dysarthria, or social cognition difficulties (Fraas & Calvert, 2007).

There may also be very recent relationships to hear about—that is, points of contact made in the minutes before the clinical session. Perhaps the client has met another client in the waiting room, stories were shared, points of contact and resonances made, normalisation, validation, and preliminary membership of a new community established. Perhaps the clinician is then confronted with a choice as to how far to embrace and support such meetings as an essential component of brain injury services, be these face to face or through dedicated online and social networking resources (e.g., www.healthtalkonline.org.) And, perhaps, also be mindful of potential associated risks, however small.

Finally, the current or past relationships between ABI clients and the professionals and organisations they interact with involve a diversity of locations, professional practices, world views, values, understanding, and cultural patterns. Clients will provide accounts of their experiences of these previous relationships, including positive stories of support and trust, in addition to recollections of unhelpful encounters. Each of these previous relationships will contribute to the clients' expectations, fears, and hopes for the relationship they might have with us and with our services. It is important, then, to understand the setting events that have occurred previously so that the current work can be situated and the meaning of professional trust understood and respected.

The first and subsequent points of contact

The first point of contact between a service and a client may be an admission (in an acute service) or the receipt of a referral letter (in an outpatient or community setting).

In the inpatient (sub-acute/post-acute) setting, the injured person might be admitted for further rehabilitation within weeks of sustaining their injury. Some might be improving rapidly, and this is typically accompanied by hope (in them and their families) of positive outcomes; others, however, might be at the very earliest stages of a slow and uncertain journey and they and their significant others might be hesitant, fearful, and unsure of what lies ahead for them. The outpatient setting typically allows some time for discussion of a referral and some decisions to be made about who to invite to initial meetings. Unfortunately, the acute setting often offers little time to prepare or deliberate about which people close to the client are seen. Family members, and sometimes their close friends, are typically close by at all times—they are part of "the package". As such, the rehabilitation team must find some point of connection and engagement with the network of people who stand literally around the client's bedside. Emotions and expectations can run high. Fears and anxieties are often voiced loudly. To complicate this, clients and their families might arrive in the unit with labels or "reputations" from previous staff groups who have worked with them. These descriptions offer the team useful, but also potentially misleading, clues about the nature and quality of their relationships (within the family, for example "they are a very close and supportive family", or "they have visited rarely . . . they don't seem to be interested", and with staff, for example, "they are difficult family . . . obstructive"). Some of these labels obviously present the team with immediate challenges and might lead us to pre-judge the relational issues that might arise.

An important point about this early contact with families is that child relatives might become "visible" only at the post-acute stage (typically, many ITU settings have strict policies about children, especially those under the age of twelve, not visiting the ward, so many children might have had no or limited contact with their injured relative). This itself has relational implications, as discussed in Chapter Twelve (by Rachel Skippon, concerning parenting) in this volume. For very young children, this separation can affect attachments, disrupt bonds, and lead children to believe that the parent has left them, or has died; there might be signs that these children have already begun grieving the lost parent. Older children typically express resentment because of having had contact with the relative and key information withheld. They might also express fears that their relative chose not to see them, feel anger about this, and refuse to visit them. While the less hospital-like setting of the post-acute rehabilitation unit might well be more openly welcoming of children, the staff might not be prepared or able to manage their distress as it presents. Many rehabilitation units around the country, however, are becoming increasingly more child friendly and focused, and this is a positive development.

Focusing directly on relationship work early in a client's admission to a post-acute unit is rarely a priority or appropriate unless this is specifically requested by the family. Typically, clients are very self-focused. Similarly, close friends and relatives tend to concentrate on the immediate individual needs and concerns of their injured relative ("Is he receiving enough physiotherapy? When will his medication be reduced?", and so on). However, early whole family education (including child relatives), particularly to reveal and later address brain injury myths, and involving families in planning goals with the resumption of meaningful life roles and activities in mind, provide the cornerstones on which to build later, more direct, relational resilience-focused work. Early direct enquiries about the wellbeing of children in the family and other relatives or close friends frames the ABI as having a systemic (and not solely an individual) impact. In addition, genograms (i.e., relational family tree diagrams, see Chapter Three in this volume for an example) can be drawn up at an early stage. This can enable us to identify sources of support for families as they manage the relational shifts that might lie ahead.

As the initial shock of the injury, accident, or illness wanes, clients and the people close to them often naturally and intuitively try to embark on a journey that tries to reconstruct their old self or the family "as it was". The signposts of this are often the relational conversations, concerns, and worries that clients and their concerned others have with clinicians. We might be asked, "Is he going to be the same man I married . . . he's changed . . . is the old person ever going to come back?" A partner of a man who had sustained an ABI in a car accident and remained in a low awareness state for many months said, from even very early on in his rehabilitation, that she needed to focus only on each day ahead. She needed to focus on understanding his assessment results, his treatment regime, and could not contemplate thoughts about the future. She told us that she had "allowed herself", only once, to "go there" and consider what would happen if her husband made no further recovery. She had opened herself up to this possibility and had been faced with a barrage of relational issues and dilemmas such as "What kind of husband will he be . . . what will it mean to be married to him, how can he still be a good father to our three children?" Considering (even briefly) the relational impact of his ABI had literally overwhelmed her to the point of being unable to allow herself access to these thoughts.

Clearly, the timing of discussions as outlined above, is crucial and will be different for each family and each individual family member. Collicut-McGrath (2007) discusses the ethical issues for the clinician surrounding such relational dilemmas and family concerns.

In an outpatient or community service, things often start via an exchange of correspondence between referrer, service, and client. The referral letter might name, or allude to, significant others, to the nature of the referral, the description of relevant problems, and could prompt the clinician to start thinking about the impact on all those around the client. This can be a continual process lasting the entire duration of the work with the client, a continuous 360-degree sweep of problems and issues from the perspective of all those connected with the client, adding on more people as you hear about them.

The response by the service, often a letter to invite the client to an initial assessment meeting, does require some thinking about. A brain injury service (and perhaps the wording of the trust/organisational name) might set up specific expectations for clients on receipt of an appointment letter, before any face-to-face meeting. Words such as "brain injury", "neuro", "medical" may all establish an expected focus on the individual client and their brain. More detailed letters might also establish a focus on physical and maybe cognitive or emotional functioning. All roads could point to a reductionist encounter at this early point, where contextual factors such as relationships, communication between people, power inequalities, and important family stories that have a bearing on current experiences are not on the agenda. Is there a way of highlighting this more? An alternative focus for the letter could be an invitation to a gathering, asking the client and their family to decide together who should come, perhaps with an indication that large groups or extended families would be welcome, if the service can support such a meeting. Powerful cultural trends are influential at this point: a Western medical framing of a one-to-one consultation with an expert to report physical symptoms and receive some form of dosage response treatment can be contrasted

WORKING WITH RELATIONSHIPS IN STANDARD NEURO-REHABILITATION   281

with those cultures that convene the first discussion of an illness or disability as a community gathering (Ogden, Cooper, & Dudley, 2003).

If such invitations have been made, the first minute of the actual assessment meeting is very informative. Who is present? Who is absent? A discussion about who is in the client's life, past and present, is as useful a conversation (and often leads to the same problem-orientated topics) as a historical review of the brain injury and rehabilitation to date. In addition to the genogram work mentioned earlier, the visual mapping of relationships beyond the family, including relationships to different agencies or services, is a useful process. Hartman (1995) describes the process of "eco-mapping", the deliberate inclusion of visual prompts on a genogram to stimulate reflexive questions such as "Who else is working with this individual or family that I don't know about?" "How are things described and prioritised in those conversations, and what action on my part would differences of this nature stimulate?" (see Figure 11.1).

Useful relational information can also be obtained from children in families (if it is agreed that they will be included in some sessions/ meetings). Talking to children about family relationships can be helpful for both the therapist and the other relatives to gain an alternative perspective on issues and changes in relationships. The Heart Strings

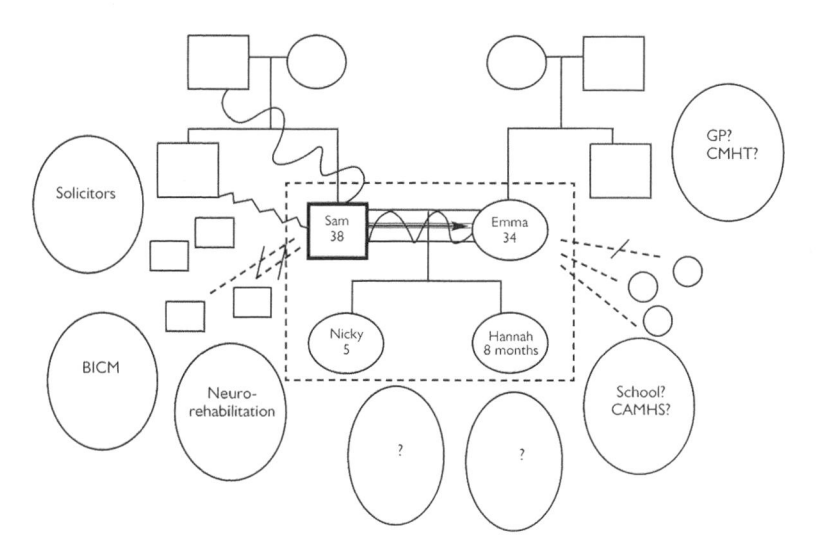

Figure 11.1. Eco-mapping (Hartman, 1995).

exercise (Hobday & Ollier, 1998) can be a useful way to support such discussions and to gain insights into children's perceptions of these relationship changes. This activity involves the child drawing a heart in the centre of a sheet of paper. Circles are then drawn around the heart and the child is asked to place names of those who are closest to them in the circle nearest the heart. People whom the child judges to be less close are placed in circles further away from the heart. This is undertaken to map out relationships both before the ABI and afterwards, and the children are encouraged to talk about these changes as they are drawn on the Heartstrings. This is a simple and straightforward activity that can yield powerful and moving information about relational changes from a child's perspective (Lloyd-Williams, 2012).

The conclusion of an assessment session is often a joint oral and/or written decision about how the relationship between the client and service should ideally proceed. This decision will be organised by the agreed priorities and will comprise the agreed pieces of work. All of these organising decisions will involve the presence or absence of significant others, perhaps in differing combinations across time (e.g., certain family members attending some sessions with the client, relative-only sessions, group sessions involving clients or relatives only). These are important decisions to decide in collaboration with those present in the initial meeting and are also influenced by service practices and capacity. Decisions need to be made about how those absent should be contacted or included in such thinking (via a subsequent phone call, or an assessment letter addressed to people present and absent in the initial session).

Individual work with clients with relationships in mind

From the above, we suggest that the individual client carries around an internal community of relationships. These are the interrelationships between different parts of their self (past and present) and both present and absent internalised figures of important others in their life. Following from this, even an individual session with a client will be a busy, crowded place, with lots of influential voices and perspectives. Engaging with this invisible community and getting a conversation going between these voices is always a productive, useful, and sometimes moving process, regardless of the clinician's profession or the rehabilitation goal.

How can this conversation get started? Question types inviting others' points of view can be used at any time. For example, setting a goal around leisure activities or return to work considerations, questions such as "What would the old Stephen think about that idea? What would you say now in response?" would be useful in fleshing out the meaning of an activity in relation to identity, adjustment, and so on. The outward identity of a client, their pre-injury public persona, and their anticipated sense of friends' and associates' responses to who they are now/what they are doing is a critical dimension. Ylvisaker and Feeney (2000) have drawn attention to their identity mapping, using these elements to establish and maintain rehabilitation engagement with very complex clients. It is also important to listen out for how the person speaks about himself, how he experiences and perceives himself, and what or who has influenced this viewpoint. It is important to see if there is an active "I" in the injured person's storytelling—often people will say when asked how they managed a situation, "You just cope, don't you" or "People just cope, don't they", rather than "I just coped, didn't I". Who else does the patient speak of? What are the barriers to these relationships; how does the person speak about the relationships with those around him. In some cases, this narrative in the second person might have a function to create distance between the self and what must be very painful, especially in a family context where there is lots of informal feedback and reminding of the brain injury.

Those questions about aspects of self and important others are somewhat "out in the ether", requiring visualisation, imagery, and creative faculties that might be lost post injury. To add a dimension of immediacy and concreteness into the discussion, approaches such as the Gestalt empty chair technique can be very evocative. This has long been used in psychotherapy to bring absent figures and relationships into the room. A client is directed to address an empty chair as if a significant figure was sitting there, and begin a conversation about an emotional issue. In the middle of a poignant account by a client relating to someone else, he or she may be suddenly asked to turn to the empty chair and direct a statement to the imagined figure. The same approach can be used with different parts of the client's self. A useful resource describing these and other techniques that bring relationships into individual sessions can be found in Boscolo and Bertrando (1996).

Narrative therapy approaches (White & Epston, 1990, see also Stephen Weatherhead's section in the Psychotherapy chapter within this volume) would take this a stage further and imagine whole gatherings and communities in the room at certain points, turning the isolated sufferer into an emissary for a larger collective of aggrieved people. Questions of this kind include, "What would you say to a whole group of other clients regarding this issue? In turn, as a group what would you all say to a smaller group of uninformed bystanders about this issue?"

More practical aspects of rehabilitation can also support relationships. For example, an occupational therapist could use a leisure-focused session to help a parent make a toy for their child, while physiotherapy could attend to helping a parent learn to sit on the floor safely to play with children or to change a baby's nappy. Such work should also concentrate on the management of "symptoms" that are most problematic for children. Much of this work is often carried out very expertly by rehabilitation professionals, but perhaps without a clear realisation that they are, in fact, addressing relational issues. More relational-focused training of rehabilitation teams could help take this work a stage further, so that while these more practical activities are being undertaken, a conversation can be opened up which might encourage the client to begin to talk about changes in relationships.

Finally, the other person in the room in individual sessions is the clinician, and the crucial relationship that is formed and maintained between clinician and client. Michael Schönberger (Schönberger, Humle, & Teasdale, 2006) has published a series of studies that demonstrate the significance of the working alliance between clinicians/ services and clients for the latter's awareness of disability and rehabilitation outcome. Clinicians and their team, therefore, have a responsibility to maximise engagement where possible, given the initial awareness position of the client at the point of service contact. This might call for a creative and flexible stance on the part of the clinician, working to find points of common ground and short-term rationales for pieces of rehabilitative work, even if longer-term expectations differ between client and clinician. Often, clinicians hold an assumption (or an unmodified trend in their practice) that the provision of feedback regarding the client's impairments will be enough to create a collaborative basis for work. Such feedback is, indeed, often not sufficient, and commonly evokes a confused and/or defensive reaction in clients. When such a reaction ensues, any resultant stand-off can erode working alliances and restrict opportunities for future rehabilitative gains, or, worse still, contribute to the client disengaging from the service. Gorske and Smith (2009) offer a useful framework for providing feedback to people with ABI about neuropsychological assessment results (based on principles of motivational interviewing and Rogerian counselling techniques).

Many schools of psychotherapy emphasise the need for a positive working or therapeutic alliance as a necessary precursor to any technical or educational phase of the intervention. In terms of attachment theory, this is the creation of a secure emotional base, from which steps into the unknown can be attempted with an increased sense of safety. These steps can include facing one's difficulties, making sense of confusing and anxiety-provoking experiences, trying something new, and running the risk of failure. Fundamentally, such work could be seen as a reconnection with profound and necessary sequences present in all aspects and stages of normal development and life. A secure emotional base can also serve as a safe platform from which to experiment with new or different behaviours and emotions, before proceeding to the much riskier stage of generalisation out there in the real world where our clients live, love, and engage in meaningful activities.

Inviting others into sessions

Given that individual work informed by a relational focus can offer all of the aforementioned avenues, the possibilities are boundless when others are brought into rehabilitation settings: partners, relatives, friends, employers/work colleagues, together with the formation of new communities such as a group of ABI clients or relatives themselves. At the same time, the intensity and speed of dynamics in communication between these can be overwhelming, distracting, daunting, and, at times, can inhibit the potential for a useful meeting or conversation. The need for specialist couples, family, and group process skills is, therefore, clear. However, the following suggestions might create opportunities for useful conversations and pieces of work accessible to most, without the need to wade into a formal psychotherapy or emotion-fuelled discussion.

Given the established vulnerability of the couple relationship following ABI, the need for inclusion of couples work within neurorehabilitation has long been stated in the literature, yet rarely provided. Specific ideas and directions for couples therapy itself have been recently stated elsewhere (Bowen, Yeates, & Palmer, 2010; Yeates, 2011). Here, however, it is important to consider how other interventions may offer benefits for the couple and closeness in their relationship. The importance of mutual loss or unwanted change of roles in the couple and the wider family following injury has long been recognised, and, consequently, the need for role re-negotiation has been suggested (Maitz & Sachs, 1995). In addition to a piece of specific couples psychotherapeutic work, occupational therapists have described their work on creating leisure and functional opportunities for couples to redefine who does what, and what can be done together (Eriksson, Tham, & Fugl-Meyer, 2005; Hallet, Zasler, & Cash, 1994). The result of this very pragmatic work (which would entail having a joint session with both partners rather than activity scheduling with the client alone) can often be a reduction in burden for the non-injured partner (as some of their assumed responsibilities are shared out, making them more free) and an increased closeness between partners.

We need to build balanced alliances with families and within families; the aim is always to work towards reducing negativity and blame and creating a family (relational) focus for solving problems. Family members can find taking this perspective challenging (at least in the initial stages, where their explanations and attributions for problems are well developed). It can be helpful in these instances to try to focus on the family member who perhaps appears most hopeless or negative, least hopeful, or who can see no solutions, as these are the people most likely to hinder progress and change. However, the balance required to secure engagement and protection of one member while preventing alienation of another family member(s) can be quite precarious and requires considerable clinical skill. Therapists, in addition to being aware of the clinical and other data continually unfolding before their eyes, also need to stay in tune with the overall, dynamic therapeutic process simultaneously and continually occurring in the background.

Beyond the couple, other family members can be involved in many avenues of core rehabilitative practice. Children of clients can be included in rehabilitation activities as a means of helping children and adults maintain their previous closeness and contact. This could range from a child observing a parent in a physiotherapy session, to undertaking joint activities (such as baking with the injured parent in an OT session), or learning to use a communication aid (Daisley & Webster, 2008 for an overview of child-focused interventions in the context of familial ABI). There are few good published child-focused ABI materials (so, as a clinician, you will need to get creative when trying to meet child relatives' information and support needs). The Brain Injury Rehabilitation Trust (BIRT) has recently started to support the development of some booklets for children (e.g., *My Parent's Had A Brain Injury* by Jo Johnson—contact BIRT at info@thedtgroup.org.). It can also be very helpful to support and encourage families to work together to make a scrapbook to document their journey through the rehabilitation/recovery process. This has been shown to have very positive therapeutic benefits in other family illness contexts (McCarthy & Sebough, 2011).

In addition, research on parents with other types of illness, such as mental health problems, suggests that to foster relational resilience between parents and children it is important to actively encourage the ill person to talk openly with their children about the emotional impact of the parent's illness on the child. Focht-Bikerts and Beardslee (2000) noted that families who restricted such discussion and displays of affect were more at risk of developing depression than those who were able to speak openly about the challenges they had faced. The key to this all this work is careful planning of what relational issues we are trying to address, what we want the parent and child to achieve, can we safeguard children from being exposed to a markedly changed parent (in how they relate to them), as well as "protecting" the injured adult from being overtaken by cognitively more able children. If we are not mindful to manage such situations the parent–child relationship can experience tremendous cracks in it as the gulf between them widens.

The sibling relationship is typically the most enduring and long-lasting family relationship one can have and it could reasonably be expected that the adult and child siblings of people with ABI might also be affected by this experience. There is little research on adult siblings, but the few studies that do exist attest to this. Gills and Wells (2000) looked at the experiences of eight adult siblings of people with ABI (all ABI clients were younger than their non-injured siblings in this study) and found that non-injured siblings reported a strong sense of duty to maintain the family by taking on a carer role in relation to their sibling. Given the chronicity of ABI symptoms, this has long-term implications. These care duties are likely to extend across the life span and might become more intensified as the injured person's aging parents become less able to maintain their carer role. Wetters (2011) examined the types of social support adult siblings provided for their injured siblings and found that affective forms of care (such as providing general emotional support and companionship) outweighed more instrumental types of support (such as providing transport, managing finances, etc.). In addition, Degeneffe and Olney (2010) found that siblings experienced increased relationship difficulties with other family members as well as increased marital discord following their sibling's ABI. Such studies demonstrate that siblings of all ages, like other family members, experience relational difficulties and distress, are likely to be actively involved in supporting their brain injured sibling, but that this support might not be readily seen or acknowledged by services. In our experience, they are often not invited to contact meetings with services and are the family members least likely to attend if they are invited. The reasons for this are not clear, and might be circular and complex (e.g., fewer invitations to connect with services leading to fewer opportunities for sensemaking, despite unique adjustment challenges such as role inversion and negative relationships with parents as an indirect result (Bowen, Yeates, & Palmer, 2010)). It seems important for rehabilitation professionals to bear siblings in mind when considering the impact of ABI on family members with programmes of intervention designed specifically to target the unique issues faced by them. There have been considerable developments in such work with younger (children and adolescents) siblings of children with ABI and other types of disabilities (Lobato, 1990).

Ogden, Cooper, and Dudley (2003) describe how community brain injury work with Maori cultures in New Zealand necessitates a common engagement and liaison with large extended families and community elders. Any rehabilitation planning takes place inside the *wharenui*, the community building, with all those connected to the client present, and decisions are made through a collective process. While this is a fascinating point of cross-cultural comparison, this is radical community neuro-rehabilitation in action and of value to any brain injury service anywhere else in the world. Similarly, the African concept of *ubuntu*, where the wellbeing of the group is thought to be much more important than that of the individual, has obvious implications. Following the example of the systemic and narrative therapies, the impetus is on the service to extend open invitations to the client and those around them, to encourage a broadening of the radar to include (as potential resources) those family members and friends not initially considered to be relevant to the rehabilitative endeavour, and constantly be asking the question, "Who else do we need to get involved to make this a useful conversation/process/piece of work?"

A community brain injury service can work creatively and fruitfully with other organisations in the community, such as ABI-related charities (in the UK, Headway, Different Strokes, Stroke Association, and Encephalitis Society, to name a few). Also, corporate organisations pursing community social responsibility schemes, and perhaps even the creation of a social enterprise venture that provides a service for the local community around the brain injury service, might be fruitful ways forward. These can create job opportunities for clients and forge close links between clients and community members who would ordinarily know nothing about ABI at all. For example, the Help group in Buckinghamshire in the UK is a group of clients who have established themselves as a horticultural business that provides services to their local community. This is done at both cost and at no charge, depending on the client. This venture is providing some employment opportunity, skills building/maintenance, and experience and networking opportunities for these clients in a vastly restricted job market. In a related sense, vocational rehabilitation itself requires a significant investment by services in relationships with employers and placement providers, to support an understanding and tolerance of ABI and its consequences in a group of colleagues who did not seek initially to work with brain injury, and who face the difficult task of offering support and opportunities to clients while managing the wellbeing of other staff. When successful, a viable paid or voluntary work position can offer an answer to the question, "What do you do then?", a source of identity and confidence, enhanced mental health and wellbeing, and broader material and psychological benefits for others connected to the client (Vanderploeg, Curtiss, Duchnick, & Luis, 2003).

Then there is the creation of communities of clients themselves, if only for five minutes, while making a cup of coffee in the service waiting room and sharing stories of similar experiences. Such interactions can be encouraged and organised as a central feature of any ABI service delivery, orientated to a "therapeutic milieu". This could be achieved via the provision of educational groups, providing opportunities for clients to meet informally, and the specialist provision of psychotherapy groups. Examples of groups of this nature are discussed in Chapter Nine, by Walsh, Weatherhead, Calvert, and Newby, in this volume. Such peer processes might be happening informally within a service that provides no such formal avenues, so it could be a small step to extend the potential value of this further. A parallel process is often provided by services for relatives, to allow conversations to emerge about difficult feelings, without fear of judgement from others who would not understand.

In 2012 and beyond, the notion of community itself no longer requires face-to-face contact, but is often in cyberspace, through social networking (e.g., Facebook, Twitter, Myspace, Skype, etc.), emailing, and texting examples. (See Newby and Coetzer's chapter in this volume for further discussion). This cultural and technological development offers new opportunities for the formation of relationships around the client. Physical mobility and financial barriers to contact are removed through online communities. Acquired communication difficulties, in all their forms, can be managed more systematically, as clients can choose how to communicate and receive communication online (to read, to listen, or watch streaming audio/video, to access information in structured and themed forms). The Internet is not without its own barriers to accessibility for clients (Elman, Parr, & Moss, 2003; Moss, Parr, Byng, & Petheram, 2004; Newby & Groom, 2010; Parr, Watson, & Woods, 2006; see www.ukconnect.org/research_221.aspx), but careful responses to this via collaborative venture between clients, clinicians, and web designers can produce useful, brain injury friendly online social resources (e.g., www.healthtalkonline.org, which offers access to survivors' subjective accounts of injury as text, video, or audio, organised and divided under themes, or as whole narratives, all with links to social networking discussion groups and information sections). Readers might also wish to look at www.

relationalwoesofatbisurvivor.blogspot.com, which is a blog written by a young man with ABI about the relational issues he faces following his injury.

Conclusions

As research on family outcomes after ABI increasingly points towards the reciprocal relationship between family adjustment and client outcomes (Harris, Godfrey, Partridge, & Knight, 2001), it is clear that relationships must be the organising framework for facilitating change and promoting resilience. An often overlooked point is that without social integration generally, and, more specifically, family adjustment, the generalisation of individual therapeutic gains is vulnerable, or might not even happen at all, in many cases. As such, professionals must prioritise supporting the connections that an ABI client has with those close to them through more relationship-focused rehabilitation activities. We hope that this chapter has opened up some of the possibilities for incorporating or increasing a focus on relationships within routine rehabilitation practice.

Note

1. Originally a concept nested within personal construct therapy, Mair (1977) is referring here to the plurality of internal voices, perspectives, and facets of ourselves that we become aware of when we relate to others in social settings and perceive how others see us. This can be a here and now experience, or a remembered phenomenon as we tell stories about ourselves in relation to others.

References

Boscolo, L., & Bertrando, P. (1996). *Systemic Therapy with Individuals*. London: Karnac.

Bowen, C., Yeates, G., & Palmer, S. (2010). *A Relational Approach to Rehabilitation: Thinking about Relationships after Brain Injury*. London: Karnac.

Collicut-McGrath, J. (2007). *Ethical Practice in Brain Injury Rehabilitation.* Oxford: Oxford University Press.

Daisley, A., & Webster, G. (2008). Familial brain injury: impact and interventions with children. In: A. Tyerman & N. King (Eds.), *Psychological Approaches to Rehabilitation after Traumatic Brain Injury* (pp. 475–508). Oxford: BPS Blackwell.

Degeneffe, C. E., & Olney, M. F. (2010). "We are the forgotten victims": perspectives of adult siblings of persons with traumatic brain injury. *Brain Injury*, 24(12): 1416–1427.

Edwards, A. (2011). The experience of being a parent with an acquired brain injury. Unpublished Doctoral thesis, Oxford University.

Elman, R. J., Parr, S., & Moss, B. (2003). The Internet and aphasia: crossing the digital divide. In: S. Parr, J. Duchan, & C. Pound (Eds.), *Aphasia Inside Out: Reflections on Communication Disability* (pp. 00–00). Maidenhead: Open University Press.

Elsass, L., & Kinsella, G. (1987). Social interaction following severe closed head injury. *Psychological Medicine*, 17(1): 67–78.

Eriksson, G., Tham, K., & Fugl-Meyer, A. R. (2005). Couples' happiness and its relationship to functioning in everyday life after acquired brain injury. *Scandinavian Journal of Occupational Therapy*, 12: 40–48.

Focht-Bikerts, L., & Beardslee, W. R. (2000). A child's experience of parental depression: encouraging relational resilience in families with affective illness. *Family Process*, 39: 417–434.

Fraas, M. R., & Calvert, M. (2007). Oral histories: bridging misconceptions and reality in brain injury recovery. *Disability and Rehabilitation*, 29: 1449–1455.

Gills, D. J., & Wells, D. L. (2000). Forever different: the experiences of living with a sibling who has a traumatic brain injury. *Rehabilitation Nursing*, 25: 48–53.

Godwin, E. E., Kreutzer, J. S., Arango-Lasprilla, J. C., & Lehan, T. (2011). Marriage after brain injury: review, analysis and research recommendations. *Journal of Head Trauma Rehabilitation*, 26(1): 43–55.

Gorske, T.T., & Smith, S. R. (2009). *Collaborative Therapeutic Neuropsychological Assessment.* New York: Springer.

Gracey, F., & Ownsworth T. (Eds.) (2008). The self and identity in rehabilitation. of *Neuropsychological Rehabilitation* (Special Issue), 18(5–6).

Hallet, J. D., Zasler, N. D., & Cash, S. (1994). Role change after traumatic brain injury. *American Journal of Occupational Therapy*, 48(3): 241–246.

Harris, J., Godfrey, H., Partridge, F., & Knight, P. (2001). Care giver depression following TBI: a consequence of adverse effects on family members? *Brain Injury*, 15(3): 223–238.

Hartman, A. (1995). Diagrammatic assessment of family relationships. *Families in Society*, 76: 111–122.
Hobday, A., & Ollier, K. (1998). *Creative Therapy: Activities with Children and Adolescents*. Leicester: BPS Books.
Lloyd-Williams, K. (2012). A qualitative study of children's relationships and how they change when a parent acquires a brain injury. Unpublished Doctoral Thesis, University of Coventry & Warwick.
Lobato, D. J. (1990). *Brothers and Sisters and Special Needs: Information and Activities for Helping Young Siblings of Children with Chronic Ilnesses and Developmental Disabilities*. Baltimore, MD: Paul H. Brookes.
Mair, J. M. M. (1977). The community of self. In: D. Bannister (Ed.), *New Perspectives in Personal Construct Theory* (pp. 125–149). London : Academic Press.
Maitz, E. A., & Sachs, P. P. (1995). Treating families of individuals with traumatic brain injury from a family systems perspective. *Journal of Head Trauma Rehabilitation*, 10: 1–11.
McCarthy, P., & Sebough, J. (2011). Therapeutic scrapbooking: a technique to promote positive coping and emotional strength in parents of paediatric oncology patients. *Journal of Psychosocial Oncology*, 29(2): 215–230.
Minnes, P., Woodford, L., Carlson, P., Johnston, J., & McCall, M. A. (2010). The needs of aging parents caring for an adult with acquired brain injury. *Canadian Journal of Ageing*, 29: 185–192.
Morton, M. V., & Wehman, P. (1995). Psychosocial and emotional sequelae of individuals with traumatic brain injury: a literature review and recommendations. *Brain Injury*, 9(1): 81–92.
Moss, B., Parr, S., Byng, S., & Petheram, B. (2004). 'Pick me up and not a down down, up up': how are the identities of people with aphasia represented in aphasia, stroke and disability websites? *Disability & Society*, 19(7): 753–768.
Newby, G., & Groom, C. (2010). Evaluating the usability of a single brain injury (ABI) rehabilitation service website: implications for research methodology and website design. *Neuropsychological Rehabilitation*, 20(2): 264–288.
Ogden, J., Cooper, E., & Dudley, M. (2003). Adapting neuropsychological assessments for minority groups: a study comparing white and Maori New Zealanders. *Brain Impairment*, 4(2): 122–134.
Orsillo, S. M., & McCaffrey, R. J. (1993). Siblings of head-injured people: a population at risk. *Journal of Head Trauma Rehabilitation*, 8: 102–115
Parr, S., Watson, N., & Woods, B. (2006). Access, agency and normality: the wheelchair and the Internet as mediators of disability. In:

A. Webster (Ed.), *Innovative Health Technologies: New Perspectives, Challenge and Change* (pp. 161–174). London: Palgrave Macmillan.

Pessar, L., Coad, M., Linn, R., & Willer, B. (1993). The effects of parental traumatic brain injury on the behaviour of parents and children. *Brain Injury*, 7(3): 231–340.

Rintala, D. H, Howard, C. A., Nosek, M. A., Bennett, J. L., Young, M. E., Foley, C. C., Rossi, C. D., & Chanpong, G. (1997). Dating issues for women with physical disabilities. *Sexuality and Disability*, 15(4): 219–242.

Schönberger, M., Humle, K., & Teasdale, T. W. (2006). The development of the therapeutic working alliance, patients' awareness and their compliance during the process of brain injury rehabilitation. *Brain Injury*, 20(4): 445–454.

Tyerman, A., & Humphrey, M. (1984). Changes in self-concept following severe head injury. *International Journal of Rehabilitation Research*, 7: 11–23.

Tyerman, A. T., & King, N. S. (Eds.) (2008). *Psychological Approaches to Rehabilitation following Traumatic Brain Injury*. Oxford: Blackwell.

Uysal, S., Hibbard, M., Robillard, D., Pappadopulus, E., & Jaffe, M. (1998). The effects of parental traumatic brain injury on parenting and child behaviour. *Journal of Head Trauma Rehabilitation*, 13(6): 289–295.

Vanderploeg, R. D., Curtiss, G., Duchnick, G. C., & Luis, C. A. (2003). Demographic, medical, and psychiatric factors in work and marital status after mild head injury. *Journal of Head Trauma Rehabilitation*, 18: 148–163.

Walsh, F. (2006). *Strengthening Family Resilience* (2nd edn). New York: Guilford Press.

Webster, G., & Daisley, A. (2007). Including children in family focused acquired brain injury rehabilitation: a national survey of practice. *Clinical Rehabilitation*, 21(12): 1097–1109.

Wetters, K. (2011). Traumatic brain injury and sibling caregivers. Right at home blog page: www.rightathome.net/chiswsuburbs/blog/traumatic-brain-injury-and-sibling-caregivers/. Accessed 31 May 2012.

White, M., & Epston, D. (1990). *Narrative Means to Therapeutic Ends*. Adelaide: Dulwich.

Yeates, G. N. (2011). Working with the vulnerable couple after acquired brain injury. *Clinical Psychology Forum*, 219: 23–27.

Ylvisaker, M., & Feeney, T. (2000). Reconstruction of identity following brain injury. *Brain Impairment*, 1: 12–28.

CHAPTER TWELVE

Supporting families and parenting after parental brain injury

Rachel Skippon

Introduction

The consequences of acquired brain injury (ABI) for the *individual* can be diverse, and affect all areas of life. But parental ABI can change life for families immensely, too. A US study (Urbach & Culbert, 1991) found that around 30–40% of people with ABI had dependent children, and we might reasonably speculate that figures for the present UK population are broadly similar.

It has become a priority for the NHS to base services on the wishes, needs, and expectations of families as well as patients (Department of Health, 2001). For instance, the *National Service Framework for Long-term Conditions* requires providers to build family support into services for people with long-term disabilities (Department of Health, 2005). As professionals working in the field of brain injury rehabilitation, we need, therefore, to consider the wider impact that an ABI can have on the family. However, working with clients who are parents can be challenging for ABI professionals, as there is little published work to guide practice in these areas (Webster & Daisley, 2005, 2007).

There are many ways in which families might be affected by parental ABI, and cognitive and physical impairments in particular have an impact on the day-to-day requirements of parenting small children. We can imagine practical difficulties in getting children washed, dressed, and fed in time for school, an inability to drive them to school, and memory problems that mean the parent cannot keep on top of all the usual reminders about the PE kit, homework, and so on. But there are many more subtle challenges that an injured parent and his/her family face. Relationships, and their changing dynamics, are the essence of family life. When one member of the family changes dramatically, it has a knock-on effect on all the other members. Roles are changed, expectations are no longer met; the secure confidence that comes from the predictability of family life is shaken.

Partner relationship breakdown might be more common after ABI. A recent US study (Arango et al., 2008) found that, among people who were married on initial hospital admission for ABI, around 15% were separated or divorced after two years. Older studies have found higher rates of relationship breakdown, in the range 40–55%, at longer intervals after ABI, between five and eight years (Oddy, Coughlan, Tyerman, & Jenkins, 1985; Tate, Lulham, Broe, Strettles, & Pfaff, 1989; Wood & Yurdakul, 1997). A more recent US study found relationship breakdown rates averaging 25% over a range of intervals from three to eight years post-ABI (Kreutzer, Marwitz, Hsu, Williams, & Riddick, 2007).

Even if the relationship with a partner is maintained, loss of other social support, inability to return to previous activities or employment, emotional (in)sensitivity, and new difficulties in perceiving how others are feeling can all impact on the ability of the adult with an ABI to manage the demands of parenting. Often, the loss of employment can significantly increase the amount of time that a parent spends with their children. This can be a challenging situation for all, but also has the potential to enable more fulfilling close relationships to develop.

It is not only the trajectory of recovery of the brain-injured parent that affects the challenges faced by the family, but also the developmental stage of the children, and the consequent changing dynamics within the family. For example, in a family where Dad has sustained an acquired brain injury when his two daughters are aged two and six years, the challenges might be mainly around practical management, helping the children to understand the injury in simple terms, reducing fear, and managing risk. However, in ten years' time, when the daughters are twelve and sixteen, the challenges are new, even if the impact of the ABI itself might not be very different. The explanation of the impact of brain injury that was appropriate ten years ago requires an upgrade, as do the strategies and support offered to Dad to enable him to parent his children through adolescence. Supporting families after parental brain injury requires an approach that recognises the effect of time and life stage, not only of the referred individual, but the family as a whole.

This chapter will:

- consider how to make the organisations we work for welcoming, accepting and supportive of families;
- demonstrate the ways in which parental identity may be affected by ABI and outline ways to support a new beginning for those facing them;
- explore ways in which strains in spousal/partner relationships might affect the parenting dynamic, and consider ways to address these difficulties;
- help to identify the ways younger children, older children, and young people might be affected by parental ABI and consider how to support them.

Start with a family-ready service

I shall begin by considering four levels at which services need to develop a family focus: the overall ethos of the service, its organisational set-up, day-to-day practice, and risk assessment.

Service ethos: working to sustain a resilient family system

Families who achieve better outcomes in the face of difficulties demonstrate certain characteristics that can be described as *resilience*. Resilient families tend to have mutually supportive interrelationships, and authoritative parenting styles. These are the underpinnings of secure, close attachment relationships that confer resilience on the individuals and on the family as a whole (Crittenden, 2006, 2008; Crittenden & Dallos, 2009). Resilience can also be located in the wider social environment, and this is where the service comes in: resilient individuals and families tend to be situated in supportive social networks, and have access to supportive health, social, and educational services.

There is little research on the experiences of families living with parental ABI, but we can learn from research on parenting with other difficulties, such as mental health problems or learning difficulties. As with ABI, the challenges faced in these families go beyond the proximate consequences of individual difficulties: many are constructed socially, in the ways that society and services respond. The *social model of disability* proposes that if appropriate supports were in place, there would not be a disability. Despite this, research highlights multiple problems in the typical approach of services (that might be inadvertently reinforcing the disability rather than removing it). In practice, services tend to focus either on the needs of the adult as an individual, typically adopting a deficit-based model, or on the needs of the children, typically adopting a risk-based model. There is usually little integration between adult and child services. Service users often face prejudice and stigmatisation, not just in their social environments, but also from service staff themselves, who make assumptions of incompetence in parenting, often without appropriate justification.

There is, however, evidence for the efficacy of a strengths-based resilience approach in supporting these families. Such an approach is grounded in the three main dimensions of resilience, focusing on (1) identifying and developing resilience factors within the individual parents and children (such as flexibility and coping strategies); (2) resilience factors within the family (such as attachment relationships); (3) supporting the family in maintaining social integration and networks. Interventions using this approach seek to develop existing strengths to the point where parenting is good enough to yield positive outcomes.

Health and social care policy-making has moved towards this kind of approach (Commission for Social Care Inspection, 2006; McGaw & Newman, 2005; Morris, 2003). The Think Family initiative, in particular (Social Exclusion Task Force, 2007), provided strong support for a resilience focus. Its report encouraged services to work together in an integrated way to provide seamless services to support families affected by multiple problems. Think Family advocated that services should no longer consider individual service-users in isolation, but "think family" and see individuals in context as members of their family unit. This led to the radical concept that the family, rather than the individual, should become the client. Thus, the starting point for services working with parents with ABI is the adoption of a resilience-focused, "think family" ethos.

Organisational set up

Build a system to identify and provide appropriate support for clients who are parents, right at the start.

In order to offer timely and appropriate support to parents and their families, it is essential that they are identified as soon as they enter the service. From the point of referral, information needs to be gathered.

- Is the client a parent?
- What are the ages of the children?
- Do the children have any particular support needs?
- Do the children live with the client?
- Does anyone else live with them?
- Who has day-to-day care/parental responsibility for the children?

These questions can be raised on a referral form or during an initial assessment.

It is also important that service-users are made aware at an early stage, in a sensitive, comforting manner, that the service addresses family issues and parenting concerns. There are two things to watch out for here, however.

1. At the mention of parenting support, some parents might be worried that you have a safeguarding concern about their children, or that you might try to remove the children from their care.
2. Adjusting to an ABI is a long and bumpy journey, and families vary in the timing of their readiness to address different issues.

Given these issues to be mindful of, professionals should take time to explain that support for parenting is offered universally across the service, and consideration should be given to the timing of delivering and reminding families of this information.

If you are working within a residential setting for those with ABI, it is important to have clear and carefully thought-through policies regarding child visiting to the unit and parenting support for parents with an ABI. Much of this chapter will consider issues salient to the development of such guidelines.

Provide specialist ABI-experienced parenting support

The key to implementing a "think-family" ethos within the organisation is to recognise the need for specialist ABI-experienced parenting support. Policymakers have recognised that, where support for families and parenting is concerned, there is often a significant skills deficit in adults' services. Staff can "lack confidence and experience in addressing the needs of parents" (Morris & Wates, 2006, p. 6).

Parenting training would be particularly valuable for clients who spend more time with their children post-ABI—for instance, if they are no longer working. While parenting support is available, for instance, from Children's Centres, it is typically offered by childcare professionals who have no experience of ABI. On the other hand, brain injury services, which have specialist skills in supporting individuals with ABI, are less experienced in delivering parenting support (but see Weatherhead & Newby, 2008 for a small scale group-based example, and see Walsh, Weatherhead, Calvert, & Newby's Chapter Nine, on group working, in this volume).

One way to address this problem is to build links with local children's services. A good way to begin is to offer to deliver some training on the effects of ABI, so that their staff will be more aware of the issues should they work with a family in this situation. It might then be possible to request some training in return, on ways to support children or young people in distress at different developmental stages. This kind of reciprocal training not only develops knowledge and skills, it also builds inter-service relationships and develops awareness of the services available on both sides.

Develop a network of family/parenting expert patients to demonstrate positive changes in families after ABI

Parents with an ABI find it helpful to hear about or meet other parents who have experienced something similar. There is significant value in facilitating groups for parents with an ABI. They enable parents to share their fears, to see that others have experienced similar fears, and to see that others are getting through them. Recruiting "expert patient" families (those feeling more confident in managing the challenges, and happy to support others by sharing their experience) can provide an effective resource.

Day-to-day practice

Facilitating peer support between service-users (using the "network of expert patient families")

Service users benefit from spending time together. Those in the early stages of recovery often feel comforted by seeing that positive change, adaptation, and growth are all possible, and feel boosted by gaining ideas about how to get there. Those in the later stages often gain fulfilment from helping others, and from recalling how far they have come in the recovery process. This can take place in the context of informal, opportunistic get-togethers (see Yeates & Daisley, Chapter Eleven in this volume), group sessions, or facilitated pair meetings.

Sometimes, particularly in the earlier stages of recovery, service-users might not feel ready for meeting face to face, but would still benefit from hearing about the experiences of others in another way. The stories of "expert patients" can be provided as written information, or even as short films on DVD or the service's website.

These activities do not require large resources or significant time involvement relative to the benefits they provide, so they are ideal approaches for small community services. They are often the aspects of support that service users report the most benefit from.

Changing the type of support as needs change over time

As we know, supporting individuals with ABI is not like treating a broken leg. A broken leg might require surgery, and then physiotherapy, but there comes a point when the leg is relatively fixed and formal care is no longer needed. The road towards recovery from ABI could not be more different. When we first meet our service users, we might be supporting them to communicate, to manage basic physical manoeuvres, and to understand what has happened to them. Subsequently, we might be supporting them in accessing benefits, adjusting to life without driving, and devising strategies to deal with cognitive deficits. Later still, we might find ourselves supporting a client who has returned to work, but has just acquired a new boss who does not accept their particular needs at work.

We accept that this type of work does not follow a regular pattern. Community neuro-rehabilitation services may often operate an open-door policy for former service users who are discharged but later require some further support for one reason or another.[1] This is often a necessity due to the residual problem-solving difficulties suffered by clients: problems build up, are not solved, and can lead to periodic crises for some. Such an open-door approach is also ideal for *families* affected by parental brain injury. Just as the individual with ABI needs different support at different points in the recovery process, so, too, do families affected by parental brain injury. This is not just in relation to the process of the parent's recovery, but also due to the changing developmental needs of children and young people and family units over time.

In my research exploring participants' experiences of being a parent with ABI, families sharing their stories with me have demonstrated some of the changing developmental needs within families affected by brain injury (Skippon, Newby, & Simpson, n.d.). These findings illustrate the complex interactions between needs relating to the individual's recovery process after ABI, those of the family's developmental stage, and the impact of changes in all these needs over time.

James' story[2] serves as an example. James talked to me about his experiences of parenting after an acquired injury at work. He found it more difficult to deal with his ABI as his children became older, as he felt cognitively "outstripped" by them. The children had been pre-school- and primary school-aged at the time of James' brain injury. Despite his ABI, he had initially still felt able to assist them in schoolwork, and undertake general parenting through support, instruction, and advice. However, as his children entered their teens, James reported feeling he could no longer offer that level of practical support as he felt his children were more "able" than he was in their thinking skills. James gave a number of examples:

- The children became better able than James to weigh up complex information, such as deciding which GCSE options to choose. James found it difficult to remember the different options, to

evaluate their pros and cons, and to think about the consequences of the decisions.
- The children became more able than James to remember and integrate prior knowledge and new information. On one occasion, they were travelling to a new place as a family, and became lost *en route*. Prior to his ABI, James would have prided himself on being best placed within the family to resolve this. However, post ABI, he felt panicked and overwhelmed. By contrast, his teenage children proved more skilled at remembering signs they had seen, used their mobile phones to find directions, and synthesised all of the information to find the destination.
- James also noticed the skills of his children eclipsing his own in following and managing sophisticated social interactions, especially at wider family get-togethers and in using social media.

Initially, the impact of all this, as James struggled to find a way to remain meaningfully involved in parenting, was that he tried to impose more of what he *could* offer upon the children. This took the form of more authoritarian parenting, becoming more focused on discipline, and limiting the children's independence. However, as the children reached the ages at which young people seek to develop more independence and define their own identities outside of the family, this approach to parenting began to conflict with their changing needs.

Over time, James and his family were helped by his community rehabilitation team to understand these changes. With their help, he found alternative ways in which he could fulfil a meaningful father role that was appropriate to the developmental stages of his children. He found that his children valued the personal qualities and strategies that he had demonstrated in coping with his ABI (determination, focus on goals, not dwelling on the past, sense of humour, treating challenges as an adventure). By finding ways to share and instil these qualities and skills in his children in the context of their own lives, James found he could strengthen his relationships with them and offer a different kind of parenting that was both helpful and meaningful for all.

I shall return to these issues later in the chapter, but a first step for clinicians is to understand that parents' and families' needs for support will not follow a predictable linear path, and to prepare to adapt their practice flexibly accordingly.

Risk Assessment

Resilience focus supports effective risk assessment

In supporting families affected by parental brain injury, professionals will often be called on to consider risk assessments in terms of the family situation, most commonly being asked to comment on an ABI person's parenting capacity. Assessment of capacity has been discussed elsewhere in this book, but requires mention here, as parenting is a complex activity, is not easy to assess, and might risk compromising the therapeutic relationship. There is little published guidance on how to carry out parenting capacity assessments in the context of ABI. Edwards (2011) carried out a systematic review of the ABI clinical and research literature to see what could be gleaned to inform practice in this complex area. Not surprisingly, he concluded that there was no one, single, comprehensive tool for assessing parenting capacity in the context of ABI and that many different assessment tools were employed (including standardised neuropsychological tests, various popular mood scales, and a range of family assessment schedules). He recommended that the overall approach to assessment should be systemic and that the individual members of the family, as well as the family as a whole, should be considered within the different contexts in which they function. This requires an assessment of how the parents themselves function (impairments and strengths), children's functioning (advice from local child and adult mental health services/paediatrics might be required), how the family as a whole is managing, their social context, and the support and resources available to them.

Current policy dictates that parental needs relating to their difficulties should be addressed before making judgements about parenting capacity (Morris & Wates, 2006). The issue should be whether the parent has capacity to parent effectively *if supported appropriately*. Assessing parenting skills *without* appropriate support being in place prior to the assessment, particularly where this might influence the residency of a child, is probably unethical. In the context of brain injury services, this means that when we undertake any risk assessment of the likely impact of parental brain injury on the children, this should follow on from the provision of appropriate support for the family. For example, a parent with an ABI who has difficulties with organising day-to-day activities and remembering important information should be helped to develop effective strategies and systems around the home and further afield (using mobile phone reminders/ alarms, timetables, diaries/planners, visual cues by the front door to remember to lock up and take keys, etc.). All of this should be supported to be developed, implemented, and road-tested *prior to* an assessment of their parenting ability.

In families affected by parental disability, children often will not disclose their own needs, or their caring roles, for fear of removal to local authority care. Developing a trusting relationship with both parents and children enables the clinician to demonstrate that their service supports the family as a whole. In this environment, the family members are more likely to be open about the extent to which they need support, and be more accepting of its provision. In turn, this will facilitate a more accurate risk assessment, which will serve to protect each of the family members and the family as a whole.

Identity as a parent

I now turn to some of the specific issues that can affect a person with ABI who is also a parent.

Practical difficulties

Practical difficulties can present a significant barrier to parents with ABI being able to fulfil a meaningful parenting role with their children. However, barriers can be overcome, or the task adapted slightly. Forward planning or structuring the activities can often be enough to make them more manageable. It is important to explore all avenues creatively before accepting defeat on parental involvement (for example, if the parent cannot drive, is the bus, train, or walking possible? Even if it is just for one journey per week, it could be rewarding for both the child and parent to facilitate involvement in the school run).

Case managers are now commonly involved in the care of people with an ABI. Where this is the case, they have a duty to support any parenting role that individual might have. For instance, provision and funding can be made available to ease many practical aspects of parenting. This can be from a one-off purchase for adapted equipment to the provision of parent-directed nanny/*au pair* support to help the parent continue to live with and maintain involvement in the care of their child, even when there are significant practical barriers to this.

Voluntary and local statutory agencies such as Sure Start (where available) can also sometimes offer practical help to families to enable them to stay together and facilitate effective parenting. For example, such agencies might be able to provide a support worker who could do household chores such as washing and ironing for a few hours per week that would enable the parent with brain injury to manage their fatigue and be more available to their children.

This is another good reason for developing and maintaining good links with local agencies, so you will be familiar with, and more successful in, accessing the support available for parents with ABI in your area.

What does it mean to be a parent?

Becoming a parent can be one of the most exciting, daunting, talked about, looked-forward-to aspects of human experience. We all have expectations about what being a parent should be like, and our own personal idea about the type of parent we want to be.

Parents-to-be often fantasise about the life of their child and the role they will play within it. This might be playing football together in the park, reading stories at bedtime, or proudly making a speech at the child's wedding in the distant future. When the fulfilment of these expectations becomes threatened through ABI, the very idea of what it means to be a parent might be called into question. Parents with ABI who feel they fall short of their prior expectations of the parenting role are at risk of depression, and isolation from family life. To support families, it is essential that we recognise the importance of these individualised expectations of parenting, and the impact they might be having.

The route to the best outcomes for both parents and children is a meaningful re-engagement with, and redefinition of, the parenting role. This can be achieved by re-exploring the fundamentals of what is important in being a parent. A father of two young children, who was finding it difficult to adjust to his altered parenting role post ABI, particularly in relation to some physical limitations he was experiencing, told me, "To me, teaching her to ride a bike *is* Dad."

It struck me how profoundly and specifically his idea of the role of Dad was embedded in his thinking. His distress was centred not on the fact of his physical limitations, but on the effect they had on his ability to fulfil the role he felt he should play.

Addressing these kinds of issues requires sensitivity and creativity. Understanding what an activity represents can often be the key to finding an alternative that could represent the same component of parenting. For example, underneath the story of not being able to teach his daughter to ride her bike, we might discover that this act represents the belief that Dads should help their children have a sense of adventure. Knowing this, it might be possible to find other activities that this Dad could do with his daughter that reflect this broader goal: camping, or having a barbecue on the beach, or identifying insects while pond dipping. The possibilities are endless, if you are willing to be creative. The key point is to get to the heart of the *personal individual meaning* of the role of parent.

Parenting positives after brain injury

Families who are able to address the types of issues described above, and who are able to work together to develop resilience within the family, often report benefits and growth that would not have occurred without the experience of ABI. In the limited research that has been conducted on this subject, some families have reported deeper levels of connectedness and warmth in their relationships following parental brain injury. (Charles, Butera-Prinzi, & Perlesz 2007; Skippon, Newby, & Simpson, n.d.). Similar experiences of a positive side have been reported in other populations who have experienced adversity (Cordova, Cunningham, Carlson, & Andrykowski, 2001; Lundwall, 2002; Mohr et al., 1999; Pollard & Kennedy, 2007; Powell, Ekin-Wood, & Collin, 2007).

We can understand this in a number of ways.

1. Post-trauma growth: the brain injured parent and those around them, having had a brush with fear and loss, appreciate more keenly what they have. This might lead to family members acting more appreciatively to each other.
2. The process of having to think about family interactions and communicate more openly, necessitated by working on rehabilitation,

can lead to more trusting, authentic, and co-operative family relationships.
3. Families might gain a new-found appreciation and respect for one another by recognising how each has marshalled their own inner resources to manage their personal share of the challenges faced by the family. This might lead to an altered style of interacting based on the new-found level of respect.
4. It might be that, owing to changes in occupation or daily activity, family members are thrust into spending more time together. This might lead to enjoying being able to share more of their lives together.
5. Getting creative about how to redefine the role of parent in a way that fits with the strengths and difficulties of the parent post ABI can lead to more fun and emphasis on doing meaningful things together.

Each of these might, in turn, lead to closer relationships and a more satisfying and comforting family environment.

Enabling parents with ABI and their families to learn about the positive possibilities post ABI can be crucial in setting them on to the path to a brighter future. As discussed elsewhere in this chapter, sharing the stories of others who have travelled a similar path can be the best way to do this.

Supporting partners and the parenting dynamic

Issues can also arise for the partner of the parent with ABI, or in the relationship between them. As part of the resilience-focused, think-family approach, we need to be alert to the needs of partners and the role they play in the family post brain injury.

Good enough parenting

Healthy and successful parenting is often a function of the delicate balance achieved between recognising one's limitations and trying to achieve parenting goals resiliently and determinedly, despite any difficulties. The concept of "good enough parenting", first developed by

Winnicott (1965) in the context of mother–infant interactions, and subsequently expanded to parenting of older children, reflects this idea. In Winnicott's picture, optimal parenting involves responding to the child's immediate needs in a "good enough" way, by progressively moving away from an instant and complete response, leading to the development of healthy independence in the child. Subsequently, the concept has been developed to reflect the recognition that parents do not have to be perfect, or to be able to meet every need the child has, every time, in order to parent effectively. This is important for families where parents have additional needs such as ABI. The family needs to have, or be supported to attain, sufficient resilience to enable good enough parenting despite the additional needs that the ABI causes.

Understanding and working with partners' concerns, supporting risk assessment

At times, partners might have concerns about the ability of the injured parent to care for their children, or even concerns about the safety of the children. It is always important to listen to partners: often they have the most accurate information available, and they are the ones on hand to deal with the consequences of any problems. Information from them is vital to an accurate assessment and development of a package of support for the family.

However, it is unsurprising that the shock of seeing a loved one experience ABI, and witnessing the variety of physical and cognitive challenges they then face, can make partners anxious about the safety of children left alone with an injured partner. Normal expectations of "good enough parenting" might be replaced by higher than normal standards, "just in case", to "make sure, given everything" that the children are safe.

Supporting partners to develop an informed judgement of both the limitations and the preserved skills of their loved one can enable the injured parent to continue to have a meaningful parenting role, while reassuring the partner. We can do this by working with both parents to identify and address specific concerns. For example, a partner might say, "He forgets to turn the oven off after using it". A specific plan could be offered to address the issue, such as using an oven timer, and a reminder flash card to turn the oven off when the alarm sounds. Using this method, we are reassuring the partner or carer with a structured, systematic method, which can be tested out, and we are also enabling the injured parent to demonstrate and build on their preserved skills in order to fulfil a meaningful parenting role. Crucially, such approaches can also safeguard children against becoming "parent watchers" (perhaps from having to report back to the non-injured parent on how the injured parent had been "performing") and, thus, maintaining appropriate family hierarchies and the balance of power, authority, and responsibility.

Partner burnout

The stresses on partners of parents with ABI can be high. Often they are responsible for caring for the injured individual, caring for the children, and managing the emotional distress of each, and they might have rapidly become the sole breadwinner for the family and be juggling with financial difficulties. Because of all the extra responsibilities, and because friends and wider family might be unsure how to support them, the partner could be left socially isolated, with limited opportunities for personal emotional support.

Carer assessments should be standard practice and regularly reviewed. There are also practical ways in which partners can be supported.

- Provision of timely, accurate information about the nature of the ABI, its effects, and the potential challenges on the path to recovery.
- Involving them in transparent, collaborative risk assessment.
- Signposting to other relevant services, for example, Citizens Advice Bureau, for support in accessing benefits, etc.
- Encouraging independent activities away from the family responsibilities and other forms of self-care; the effect of being given "permission" to care for themselves can be significant.
- Facilitating access to carer groups or meetings for peer support.
- If needed, suggesting a visit to the GP to access counselling or other talking therapies, which might help the individual cope with their situation.

Managing parenting after relationship breakdown

Separation or divorce is not uncommon after ABI. When relationships break down, ex-partners might behave towards each other in ways that are not pleasant, and that can lead to difficulties in managing contact arrangements with children. Some parents with ABI experience significant problems with negative behaviours from their ex-partners, and exploitation of their injury-related difficulties.

Services can provide appropriate interventions that can smooth the transition for both the injured parent and the children affected by the break-up. For example, a service might support the injured parent with strategies to manage the practicalities of contact arrangements with the children. A trusting and open relationship between services and families can increase the likelihood that such interventions are possible, and successful.

Supporting families affected by parental ABI through relationship breakdowns can, however, be stressful for the clinicians involved. They might find themselves torn between the separating couple, or feel pressure to become involved in issues outside of their professional remit. It is essential that the services manage this risk to its clinicians. Such issues should be addressed in clinical supervision, and supervisors should be alert to the need to address them. It might also be helpful to have one member of the team focusing on the rehabilitation needs of the individual, and another focusing on the family needs. Strategies such as these can help to remove or share the emotional burden (Webster, Daisley, & King, 1999).

Working with younger children

Working with children who have been affected by parental ABI can be daunting; most services (and ABI professionals' training) are predominantly adult focused and, without adequate published guidelines, it can be difficult to know where to begin. Readers who wish to know more are signposted towards the useful overview provided by Daisley and Webster (2008).

Supporting younger children affected by parental brain injury brings with it specific challenges and opportunities. This section will consider how best to work with these in order to support the whole family optimally.

Safeguarding the attachment relationship

Attachment relationships are central to effective emotional development and stability. We can support attachment relationships with the injured parent by minimising separation. Where prolonged separation is inevitable—for instance, where a parent might be in a residential rehabilitation setting—services can enable the child to find meaningful ways to stay in touch with their injured parent, or to feel involved and acknowledged when visiting. This can be achieved, for example, using rehabilitation activities such as writing a letter or email to the child, telephoning/texting, or even sending photos of the parent undertaking their rehabilitation activities.

Separation between child and parent can also mean that the child is cared for by a range of people. While there might be some benefits to this (the child might get special treats or trips out and the uninjured parent might get some respite), it can also lead to the child feeling confused and unsafe. When it is necessary, we could encourage families to consider limiting the number of others involved as far as possible.

Families could also be encouraged to maintain a regular routine for the child. This will enable the child to cope better with the changes happening within the family, because some things about their life remain calm and predictable. Even if the family environment was somewhat unstructured before, it is a good time to bring about a regular routine, as this will also aid the parent with the brain injury.

Children of all ages have been found to benefit from taking small amounts of responsibility within the family and receiving praise when they fulfil their role or duty. The consequent sense of accomplishment, belonging, and independence helps them to develop a healthy self-esteem and sense of identity. It can be helpful to involve the child in the rehabilitation activities of the brain injured parent and the organisation of the household. This can be introduced in many ways. For example, the child could be given a regular household task to complete with the injured parent: something as simple as planning the evening meals for the week and writing them up on a whiteboard (as part of memory strategies for the parent). This could be combined with checking the child's homework planner and organising things such as what day they need to take their sports kit to school. In this way, the child would be involved in the rehabilitation of their parent in a manner that is normalised, and the parent is consolidating their rehabilitation in a relevant parenting task.

However, it is also important to be mindful of the potential for children to become overwhelmed by their role as young carers. Children's responses to involvement should be carefully monitored, and we should sensitively explore their involvement in terms of frequency, duration, and impact on other activities in their lives.

Individual attention is often lost at times of crisis within families. Encouraging both parents to make time for one-to-one attention for each child can help to maintain close bonds between parent and child, and limit feelings of loss and fear. Even a small amount of time to read a story or play with them can yield large rewards in this respect. Beyond this, clinicians could also consider helping such children make contact with young carer support groups if they are locally available (see below).

Understanding the impact of ABI on the parent through the eyes of the child

As well as the commonly recognised difficulties following ABI, such as problems with memory and organisational skills, some cognitive impairments can have a profound impact on children, and might be particularly difficult for them to understand. For example,

- decreased sensitivity in interactions (difficulty turn-taking in conversations, problems recognising emotional tone in others' speech, for instance);
- limited tolerance for noise, disruption, and demands of others;
- difficulty in self-monitoring: for example, speaking in a loud voice that children might believe indicates they are angry.

Rehabilitation professionals will often recognise these issues and begin to address them as part of wider rehabilitation. However, when we are aware that a client is a parent, we should also consider the likely effects of these problems on the children and prioritise their needs.

Children whose parents have had a brain injury might feel scared when they first come back into contact. They might have fears that the injury was their fault, or that it might happen again. They might feel fearful or anxious about physical differences they witness in the parent. Provision of age-appropriate information about ABI will help, but some of these concerns can also be addressed by helping the child to connect the changed parent before them with the parent they remember. It is often difficult to find this kind of accessible information and we are often best placed to create it ourselves; in this way, it can be tailored specifically to the needs of the individual child.

It can be helpful to enable a physical connector to the remembered parent to be paired with the parent that is present. For example, the parent can wear clothes that are familiar to the child, or their regular perfume or deodorant, or have on music that the child associates with the parent. These seemingly inconsequential details form the fabric of the security of home and family for children. However, they often become disrupted or changed following the upheaval of brain injury within the family. Professionals supporting such families can unpick them by gently exploring with the family and can explain how familiarity might be helpful for the children.

Supporting the child's emotional reactions and social encounters

Providing accurate, truthful, age-appropriate information about ABI is an important aspect of supporting the emotional wellbeing of children. Children are often more insightful and aware than adults give them credit for, so presentation of information needs to carefully thought out. It is helpful to collaborate with parents and partners, and prepare information that they can deliver either by themselves, or together with the clinician. As children develop, their information needs will change, and the depth and complexity of explanation required increases. We need to be aware of this, and update the information they receive appropriately.

Information might also need to be provided to other social systems in the child's life, for instance, to their school class and teacher, or in social/leisure activity settings that the child might attend (e.g., sports clubs). This can fulfil several purposes: it might help to deal with the barrage of questions and inappropriate comments the child might receive from inquisitive peers, it might increase the likelihood that the child will be able to access peer and adult support when needed, and it might reduce some of the embarrassment or fear that could arise, in both the child and parents, about the injured parent participating in school life (e.g., by attending parent's evenings or school concerts etc.).

The more creatively this is engaged in, the more effective it can be. It might be appropriate for the ABI professional to give a short informal talk about ABI and its effects. Alternatively, the child could be the one, with support, to talk about the ABI experienced by their parent, and perhaps this could be in conjunction with the parent. The possibilities are endless and the potential for gains high. As long as care is taken by the ABI professional to carefully explore families' contexts and regard the feelings of those involved, creative joint therapeutic activities can engender strong senses of ownership and empowerment in participants.

Many children will still find their experience emotionally overwhelming at one time or another. At these times, children should be able to have the space to express their feelings in a calm, sensitive, and encouraging environment. This is not necessarily a role for health professionals. A family member, teacher, or friend is often best placed to enable the child to talk through and make sense of their feelings, which might include guilt, embarrassment, fear, self-blame, resentment, anxiety, loss, isolation, depression, or confusion. However, when clinicians are able to develop trusting relationships with families, they might be able to provide this space for children if it is not available elsewhere. Often, just the experience of expressing feelings, being listened to and not judged, will be enough to help the child work through their difficulties and move forward. If their difficulties are sustained, it might be necessary to access further support from the school counsellor (if available) or to refer the child (via the GP) to their local child and adolescent mental health service (CAMHS) to receive more comprehensive support.

Peer support groups can also be helpful for children coping with their family circumstances. In fact, children might benefit even more than adults, given that peer socialisation is often more salient to children. A neuro-rehabilitation service could provide a group for the children of its service users, or there are many groups already in existence that enable children who are experiencing challenges at home to meet up, have fun, and access peer support. Young carers groups, for example, might offer a variety of activities and opportunities for children of different ages. Children's centres, youth groups, and social services can often put you in touch with these types of services.

Working with older children and young people

Different issues can arise for older children and young people in the family affected by parental brain injury. We will consider here how these challenges can be addressed.

Changing family roles

Older children and young people can often find that their role within the family changes the most. They might find the caring/cared-for relationship between themselves and their injured parent is reversed. However, when caring is inappropriate to a child's level of maturity, there can be adverse consequences. Children might become focused on other people's needs, and less able to attend to their own.

Situations where an older child becomes "parentified" often result from burnout and social isolation in the injured parent's partner. The partner might be seeking the comfort and understanding from the older child that they would have received from the injured parent prior to the ABI. Recognising these issues and enabling both the partner and the older child to access appropriate social support is essential. Young carers' organisations can provide relief, understanding, and peer support for older children and young people.

As with younger children, it is important to work creatively to support the injured parent to find meaningful ways to fulfil a parenting role for the older child or young person. Often, the opportunity for regular one-to-one conversation will be valuable. One-to-one parental attention for children of all ages remains the same after ABI; it is universally welcomed.

The job of being a teenager

Adolescence is a period of identity formation and moving towards independence. It is a time for challenging boundaries, defining new rules, searching for your place, and finding where you fit. These tasks are challenging enough for any teenager and the parents who support them. Success in these endeavours is often dependent on having a secure base to step from and retreat to.

After parental brain injury, it might be that the family no longer feels like a dependable and secure base, or it might no longer feel like a place that it is safe to leave. Young people often feel a sense of responsibility to remain at home in caring roles, sometimes taking life-changing decisions, such as getting a job rather than going to university, to provide financial support at home or to remain living at home when they previously planned to move in with friends. However, they might also experience feelings of resentment at the loss of the life they could have had.

Other challenging emotions that may be experienced by young people include frustration, guilt, and embarrassment. If the young person has limited ways to express these feelings, they might become stressed, low in mood, or their behaviour might become more challenging. Sometimes, they might take advantage of the limitations of their injured parent in order to push boundaries; parents can often find this a very difficult challenge.

The most effective route to managing these difficulties is early identification and maintaining open communication. Regularly exploring the young person's thinking about, and understanding of, the family situation can help with this. Facilitating access to emotional and social support can provide a safe place for young people to think through their future plans, hopes, and expectations. Also, one-step-removed modes, such as emailing, can allow children to express difficult thoughts and feelings at a time of their choosing and in a familiar language and context (see Newby and Coetzer's chapter on electronic media in this volume).

It can also help families to normalise their older child's responses. We could ask, "Would this be happening anyway in our family given the stage we are at/the age of the children etc.?" It is important to help families avoid falling into the situation of viewing all issues through the lens of the parental brain injury.

Explaining, explaining, and revisiting explaining

As with younger children, older children and young people need developmentally appropriate updates to the information and explanation they have about their parent's ABI. Cognitive functions and social competence increase rapidly during adolescence, so, in a short interval, the information needs of the young person could change several times. The rehabilitation professional should be alert to the likelihood of these changes and support the family through them. It is important to remember that emotional distress will reduce the ability of children and young people to take in and act on information they receive. This issue needs to be carefully considered and explored by the professional supporting the family.

Similarly, as young people get older, their wishes and expectations of the support they desire from their parents changes, too. As with parents, it is important to explore the specific personal meaning of being a parent for the young person, in order to support the injured parent to fulfil these wishes in the best way possible.

Conclusion

Working with families affected by parental brain injury can be complex and challenging. However, it also has the potential to make a significant difference to the wellbeing and life course of many. It is hoped that this chapter has provided food for thought in terms of developing awareness of the probable challenges that might be faced, and offered some ideas to start the process of getting stuck in with supporting families.

Notes

1. However, we are aware that in these financially-straightened times, many services are being pushed to discharge clients more quickly and to limit care episodes.
2. "James" is a pseudonym.

Resources

Headway (2009). *Parenting After Brain Injury*. Nottingham: Headway

References

Arango, J., Ketchum, J., Dezfulian, T., Kreutzer, J., O'Neil-Pirozzi, H. F., & Jha, A. (2008). Predictors of marital stability two years following brain injury. *Brain Injury*, 22(7–8): 565–574.

Charles, N., Butera-Prinzi, F., & Perlesz, A. (2007). Families living with acquired brain injury: a multiple family group experience. *Neuro-Rehabilitation, 22*: 61–76.
Commission for Social Care Inspection (2006). *Supporting Parents, Safeguarding Children: Meeting the Needs of Parents with Children on the Child Protection Register*. Newcastle: Commission for Social Care Inspection.
Cordova, M. J., Cunningham, L. L., Carlson, C. R., & Andrykowski, M. A. (2001). Posttraumatic growth following breast cancer: a controlled comparison study. *Health Psychology, 20*(3):176–185.
Crittenden, P. M. (2006). A dynamic–maturational model of attachment. *Australian and New Zealand Journal of Family Therapy, 27*: 105–115.
Crittenden, P. M. (2008). *Raising Parents: Attachment, Parenting, and Child Safety*. Cullompton, Devon: Willan.
Crittenden, P. M., & Dallos, R. (2009). All in the family: integrating attachment and family systems theories. *Clinical Child Psychology and Psychiatry, 14*(3): 389–409.
Daisley, A., & Webster, G. (2008). Familial brain injury: impact and interventions with children. In: A. Tyerman & N. King (Eds.), *Psychological Approaches to Rehabilitation after Traumatic Brain Injury* (pp. 475–508) Oxford: Blackwell.
Department of Health (2001). *Making the Change: A Strategy for the Professions in Healthcare Science*. London: NHS Executive.
Department of Health (2005). *The National Service Framework for Long-Term Conditions*. London: DoH Publications.
Edwards, A. (2011). Parenting capacity after acquired brain injury: a systematic review. Unpublished Doctoral Thesis, Oxford University
Kreutzer, J., Marwitz, J., Hsu, N., Williams, J., & Riddick, A. (2007). Marital stability after brain injury: an investigation and analysis. *NeuroRehabilitation, 22*(1): 53–59.
Lundwall, R. (2002). Parents' perceptions of the impact of their chronic illness or disability on their functioning as parents and on their relationships with their children. *The Family Journal: Counselling and Therapy for Couples and Families, 10*(3): 300–307.
McGaw, S., & Newman, T. (2005). *What Works for Parents with Learning Disabilities*. London: Barnardo's.
Mohr, D. C., Dick, L. P., Russo, D., Pinn, J., Boudewyn, A. C., Likosky, W., & Goodkin, D. E. (1999). The psychosocial impact of multiple sclerosis: exploring the patient's perspective. *Health Psychology, 18*(4): 376–382.

Morris, J. (2003). *The Right Support: Report of the Task Force on Supporting Disabled Parents in their Parenting Role.* York: Joseph Rowntree Foundation.

Morris, J., & Wates, M. (2006). *Supporting Disabled Parents and Parents with Additional Support Needs.* London: Social Care Institute for Excellence.

Oddy, M., Coughlan, T., Tyerman, A., & Jenkins, D. (1985). Social adjustment after closed head injury: a further follow-up seven years after injury. *Journal of Neurology, Neurosurgery and Psychiatry, 48*: 564–568.

Pollard, C., & Kennedy, P. (2007). A longitudinal analysis of emotional impact, coping strategies and post-traumatic psychological growth following spinal cord injury: a 10-year review. *British Journal of Health Psychology, 12*: 347–362.

Powell, T., Ekin-Wood, A., & Collin, C. (2007). Post-traumatic growth after head injury: a long-term follow-up. Brain Injury, 21(1): 31–38.

Skippon, R. H., Newby, G., & Simpson, J. (n.d). The experience of being a parent with acquired brain injury. Manuscript awaiting acceptance.

Social Exclusion Task Force (2007). *Reaching Out: Think Family. Analysis and Themes from the Families at Risk Review.* London: Cabinet Office.

Tate, R., Lulham, J. M., Broe, G. A., Strettles, B., & Pfaff, A. (1989). Psychosocial outcome for the survivors of severe blunt head injury: the result from a consecutive series of 100 patients. *Journal of Neurology, Neurosurgery and Psychiatry, 52*: 1128–1134.

Urbach, J. R., & Culbert, J. P. (1991). Head injured parents and their children: psychological consequences of a traumatic syndrome. *Psychosomatics, 32*: 24–33.

Weatherhead, S. J., & Newby, G. (2008). Supporting dads: a parenting programme for fathers with an acquired brain injury. *Clinical Psychology Forum, 182*: 36–39.

Webster, G., & Daisley, A. (2005). A family resource pack for working with children affected by familial acquired brain injury. *Clinical Psychology, 46*: 26–29.

Webster, G., & Daisley, A. (2007). Including children in family focused acquired brain injury rehabilitation: a national survey of practice. *Clinical Rehabilitation, 21*(12): 1097–1109.

Webster, G., Daisley, A., & King, N. (1999). Relationship and family breakdown following acquired brain injury: the role of the rehabilitation team. *Brain Injury, 13*(8): 593–605

Winnicott, D. W. (1965). *The Maturational Processes and the Facilitative Environment.* New York: International Universities Press.

Wood, R. L., & Yurdakul, L. K. (1997). Change in relationship status following traumatic brain injury. *Brain Injury, 11*: 491–502.

PART III

WORKING WITH PROFESSIONAL AND ORGANISATIONAL SYSTEMS

CHAPTER THIRTEEN

Leading a community acquired brain injury team: the South Cheshire experience

Beth Fisher

I ought to begin by congratulating the readers (especially the managers among you) who have turned to this chapter. This is not because I would claim that the chapter is the last word in all things managerial. Rather, I wish to congratulate you because you have found time to do some reading and self-development. Managers should lead by example. Including the often near impossible juggling skills required of those working in healthcare environments to carve out time for continuing professional development (CPD).

Having and growing a culture of continuous development for your team, comes from "walking the walk", not just "talking the talk". However, if you are also flicking through your emails and filling in your travel claim form while hanging on for a GP practice to answer the telephone at the same time as reading this, please remember that ring-fenced time for CPD (see Chapter Fourteen, by Newby and Weatherhead, in this volume) is just as important as on-the-job multi-tasking. Do you book reading or development time into your diary as a matter of course for the year ahead, or does it happen by chance? Do you (as I sometimes do) book other, usually client-related, things into that time because it is higher priority?

Bearing your time pressures in mind, I have made reference to some key ideas and have pointed readers to some key managerial texts. However, in the vein of "walking the walk", my main aim in this chapter is to lay down some of my reflections from being a manager in a community acquired brain injury service and to share some ideas, resources, and insights that I hope will help busy managers/team leaders in performing their roles.

Reflections on my initiation in acquired brain injury management

It is ten years since I was appointed to the role of Acquired Brain Injury Service Manager for South Cheshire Health Authority. I vividly recall being shown into an empty building (due to be sold for demolition) and taken up a Victorian staircase to an empty top floor room—my new office! The saving grace was that I was with Dr Richard Warburg, Consultant Neuropsychologist, who proved to be, on that first day, personable, professional, and entirely positive. We were given a list of names of patients to relocate closer to their family, some key people to speak to in commissioning and clinical services, and a budget of £80,000.

To this day, the management and leadership challenges remain the same. In retrospect, those formative first few hours encapsulated the key and recurring challenges of successful service management.

- *Recruitment.* Get the best staff you can across all grades; work hard at recruitment to get a group of enthusiastic and effective professionals.
- *Cap activity levels.* This is particularly important if you have service level agreements/contracts with key performance indicators to deliver on. Know your referral rates and expected activity levels per week for both direct and indirect contacts.
- *Find the right accommodation.* Plan for the right location, size, and accessibility. Use business continuity plans or service assurance frameworks to raise risks around accommodation. Have a specification of your ideal space to hand should the opportunity arise to relocate.

- *Show that your service can meet clients/carers needs.* Make good use of qualitative as well as quantitative outcome measures. Carry out and report on service user audits annually. Report all compliments upwards to governance teams.
- *Develop a network.* We cannot work in isolation if our services are to deliver holistic client centred goals (see Tip 17).
- *Good budget management.* Plan realistically and be cost effective. Savings can be made on skill mixing where appropriate, but do not forget to look at income generation opportunities.
- *Facilitate development.* Standing still and maintaining the status quo is not an option.

Trait theory and leadership

The National Leadership Council (NLC) Emerging Leaders Survey (2011) lists the top three leadership traits as: integrity, inspiration, and vision. It also lists the following as abilities leaders in the NHS should have:

- the ability to utilise, galvanise, and incorporate people talents, skills, and knowledge;
- a hands-on approach;
- a superior breadth of experience both inside and outside the NHS;
- a commitment to patients.

The fact that I turned up for day two goes some way to confirm a key leadership trait: leaders tend not to walk away from a challenge. I will not, however, review the plethora of leadership/management models; Hersey and Blanchard's Situational Leadership; Blake and Moutons Managerial Grid, and Fielders Contingency Model and many more can be reviewed on the Internet. A good general site to start with is 1MindTools.com (2011). I am also avoiding the management *vs.* leadership debate. The "more for less" current economic ethos probably means 99% of you will have elements of both in your working day. I also concur wholeheartedly with the following: "Good management is the art of making problems so interesting and their solutions so constructive that everyone wants to get to work to deal with them" (Hawken, 1988, p. 39).

Leading an acquired brain injury team in the modern NHS: an overview

I like the following definition of a team: "A team is a small number of people with complementary skills who are committed to a common purpose, performance goals and approach for which they hold themselves mutually accountable" (Katzenbach & Smith, 1993).

I have assumed that most readers are managing an existing team. If, however, you are starting from scratch, then use British Society of Rehabilitation Medicine Guidelines for staffing levels (British Society of Rehabilitation Medicine (BSRM), 2009). These are based on minimum staffing levels per million of population: one team leader/co-ordinator, three physiotherapists, five occupational therapists, two speech and language therapists, two clinical psychologists/neuropsychologists and 1.2 medical consultants in rehabilitation.

Many of you will no doubt be smiling ironic smiles at the idea of this being a "minimum" standard, given that many community services are staffed at well below these levels with no realistic prospect of increase in the foreseeable future. Ringfence a number of weeks for mapping patient pathways. Then invite key staff from that pathway to some workshops to prioritise areas for your team's intervention and to formally launch the service. I recommend checking last year's complaints reports to see if any major issues were raised for ABI clients. Make sure you get some direct client and carer input. Do not rush to recruit the full team at once. Recruit to two or three key roles and then involve these staff in the second tranche of recruitment some months in. You are building a team. It takes time, and senior staff like to have a say in choosing their team. Start a service database from the outset, even if it means a paper exercise until you get your IT systems in place. Finally, contact an existing brain injury service and arrange to visit. Learn from their journey.

Practical tips on leading a community acquired brain injury team

As the service manager, you are responsible for creating the collective vision of what your service is about. It used to be called your "mission statement". Now, you are more likely to have service objectives. You have to impart how your organisation's key objectives relate to your specific service, how the service functions within your organisation, and what it has to deliver on. Hold an overview, set targets, and guide how the team will move forward. Therefore, to provide a conceptual framework on leading, I have grouped my tips as follows.

- Self-management: tips 1–6.
- Leading the team: tips 7–15.
- Networking and profile: tips 16–20.

Self-management

Tip 1: Find something to praise on a daily basis

It can be the norm for managers to be involved in reactive crisis management, conflict resolution, and problem solving negative situations. You will be the "go to" person for the team with all the niggles, failures, complaints, and issues they might bring. There have been days when I asked myself, "What did I actually achieve today?" I will have spent it fire-fighting an unexpected client-related problem, listening to staff, or filling in an Excel spreadsheet that just has to be returned with a twenty-four-hour, last-minute turnaround. Proactively, look for a positive. It is good for you and it will certainly be rewarding for the recipient of your praise. A genuine "thank you "or a "well done" are never out of place, and finding a positive on some days will be a welcome pick-me-up.

Tip 2: Check your in-house learning and development programme and either start or refresh your leadership skills.

My clinical qualifications certainly did not cover managerial or leadership skills. Therefore, I highly recommend checking out your in-house training modules. Most NHS posts graded at Band 7 and above are considered for professional development, clinical leadership, and quality courses (e.g., see the NHS Institute for Innovation and Improvement (2011) website based module). Leadership training will cover recruitment and selection, staff development, continuity planning, risk assessment, complaints, sickness, and capabilities management, budget/financial management, and much more. Joint working with many local universities now means there is also a range of leadership courses that are accredited towards a postgraduate qualification. Ask your learning and development team, or check with your local university prospectus. If you are an "old hand", can you mentor a new manager? Do you need a refresher on any of the key areas? Who in the team has deputising responsibilities and have you briefed them well enough? If you do not have a deputy, ask yourself why not. How can you go about creating one or more? (See Tip 4.)

Tip 3: Do a self-assessment on the NHS leadership website

How do you personally manage/lead? Ask yourself how you deal with conflict. Who you are and what you set as standards of behaviour, work ethic, professionalism, and working atmosphere will have a direct impact and influence your team on a daily basis. Emotional intelligence is often discussed as being a key skill for good leaders: empathy, trust. Self-awareness and interpersonal insight are both key to emotional intelligence.

The psychologists among the management community have a good headstart in the area of self-awareness, but to the rest of the professions out there, do not be put off. Self-awareness is a very useful tool, and once you have taken the first step, be brave and ask your line manager, a peer, and some team members to score you (National Leadership Council, 2011). The trick here is how you keep this anonymous. The commercial world and recruitment agencies have used these 360-degree tools for a long time. How do others see us? Does your team see you as a pushover? Do your peers think you take your fair share of the management burden? Does your line manager have faith in your abilities?

The NHS Leadership Framework was launched in June 2011 (National Leadership Council, 2011) and covers demonstrating personal qualities, working with others, managing services, improving services, setting direction, creating a vision, and delivering on strategy.

Tip 4: Ask yourself what you can stop doing

Good delegation is a key skill for successful management. It will most probably be clinical team leaders that you are delegating to. Student placements can be delegated to a lead clinician, service volunteers to your lead vocational occupational therapist. Delegate tasks to team members' strengths with shadowing for staff members developing that skill set. Lots of management process tasks, such as sickness returns, equipment orders, and activity statistics can be delegated to efficient administration staff. On numerous occasions, our team secretary, Anne, has saved the day, rebooking rooms, finding case records, dealing with distraught clients or carers, liaising with consultants' secretaries, and keeping the service database operational.

Good administration staff proactively problem solve for clinicians, giving them time to treat, not type. If I have not shouted it from the rooftops yet, I will now. Identify and employ the appropriate level of skilled administration staff. Anne, our team secretary, is one of my personal key enablers. Tannenbaum and Schmidt's (1973) continuum of leadership behaviours looks at increasing team members' responsibilities and how you delegate to encourage staff development. Reviewing what and how you delegate can help highlight whether you are being too controlling, too hands off, or are using an appropriate range and level of delegation across the team. They list seven levels.

1. Manager makes the decision on a task and announces it.
2. Manager "sells" the decision to the team.
3. Manager presents decision with ideas and invites questions.
4. Manager suggests provisional decision and invites discussion.
5. Manager presents the situation, gets suggestions, and decides.
6. Manager explains, defines parameters, and asks team to decide.
7. Manager allows team to develop options and decide on action within the agreed limits.

Good delegation creates that all-precious commodity: time. It develops your team members and builds ownership. Opportunities for delegation or distributed leadership (Spillane & Diamond, 2007) should be reviewed at staff performance reviews.

As a service manager, I find myself with both a clinical and a leadership/management role. I lead from within the team and not from top dowm, and my approach is collaborative and sharing. But I can be, as Gavin, the team's consultant neuropsychologist, has told me, "robust" in my approach when necessary.

What is your management style? And how does that affect your team? Where are you physically in relation to your team? I am based in our one group office, so there is no escaping me! (The redeeming fact for the team is that I am out of the office at least a few times a week.) Are you easily accessible? Do you have an open door policy that is over used, leaving you forever involved in minor disputes, or are you there on a Monday morning and not seen again to the following week?

Tip 5: Ensure you know the key staff in your organisation who can help you in your role as leader/manager

As well as knowing who holds key organisational roles, it is really important to be able to contact them when you need to. I am sure that all of you will have had the frustration of having an introduction to Joan, the Business Development Manager, in a meeting and finding that she was really helpful with a particular issue. Then, as you leave the meeting, you realise you do not know her surname or have a means of contacting her (and, to make matters worse, she is not in the internal directory). As a simple measure, you could build up a contacts list. I have listed the roles that help me and that hold key operational control across the main function areas of my NHS Trust.

- Finance lead.
- Business development manager.
- Procurementcontracts lead.
- Recruitment team.
- Human resources link worker.
- Research and audit lead.
- Clinical governance lead.
- Complaints team.
- Essence of care lead.
- IT department service desk.
- Safeguarding team.
- Other service managers.
- Information team (collates service activity data).
- Directorate manager.
- Communications team.
- Governor.

- Non-executive director.
- Chief executive/managing director.

Being a manager can feel like that old stage act of plate spinning: too busy, pressured, and rushed. However, both the internal organisational roles listed above and external networks can work for you if proactively managed. Find out who is out there to help you in your role of manager/leader within your organisation. How often do you meet with them? Is it only reactively to a negative situation? How can you change that?

I now have monthly finance meetings, which did not happen a few years ago, and it helps to address potential overspends or, indeed, savings in a much more structured manner. It resulted, for example, in the development of our service's "Income generation budget line" and the agreement that I could fund staff training from this income stream.

Tip 6: Clearly differentiate in your diary clinical vs. *management/leadership roles and ringfence time accordingly*

There will always be more demands on your time as a manager/leader, particularly if you are also carrying a clinical caseload. Guard your management time as vehemently as your clinical time. As a clinician at heart, I struggle with this, as already confessed in the Introduction. It is, however, a very positive sign of the team's collaborative approach when my lead OT, Bernie, manages me and does not allow me to fill that management space, pointing out that I am falling into my old habits.

Time management takes up whole chapters in leadership and management books. I, however, am going to refer you again to 1Mind Tools: Essential Skills for an Excellent Career (2011). This site has a good self-assessment guide with links to easy to use tools for areas where you might not have scored well; for example, an action priority matrix or managing interruptions guide. My three top tips with regard to time management would be:

- ensure your secretary filters phone calls;
- limit yourself to review and respond to emails at set times in the day when office bound, rather than being a slave to the binging computer screen;

- declare an unavailable slot in your week where you are free from interruption.

The other time management example you have to set is that of work–life balance. Overworked, over-stressed staff will not produce quality work, and neither will the over-stretched service manager. Make use of time in lieu/compressed hours/annual leave/ flexi-time to help you find the right balance.

Tip 7: Use your "NO" vote carefully and only after active listening

This skill can be under recognised. Pacing your own and your team's activity are vital to delivering a quality service. When you are as lucky as I am to have a team that loves challenges, seeks out new opportunities, and, for the most part, embraces change, you do have to be the one that points out that new tasks/ideas are not necessarily a priority on a whole team plan or that new student placements cannot be accommodated this year owing to other clinical commitments. Having the service work-plan for the year that is shared with all staff helps them better understand the rationale for the "No" that should always be accompanied by a reason.

Team management/leadership

Tip 8: Do not assume one profession knows what and how the other works

What does it mean to manage a community brain injury team? You may be in the private sector or the NHS. You could have occupational therapists, physiotherapists, speech and language therapists, psychologists (who could be clinical, counselling, or neuropsychological by specialism), psychiatrists or other doctors, social workers, nurses, administration staff, care staff, possibly volunteers, and the list could go on. This team will undoubtedly be multi-disciplinary, maybe even inter-disciplinary. Therefore, remember the following.

- Service induction should give new starters a taster session with your key team disciplines.
- Service information leaflet/s should give a brief outline of what each profession delivers. (This is helpful not only for clients/carers, but referrers and commissioners as well.)

- Have routine profession-specific updates at team days to keep the whole team abreast of clinical developments and service delivery.
- Encourage shadowing and joint working on team projects, not just patient treatment.
- Make sure team members explain and share assessment results in a way that is meaningful to all staff. Our technical professional language can so often be used to differentiate our specialities and as a sign of authority and status. All professions have their own unique jargon, so I hope my neuropsychology colleagues do not mind me using a classic from their stable: "his delayed auditory memory falls in the first to the third percentile and he displays signs of attentional capture". I was once told to "say it so your granny would understand", therefore, a translation of the above might go something like this: *he can't remember much of what you tell him and he gets easily distracted*. The latter statement means more to the Band 4 rehabilitation assistant or the nursing auxiliary. The former merely excludes them.

Tip 9: Involve service users/carers/third sector representatives

A service user on an interview panel will provide vital feedback on soft skills and insights you will not have. Recruitment is always an interesting and challenging task. Despite the fact that job descriptions are clearly defined with competency-based key skills frameworks, which identify capability and competency levels in line with grades, I repeatedly find myself assessing the "soft skills" at interview: enthusiasm, openness, empathy, optimism, humility, and, most importantly, evidence of, or the potential for, true team working. Do you need to recruit an independent, strong character to go head to head with the hospital discharge process, or an empathetic listener to deal with family members? It is personality traits that we assess in these contexts, not just qualifications. Do you list any of these soft skills in your essential and desirable criteria on job descriptions, or ask questions at interview to elicit some insight into the candidate's soft skills?

Involving service users needs to be done in an organised and targeted fashion if it is going to be successful for both the service and the users. The NHS Modernisation Agency's top tips for effectively involving and recruiting patients and carers asks you to consider the four Rs: remit, role, relationship, and responsibilities (Department of

Health, 2009). I recommend creating a small core group of service users that you can call on for comments, meetings, talks, etc. This means they, too, then have peer support. Do not be afraid to ask; many users and carers want to give something back. Can they contribute to a "my story" piece for Brain Injury Awareness week? Would they do a video blog for your Trust's intranet? It is also useful to tap into the expertise of your third sector organisations, be that Headway, Brain and Spinal Injuries Charity, or Encephalitis Society, etc. We also undertake an annual service user survey, have final year psychology students on placement who undertake service related research with users and carers, and have a service user volunteer who supports our local user group Head Injured People in Cheshire (also see Walsh and co-authors, Chapter Nine, in this volume).

Tip 10: Ask all staff grades at interview about their experience of team working and how they would deal with a conflict situation

What is it that makes you choose X over Y when, on paper, candidates look equal in experience and expertise? The answer is not to just assess the soft skills, but also to bear in mind the dynamics of the existing team and judge how the new candidate would fit in. I am sure we can all recall from our working lives "the grafter", "the slacker", "the rumour-monger", and "the downright jobsworth". I have, in the past, recruited the wrong people to teams, and it is so pervasively destructive to the working atmosphere, morale, and team effectiveness. Therefore, to reduce the risk of placing a square peg in a round hole, consider Tip 6.

Tip 11: Do you know the answers to the following questions?

- How does my team interact?
- How does my team currently learn?
- How does my team deal with conflict?
- How does my team manage the caseload?
- How does my team deal with failure?
- How does my team deal with a deadline?
- How does my team deal with success?
- How does my team deal with a challenge?

These are my personal key questions. If you know the answers to the above, I believe you will be less likely to recruit the wrong team member and will be in an excellent position to support the new starter in any of the key areas they might find a challenge. One of my other personal monitors of my team's status is whether I hear laughter in the office on a regular basis. I am a strong believer in the ethos that a happy team is a more productive one. Hackman and Oldham (1976) state that three elements need to be present for an employee to be happy in their work.

1. Their work should draw on a variety of the person's skills and abilities.
2. The employee should complete a whole task rather than play a minor role in a big picture.
3. The employee should know that their work has a significant impact on others.

Looking more closely at the actual existing team dynamic, can you answer these questions?

- Who are your key trouble-makers?
- Who leads the anti-change brigade?
- Who is your best researcher?
- Who mediates in team disagreements?
- Who is your hardest worker?
- Who lacks motivation?

Have you ever taken ten minutes to ask yourself questions like this? Do you know who these people are? Use annual reviews to discuss pastoral and work–life balance issue as well as professional performances. Find out what makes your staff tick and have a management plan in place for those names you have put against the questions above. You can, of course, create your own questions for your team. The management plan could be brushing up on your own conflict resolution skills, or sending team members on a course. You could encourage an older team member by asking them to mentor a junior, or deal with an antagonist via peer pressure rather than managerial power. A non-threatening way of helping the team to look at its dynamics is to try Tip 12, below. This exercise does not look at grading or clinical expertise and it is a welcome change for staff members who are performance managed against key skill frameworks.

It is generally considered that teams of 5–12 members is the optimum size. Over this size, teams can become cumbersome and often break down into sub-teams (Knowledge@Whorton, 2006). In a community team, there will most probably be clinical sub-divisions. If so, make sure your project teams are multi-disciplinary: that is, ensure a team identity exists as well as a series of professional identities.

Tip 12: Do a Belbin team role exercise on a team building or training day

Belbin is a UK-based management consultancy and training organisation that has developed a well-regarded theory of team functioning and programme of team improvement exercises (Belbin, 2011). Belbin's theory lists nine key team roles and associated behaviours that might be useful for you to consider. These are outlined below.

1. *Implementer*: conservative, self-discipline, predictable.
   Positive qualities: practical action, efficient.
   Weaknesses: lack of flexibility, unresponsiveness to ideas.
2. *Co-ordinator*: calm, self-confident, controlled.
   Positive qualities: welcoming all potential contributors on their merits and without prejudice. A strong sense of objectives.
   Weaknesses: ordinary in terms of intellect or creative ability.
3. *Shaper*: highly strung, outgoing, dynamic.
   Positive qualities: a readiness to challenge inertia, ineffectiveness, complacency.
   Weaknesses: proneness to provocation, irritation, and impatience.
4. *Plant*: individualistic, serious-minded, unorthodox.
   Positive qualities: genius, imagination, intellect, knowledge.
   Weaknesses: head in the clouds, inclined to disregard practical details.
5. *Resource investigator*: extroverted, enthusiastic, curious, communicative.
   Positive qualities: a capacity for contacting people and exploring anything new. An ability to respond to challenge.
   Weaknesses: liable to lose interest once the fascination has passed.

6. *Monitor–evaluator*: sober, unemotional, prudent.
   Positive qualities: judgement, discretion, hard-headedness.
   Weaknesses: lacks inspiration or the ability to motivate others.
7. *Team worker*: socially orientated, rather mild, sensitive.
   Positive qualities: co-operation, builds team spirit.
   Weaknesses: indecisiveness at moments of crisis.
8. *Completer–finisher*: painstaking, orderly, conscientious, anxious.
   Positive qualities: a capacity for follow through, perfectionism.
   Weaknesses: a tendency to worry about small things; a reluctance to "let go".
9. *Specialist*: seeker of knowledge; single minded.
   Positive qualities: Can be called upon to make decisions based on in-depth experience.
   Weaknesses: contributes on a narrow front.

One staff member may have more than one role within the team over time, but it is interesting to see where colleagues sit and if you have any missing roles among your current staffing. It is a useful tool to help you choose members for service specific projects, either internally or to build networks in bigger organisational projects. My team, however, spotted a glaring omission from Belbin's key team roles: the tea and coffee maker!

Tip 13: Set a yearly timetable of meetings with your team leaders and review standing agenda items

Grow your own agenda. It should include supervision and staff appraisals, sickness levels, annual leave, activity levels, discharge rates, outcome measures, student placements, audit and research, policy review, and development. Check the progress of delegated tasks. Have updates on external factors such as restructuring or the introduction of other teams' new protocols. Rotate the role of chairing the meeting once you have the agenda items set. This team leader meeting is your formal peer support for staff at this grade. However, if your team is small, then ensure your brain injury team leaders have the opportunity to meet with their counterparts from other services.

Tip 14: Review your service activities

Completing business plans, or Excel spreadsheets, having monthly finance meetings, submitting activity statistics on new and discharged clients *vs.* direct and indirect contacts, over time all become quite rote activities. To step away and have a "throw everything on the table" session can be very enlightening and positive if managed well. The interlinking circles model can be used in many ways to look at interfaces between various areas or functions. I divide it up into service, service users, and commissioners when reviewing my team's activities (Figure 13.1).

Develop your own list of elements/processes and monitoring for each circle. Some things might sit in the interface between circles. For example, key performance indicators would sit between commissioners and the service, whereas service user audit would sit in the middle of all three circles. If you do not know where to start, create three subgroups with each one listing independently from the other the processes, policies, or activity for their circle. When you all come back together, overlaps should instantaneously become apparent.

As a rough guide to get you started, in the "Service" circle you could include staffing levels, accommodation, equipment, budget, staff performance reviews, research, student placements, activity reporting, clinical guidelines. In "Services users" could be triage system, risk assessment, lone worker policy, dual diagnosis policy, clinical guidelines, service information leaflets, service user audit, group treatments. In "Commissioners" you could have business continuity plan, audit reporting, service assurance frameworks, or key performance indicators.

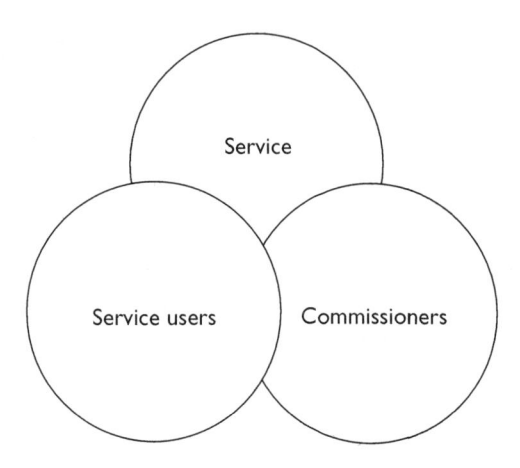

Figure 13.1. The interlinking circles model.

Have you work-streams in all three circles for the services annual work plan? Review strengths and weaknesses. This will feed into or amend your plan. Depending on the size and capacity of your team, agree a work plan with, ideally, an activity in each of the circles. If you are astute, some targets will almost certainly be sitting in the overlapping areas. For example, an audit on your team goal-setting process will sit in the overlap between service and service users. It provides the team with feedback on a clinical process that will benefit the service users. Your results can help to inform the governance committee. It will also build a team profile with the audit and research team. Identify project leads by delegating to team members' strengths. Remember your Belbin roles. Set realistic timelines, making use of Gantt Charts if necessary. Monitor progress at predetermined intervals. These are all good delegation skills. (See also Tip 4.)

Tip 15: Structure team discussions in a positive and managed way

There may be protagonists, over-optimism, or blinkered viewpoints in any team debate. I use Edward de Bono's *Six Thinking Hats* (de Bono Group, 2011) or a smaller version of his model to try to achieve a rounded picture of a situation. It helps to ensure that not only those that shout loudest are heard, and allows the whole team to hear the pros and cons of every argument.

- *White hat*: calls for information known or needed,
- *Red hat*: reports feelings hunches and intuition.
- *Black hat*: acts as devil's advocate.
- *Yellow hat*: optimism.
- *Green hat*: thinks creatively, looks at alternatives.
- *Blue hat*: manages the thinking process.

You can place staff according to their Belbin team roles (e.g., resource investigators as white hats), or purposely ask staff to assume positions that they would not naturally espouse. Assign pairs of staff members to each hat when reviewing an issue raised and keep it well-structured: 10–15 minutes for each section to generate ideas and questions. Follow this by generating feedback and prioritisation for specific actions depending on the size of the task at hand.

Tip 16: Remember to apply a model of influence to your management and decision making around your work plan

Influence is something we can exercise consciously or unconsciously. As the team leader, you should have a good working knowledge of the following six types of influence and how you apply it. Which type of influence do you use most? Should you be using a greater range of influence? "The influence model—communications skills training" outlines the following types (MindTools, 2011).

1. *Reciprocity.* "You scratch my back and I will scratch yours". Look for projects that are mutually beneficial to one or more providers. A prime example of this would be pathway development or creating a new joint working protocol.
2. *Commitment.* Ensure you display this. Get key stakeholders interested early on. You could do a trial period to prove worth, or run a pilot project. It is also vital to know when you do not have that commitment from another stakeholder. You might have to cancel or reject an idea if there is not sufficient buy-in.
3. *Social proof.* This is about creating "a buzz". Spreading the word to other key influencers in the stake holder groups who will in turn do some of the promotion for the work item in their own areas of expertise.
4. *Liking.* This is about building those relationships with fellow workers. It goes back to emotional intelligence, trust, and respect.
5. *Authority.* This is about using your role in the organisation positively to gain support or empower others.
6. *Scarcity.* This one I have used a great deal when setting up the service. Commissioners and other professionals need to know what they are missing out on. Can you do a loss leader to prove value for money/improved patient outcomes? For example, community based neuropsychologists are still a relatively rare commodity.

Networks and team profile

Tip 17: Manage community networks with other service providers

This next section looks at managing external support and networks from a wide range of non-NHS provider services. It takes multi-agency working to ensure effective management of ABI clients in the community. Who is responsible for these relationships in your team? Identify and build on existing good joint working. Find out what works well *vs.* what is a repeated sticking point. What skill/ information sharing could enhance joint working? Sharing student visits across services promotes future joint working, staff shadowing, joint client visits, formal training sessions, and so forth. These are all pragmatic tools to use for building relationships. If necessary, form a "task and finish group" to deliver on a joint working protocol. Networking facilitates win–win scenarios, it creates and strengthens your referral sources; an essential in the new commissioning driven NHS, it seeks out new opportunities and builds your service profile.

Based on client lead needs, the key joint working networks that my service positively manages are as follows.

1. Vocational occupational therapist is responsible for networking with:
   - supported education teams at our three colleges (learning support tutors, educational psychologists, classroom assistants);
   - voluntary/charity organisations (Brain and Spinal Injury Charity, Stroke Association, Encephalitis Society, Bell's Palsy Group, Head Injured People in Cheshire, Headway, Epilepsy Action, Carers Association, Brain Tumour Support Group);
   - other volunteer agencies;
   - Access to Work;
   - Job Centres (disability employment officers, third party contractors, occupational psychologists);
   - Learn Direct;
   - Benefits Agency.

2. Psychology/neuropsychology staff are responsible for networking with the:
   - Driver and Vehicle Licensing Agency (DVLA/Driving Assessment Centres);
   - Advocacy Services/Independent Mental Capacity and Mental Health Advocates (IMCAs and IMHAs);
   - police (custody sergeant, community police team, domestic violence unit);
   - probation services;

- Sure Start;
- medico–legal services;
- mental health services.

3. Case manager is responsible for networking with:
   - social services (discharge teams, access teams, children's teams, family-based care workers, direct payment advisers, carers groups);
   - army (medical officer, liaison officer, Soldiers, Sailors and Air Force Association);
   - housing associations;
   - private providers of care and rehabilitation;
   - private case managers;
   - continuing health care teams.

I try to include one or two networking goals in the service work plan (see also Tip 19). For example, we have invited occupational psychologists to present to a team training day and the team's vocational occupational therapist has run a joint art group with local college and the Stroke Association (see also Chapter Eight, by Walsh, in this regard). My clinical team is such that the liaison roles above are frequently interchangeable across staff groups or jointly managed, dependent on client needs. However, structuring the management of these networks ensures ideas do not get lost, and the most is made of the opportunities that arise.

TIP 18: Map local services and resources

Why reinvent the wheel?

In a community service, resources and staffing levels are always a challenge. Successful joint working with the range of providers above builds strong partnerships and delivers improved services for ABI clients and their families. It pays dividends to take time to map what is out there in your patch, which always seems to be an ever-changing tapestry of uncertainties. Here is a quick checklist.

- Ask your clients what they or their family go to and what other services they have access to.
- Consult the local paper and look at what groups and activities are already up and running in the community.

- Check the local library notice board for events of interest.
- Get copied in on other organisations' newsletters.
- Obtain the course outlines for your healthy living centres, leisure centres, and volunteer bureau.

The above is usually a quick task for a rehabilitation assistant or student on placement to complete. If possible, do it once or twice a year. Duplication of effort is something we all fall foul off. Having a good working knowledge of the range of services stops us reinventing the wheel. We were reviewing the option of a brain injury group for mums with babies, but discovered our local Sure Start programme could cater for this group with only a little bit of extra information from the team's neuropsychology staff. Instead, we went on to develop a parenting group for fathers with older children, an area where there was no local provision (see Weatherhead & Newby, 2008; and Chapter Nine in this volume, by Weatherhead, Walsh, Calvert & Newby, for more information about this group).

The final section in this chapter addresses operational issues, change management, and team profile. I find that time to review these areas as a team usually falls to the bottom of the "things to do" pile. We are all clinicians and clients and clinical issues come first. But, as already discussed, networks for community working are essential. Restructuring across not just health, but social services, employment, and voluntary sectors is happening at almost breakneck pace. Within health services alone, there have been the demise of Primary Care Trusts, new GP-led consortia for reworked geographical clusters, and major changes to commissioning. We are being constantly told we are in a health economy with the concept of "any willing provider" and "payment by results". This means that I am now required to look at public relations issues, marketing, and the team profile in a whole new way.

Tip 19: Create a service work plan for the year to address service profile, marketing, and development

I tend to do a work plan after staff performance and development reviews. When it comes to service profile, this needs to be considered across service users, your service/organisation, and your commissioners (see Tip 14). The private sector far outshines many NHS services in the area of public relations (PR) and marketing. But marketing and PR are vital for community brain injury teams' continued existence. There are significant pressures to skill-mix downwards and integrate teams and services. There is rarely a government directive specifically related to our part of the patient pathway; with even *The National Service Framework for Long-term Neurological Conditions* having limited success in affecting positive change for most brain injury services.

So, be proactive, as outlined below.

1. Find out in the new commissioning cluster who your local lead commissioner is and ask how and what you can usefully report on around a quality agenda and not just quantity.
2. Ensure *all* service plaudits are reported upwards.
3. Submit an article to your internal e-brief or newsletter.
4. Do a poster for the research and audit conference.
5. Present something for Brain Injury Awareness Week. Will a client share his story? Can you get in the local press or radio?
6. Do any of your team want to hold other roles in your organisation; for example, taking on the role of patient governor or equality and diversity lead.
7. Ask a commissioner/non-executive director/chairman of the board to visit the department, meet some families, and sit in on a group intervention.
8. Build service user involvement via yearly surveys, readers group, or service volunteers (see also Tip 9).
9. Promote student placements, especially where dissertations and pieces of research undertaken will benefit the service.
10. Pathway development work is very good at building your service profile with other staff groups and providers.
11. Can you build relationships with other providers by providing training events? This can have the added value of being an income generator.
12. Review and revamp service information leaflets for commissioners and referrers. Include response times, types of packages of treatment that can be delivered, and list outcome measures used.

Finally, on the point of profile, if you do not already have a business card, get one. Marketing is now in your job description as part of the new NHS health economy.

TIP 20: Foster an ethos of trust and respect

A good team watches each other's backs, helps when things get busy, supports when there are external pressures, and makes allowances for each other's deficits and errors. There should not be a culture of blame; rather, one of learning from challenges met and resolved.

Conclusions

To summarise, I feel that to be recognised externally as a good leader you need a business nose for opportunities and a profile across your referral sources that is positive and proactive. Internally, you should be known to your colleagues as someone who can deliver a quality service and who can respond to change positively. For your team to hold a positive opinion of you requires hard work, commitment, honesty, integrity, and leading by example (Kaplan, 2011). I hope the tips above have delivered on my aim of giving you some practical ideas to implement with your own team and that they will help you in developing your own leadership style and role.

References and resources

1MindTools (2011). The influence model—communications skills training. www.mindtools.com/pages/article/influence-model.htm. Accessed 23 November 2011.

Belbin (2011). Belbin team role theory. www.belbin.com/rte.asp?id=8. Accessed 23 November 2011.

British Society of Rehabilitation Medicine (2009). *BSRM Standards for Rehabilitation Services Mapped on to the National Service Framework for Long-Term Conditions*. London: BSRM.

De Bono Group (2011). De Bono's 6 Thinking Hats. www.debonogroup.com/six_thinking_hats.php. Accessed 23 November 2011.

Department of Health (2009). *The Engagement Cycle: A New way of Thinking about Patient and Public Engagement (PPE)*. www.dh.gov.uk/en/PublicationsPolicyAndGuidance/DH098658. Accessed 23 November 2011).

Hackman, J. R., & Oldham, G. R. (1976). Motivation through the design of work: test of a theory. *Organisational Behaviour and Human Performance*, 16: 250–327.

Hawken, P. (1988). *Growing a Business*. New York: Simon & Schuster.
Kaplan, R. S. (2011). *What To Ask the Person in the Mirror: Critical Questions for Becoming a More Effective Leader and Reaching your Potential*. Boston, MA: Harvard Business Press.
Katzenbach, J. R., & Smith, D. K. (1993). *The Wisdom of Teams: Creating the High Performance Organization*. Boston, MA: Harvard Business School Press.
Knowledge@Whorton (2006). Is your team too big? Too small? What's the right number? www.knowledge.whorton.upenn.edu/article.cfm?articleid=15011. Accessed 10 January 2012.
MindTools (2011). *Leadership Skills*. www.mindtools.com/fulltoolkit.htm. Accessed 10 December 2011.
National Leadership Council (2011). *NHS Leadership Module*. Web page: www.nhsleadershipframework.rightmanagement.co.uk/development-guidel. Accessed 23 November 2011.
NHS Institute for Innovation and Improvement (2011). *Leadership: Building Leadership Capability and Capacity in the NHS*. Electronic version: www.institute.nhs.uk/building_capability/general/leadership_home.html. Accessed 23 November 2011.
Spillane, J. P., & Diamond, J. B. (2007). *Distributed Leadership in Practice*. New York: Teachers College Press.
Tannenbaum, R., & Schmidt, W. H. (1973). How to choose a leadership pattern. *Harvard Business Review, May–June*: 162–180.
Weatherhead, S., & Newby, G. (2008). Supporting dads: a parenting programme for fathers with an acquired brain injury. *Clinical Psychology Forum, 182*: 36–39.

CHAPTER FOURTEEN

Thinking creatively about continuing professional development

Gavin Newby and Stephen Weatherhead

Continuing professional development (CPD) is necessary and healthy in any modern healthcare system to ensure safe, effective, and up to date practice. It is vital at any stage in anyone's career; whether you are wet behind the ears or a wizened old hack. Ensuring practitioners recognise the importance of CPD and follow auditable programmes of knowledge updating forms the backbone of professional regulation and governance. Furthermore, it helps to encourage the best possible care for the people who access our services.

It is important to accept that in the real world of the modern UK healthcare economy, CPD can seem something of a tall order. It can feel like walking a tightrope when trying to balance the "core" aspects of one's role (e.g., face-face client sessions, writing letters and reports) with fulfilling one's developmental needs and professional interests in the context of straitened financial times. This can be particularly poignant when in the "conscious incompetence" phase of Maslow's developmental model (Maslow, 1987), a phase in which perhaps most of us spend most of our time.

Our aims in this section are to consider the issues above by:

1. Defining CPD in its broadest possible sense, demonstrating that some activities which are commonly underplayed or dismissed can be important sources of CPD.
2. Presenting some individual, local, and national examples we have been involved with, which have supported our CPD, and could also support yours.

What have professional guidelines done for CPD in brain injury?

Professional membership and statutory regulation has raised the profile of neuropsychology and clinical psychology in the UK. It also raises the importance of maintaining high standards of practice through CPD. The Health and Care Professions Council (HCPC) identifies five standards that their members must fulfil in relation to CPD:

1, Maintain a continuous, up-to-date and accurate record of their CPD activities.
2. Demonstrate that their CPD activities are a mixture of learning activities relevant to current or future practice.
3. Seek to ensure that their CPD has contributed to the quality of their practice and service delivery.
4. Seek to ensure that their CPD benefits the service user.
5. Present a written profile containing evidence of their CPD upon request. (HCPC, 2012)

HCPC registration can be at stake if clinicians do not maintain their CPD activities, and the HCPC is at liberty to randomly audit any registrant's CPD profile. While a first read of the five standards might make many of us gulp, when the two of us have taken second and third looks, we have come to realise the governance system provides a helpful structure as well as a set of criteria. While many of us might not be as assiduous as we should in recording our CPD, the standards are surely an injunction to not only do CPD, but also reflect on what we have learnt and to make it relevant for our work.

A further cue for promoting the importance of CPD is the Department of Health's Knowledge and Skills Framework (KSF) that was designed, in part, to support the development of individuals working within the National Health Service to ensure employees are effective at their work. The KSF stipulates that individuals need to apply a range of knowledge and skills in a number of different dimensions in order to achieve the expectations of their post. One of these dimensions requires the psychologist to "develop oneself and contribute to the development of others".

Finally, we should also, of course, acknowledge the view of our main professional body, The British Psychological Society (BPS), and its member networks. The guidelines they produce act as drivers for service managers. The BPS states that "CPD and its impact on one's repertoire of knowledge and skills on everyday clinical practice remains a core function and responsibility of all clinical psychologists [and clinical neuropsychologists]" (BPS, 2009, p. 1).

Having considered the formal requirements, what follows are the nuts and bolts of selecting, accessing, defining, and facilitating CPD in a range of neuropsychological arenas.

CPD: what is it really for?

As discussed in the Introduction to this section and in the formal definitions above, CPD can make the professional feel it is something that you have to do to keep practising, something that is a bit of a chore but necessary—a bit like taking cod liver oil! However, we feel that CPD, to be really effective, has to be much, much more than this.

First, we strongly believe it should be enjoyable! CPD, to be truly effective, must be seen as a positive opportunity rather than an administrative threat. A great deal of this type of approach should be regarded as the personal responsibility of the recipient. This is truly about you as a professional seeking to enhance and develop your practice and vocation. It is your responsibility to make sure CPD takes place . . . it is much easier to make it happen if you see it as an exciting opportunity, rather than a waste of time or something that takes you away from the "real work". So, go to CPD with an open and enquiring mind—you will always learn something new about the job you do, and probably about yourself.

Second, make your CPD personally meaningful and organisationally relevant. This means you need to take time out to reflect on gaps in your portfolio of skills that are relevant to the job you are doing, as well as the jobs and positions you might take up in the future. What do I need to do, what is missing from my work, and how will my clients and workplace benefit? You might do this process individually, or as part of supervision, or with peers.

Third, CPD should always be about progressing, improving, and developing. There might always be something of an organisational imperative behind some CPD, for example, a management course or note-keeping standards, but again go in with an open and positive mind—such courses always open up areas you could improve on, as well as delivering news of a delightful time addition to your working day.

Fourth, it goes without saying that CPD should be governable by employers and national regulatory organs such as the Health and Care Professions Council, so do not forget to keep that CPD log (e.g., see BPS (2012) for a possible format, and Newby & Coetzer, 2012, for a more detailed discussion of the practicalities and benefits of maintaining CPD logs).

So, with a positive and wholesome attitude now embedded, how can we make CPD "do-able"?

CPD in brain injury: a broad church

Individual responsibilities and tasks

CPD starts at home, with your reflective capacity, and by celebrating the work you do. Taking time to reflect on what you have done on a regular basis can seem trivial and maybe a little blurred with supervision. Even a few minutes of quiet reflection on a regular basis can help you identify patterns in your casework . . . have I seen this before . . . mmm, never seen that before, I need to find out more. Perhaps it is nothing more than maintaining a sense of curiosity about your work. CPD can be small and fleeting, large and extended, or something in between—CPD is in the eye of the beholder. Remember there is plenty of personal reading you can do, even just reminding yourself about test instructions from a familiar manual can open you up to little mistakes that have crept into delivering that test.

Supervision must be about personal development. Most of us who supervise, and all of us who receive supervision, would recognise that there are gears to supervision. The gears might reasonably include nitty-gritty casework (i.e., reviewing letters, suggesting things to try), and meeting organisational imperatives (e.g., have you been on that mandatory course, completed that activity form?). However, it should also include education (i.e., have you read that paper or book?; after anoxia you might expect this pattern of neuropsychological difficulty), pastoral care (are you all right or are you working too hard?), and career development (what about doing that post qualification course, that Personal Constructs course, going on that conference, if you want to be a consultant, what is missing from your CV, how are we going to get you there . . .?) (see Scaife, 2009 for an extended discussion of these type of issues).

Individual CPD does not have to take the form of accessing courses and gaining accreditation. One of the ways in which we both feel that individual development can occur is through supervising research projects. We think of this as "vicarious CPD", because often it is by helping to develop others that we inevitably develop ourselves. Local clinical psychology training courses can be a perfect avenue for exploring this form of CPD. Not only do they present opportunities to collaborate on high quality service relevant research, but they also come with the distinct added value of acting as a source of ready, willing, and more than able principle investigators (in the form of trainee clinical psychologists). The trainees will usually (if not always) carry out most of the hard labour of research. At the same time, their supervisors will be doing their best to keep up with the trainee's growing knowledge base, through reading, one-to-one discussions, and engagement with the research process.

Some examples of research we have supported in our own practice, which have helped to develop us and our services, include projects looking at:

- the accessibility of an ABI website for the people who access the service (Newby & Groom, 2010);
- attitudes towards risk assessment in acquired brain injury (Weatherhead, Newby, & Skirrow, 2012);
- the experience of parenting after a brain injury (Skippon, Newby, & Simpson, n.d.);
- narratives of people who have undergone cranioplasty (Flynn, Weatherhead, & Daiches, in press).

Obviously, these projects have developed through negotiation with the relevant academic institution, and the trainees. The final project often tends to be a pragmatic evolution of the original idea. However, here are our top ten tips on how to ensure research is useful to you as a form of CPD for all involved.

1. Ensure the project has clinical relevance.
2. Disseminate "the small and the ordinary"; the often overlooked aspects of practice, research, and experience.
3. Don't get bogged down by the process.
4. Consider team meetings as a melting pot of ideas.
5. Be mindful of the scale of the project, and ensure it is "do-able".
6. Share the load; do not take responsibility for every aspect of the research.
7. Use research as a way to explore your particular interests.
8. Develop a robust research design.
9. Be prepared to compromise.
10. Ensure you have the "buy-in" of the whole service, and be aware of "research fatigue" during this process.

The role of local networks

It is surprising how easily we can overlook the expertise and support that is on our doorstep. Peer supervision is increasingly a well-recognised formal supervision and CPD format (e.g., see the *Qualification in Clinical Neuropsychology Handbook*, BPS, 2010) and can be a tremendously rich source of further information and education. We would strongly advise getting to know who is around and what their expertise is. You might want to develop a local register of expertise and interests. In our experience, the local clinical psychology training courses have something like this through their register of placements, so you might not need to reinvent the wheel. Third, do not forget (or pretend to forget) to attend any of the regular local service/organisation meetings. While local formal departments might now be a thing of the past in the main, trusts will often have a professional lead in clinical psychology that will arrange regular or *ad hoc* meetings to discuss important matters affecting the profession and can be important ways to share expertise and information.

Traditionally, within UK clinical psychology organisational frameworks, we have special interest groups (SIGs) and regional subdivisions of national organisations such as the Division of Clinical Psychology (DCP) and the Psychologists' Special Interest Group in the Elderly (PSIGE). Each organisation and geographical area will vary in the activity and presence of such groupings, but most will have several meetings per year, structured around a presentation of some sort, questions and answers along with some opportunity to network and share local/regional service developments, jobs, and other CPD opportunities. The British Psychological Society website (www.bps.org.uk) contains details of all of these networks.

The role of organisations at a national level

There are now plenty of national opportunities to receive both *ad hoc* and formally structured training days and post-qualification courses. The PSIGE national conference is a good example of relevant, well-priced specific conference setups. They are held in various locations around the UK over three days, with keynote speakers, themed seminars and lectures, along with formal and informal opportunities to network. The Division of Neuropsychology also holds regular training days, chiefly in London, and this has recently included effort testing, driving, and working with families. Other providers of excellent formal conferences include the Brain Injury Rehabilitation Trust and the British Association of Brain Injury Case Managers.

At a more structured level, there are formal courses that lead towards post-qualification accreditation. Good recent examples include the Solomon's University Course in Neuropsychology with the Elderly, and the Division of Neuropsychology's Qualification in Clinical Neuropsychology (QiCN—see below). Please also remember that many of the Postgraduate/Masters courses in Clinical Neuropsychology, which form part of the QiCN accreditation, also offer the opportunity to attend single sessions/modules as a formal framework for CPD.

Courses such as those discussed so far not only help to skill up new and aspiring practitioners but also help to further establish neuropsychological practice as highly credible and expert. Next, we present some examples of CPD opportunities that have been accessed/manufactured/developed in the areas in which we work.

Examples of CPD schemes

ABI team half days

GN has worked for a UK-based community acquired brain injury service for over seven years, and SW worked there from 2008–2011. The original service has a small staff consisting of a service manager/case manager (who is a speech and language therapist by background), consultant clinical neuropsychologist, clinical psychologist, specialist vocational OT, a rehabilitation assistant and an administrator. All of us have CPD needs and, while we have been successful in securing formal training/CPD opportunities (such as the Post Graduate Diploma in Clinical Neuropsychology at Glasgow University, a foundation course in Personal Constructs Therapy and an MSc in Vocational Therapy at Sheffield University), we also create our own CPD. Every quarter, we book out half a clinical day for team learning. Predominantly, we will research and present on an area ourselves (e.g., visual perceptual disorders and narrative therapy). We also regularly have had invited speakers on topics such as the benefits system, and occupational psychology and job centre resources.

The North West Special Interest Group in Neuropsychology

The North West Special Interest Group in Neuropsychology (known locally as the "Neuro SIG") has been well established for a number of years. Up to 2005, the group met every other month, with each meeting consisting of a presentation and questions lasting around 2–2½ hours. The presentations were usually seen as informative and were well received, with any remaining discussion being about ensuring future presentations and only limited discussion of strategic issues. The group did not act as a working body producing documents or responses to organisation/national directives. The attendance at group meetings was very variable, but tended to include a high proportion of assistants, trainees, and more junior qualified staff, rather than senior clinicians. Together, these issues made it difficult for the group to be a consistent forum for discussing strategic issues.

Members of the group were aware in 2005 of the plethora of UK government initiatives and guidelines, such as various National

Service Frameworks, the Mental Capacity Act, and expected revisions to the Mental Health Act (for details, please consult the Department of Health's website, Department of Health, 2012). The Agenda for Change process and governance agenda had raised huge issues about how our work was valued and evaluated. As a further point, we were all well aware that service provision was extremely patchy across the region, with a number of "black spots" with little or no co-ordinated specialist neuropsychological services available to clients. There were, occasionally, reports of recruitment processes occurring without the involvement of the appropriate senior clinical neuropsychologist, which could have led to inappropriate appointments.

In order to create a momentum for change, six or seven interested members of the group formed a committee consisting of a chairperson, vice chairperson, geographical convener, and secretary. We also sought geographical representation across the North West Region and specific representation from sub-disciplines of neuropsychology, including: neurosciences, adult mental health, older adults, forensic, and neuropsychological rehabilitation. We also ensured academic representation from the Lancaster, Liverpool, and Manchester training courses in clinical psychology. One of our first acts was to create clear Terms of Reference for the Committee, a Mission Statement, and a constitution. The interested reader is more than welcome to contact GN for more information on this.

In brief, we established that the committee would be a steering group that created a new strategic representative body of practitioners in neuropsychology in the North West. After formalising the terms of reference, etc., it was envisaged that the group would:

- provide opportunities for the exchange of knowledge and expertise between members;
- advise and participate in matters of teaching and training;
- facilitate the development of appropriate service provision for people with neuropsychological needs;
- stimulate research and disseminate research findings;
- act in an advisory capacity on the issues related to the psychological wellbeing and provision of care for people with neuropsychological needs;
- foster an exchange of information and ideas with other professional voluntary groups;

- promote mutual support for members, especially through the activity of geographical area groups.

The group aspired to be a representative body that commissioners and service planners could consult in the planning of neuropsychological provision. It was hoped that the committee would have a role in developing local practical responses to national guidelines such as NICE, NSFs, etc. The body could also be a driver for ensuring that there is neuropsychological representation in local implementation bodies (such as for the statute Mental Capacity Act, 2005) and developing detailed guidance on how to interpret each of the guidelines.

To date, the group has had some successes.

- In 2008, it held a one-day conference on applications of neuropsychology in modern NHS practice (with presentations on subjects such as chronic fatigue, working with asylum seekers, neuropsychotherapy, and working with commissioners), and has held further one-day workshops on neuropsychotherapy in 2010 and cross-cultural neuropsychological assessment in 2012.
- It has provided consultative input into series of regional strategic and workforce initiatives, such as ensuring senior neuropsychological involvement in recruitment, advice to Agenda for Change grading committees, and a cross-area workforce redevelopment.
- The bi-monthly presentation format has continued, with well-attended lectures and discussions on subjects such as working with the children of ABI clients and working with the Mental Capacity Act. Attendance across the year can be variable, with summer and Christmas presentations often being poorly attended. Some members have reported finding it increasingly difficult to get permission from managers to get away from face-to-face clinical work or clinics.

Neuropsychology peer support for newly qualified clinical psychologists

While attending the North West Neuro SIG described above, it was noted that the people who had recently qualified and were attending the group could benefit from some protected time specifically to discuss issues that were pertinent to beginning work in neuropsychological settings. Typical examples of these issues included transitions (from trainee to qualified clinical psychologist), further qualifications, and practice issues, such as managing expectations, teamwork, supervision, test selection, critiquing the statistical qualities of tests, and assessment feedback.

In order to foster an open, supportive forum in which to discuss issues such as this, a peer supervision scheme was set up. This was quite a long process. First, expressions of interest were gathered from members of the Neuro SIG, local contacts, and other networks. A "period of negotiation" then took place to consider some of the logistical issues, such as what day of the week it would be held on and what the location would be. Next came some of the more important aspects, such as devising the parameters of the scheme. This is particularly significant when considering issues such as clinical responsibility, the remit of the scheme, and the boundaries of confidentiality. Finally, the scheme was set up, and took place every two months.

Unfortunately, despite the planning that took place and the genuine enthusiasm held by members and potential members, the scheme ran for only eight months, with four sessions taking place in that time. The scheme was then discontinued due to low attendance rates. The four sessions were, of course, useful to attendees; very positive feedback was received. However, the primary reason for people not being able to attend regularly was that other service priorities had to take precedence, or individual line managers did not feel the scheme warranted the time away from direct clinical contact.

You might ask why we are reporting a scheme that was relatively unsuccessful. Partly, this is because we feel that while the scheme did not work here, it might be successful in other areas, but mostly it is because we feel that as much (if not more) can be learnt from failures as can be learnt from successes. Certainly much was learnt from this scheme that was the crux of later setting up another CPD scheme in Lancaster, as detailed below.

Lancaster University CPD & Peer Supervision for Newly Qualified Clinical Psychologists

We would agree that it is not the catchiest of titles, but it does what it says on the tin, and has been successful in meeting its remit for over three years. In 2009, a few of us who had earned doctorates in clinical psychology from Lancaster University discussed the potential benefits of continuing to meet regularly as a form of CPD. We discussed ways in which this could be formalised, and justified to line managers as a valuable form of CPD.

We realised that it would be important to give the scheme some formal weight, so we took three major steps in order to give the scheme the credibility needed to obtain buy-in from important stakeholders (e.g., members, hosts, facilitators, supervisors).

1. We selected a working party to manage the set-up of the scheme.
2. We liaised with Lancaster University, who agreed to host the sessions and provide refreshments free of charge. In return, we allowed current third-year trainees to attend the workshop part of the scheme.
3. We produced a "Positioning Document", which was disseminated to all potential stakeholders. The document covered the following areas:
   - the context of CPD & peer supervision;
   - the aims of the scheme;
   - the structure of the scheme.

Experience of the neuropsychology peer support scheme had taught me (SW) that it would be important to enable the scheme to be self-sustaining, and to continue to run without the input of any one individual. Therefore, the structure outlined below was proposed and accepted by the working party.

The scheme would be chaired by a recently qualified clinical psychologist, and the vice chair would be a current final-year trainee. Three additional members were also brought in from the working party to form a committee. The committee made decisions about the scheme in conjunction with members (via electronic surveys). These facets encouraged members to feel an ownership of the scheme. However, perhaps the most important aspect for the scheme achieving a sense of longevity and continuity was the following. The chair tenure would be for 12–18 months, and each year the vice chair (once qualified and embedded in post) would become the chair. A new vice chair would then be sought from the next crop of final-year trainees. Committee membership was more flexible, and selected to meet the needs of the scheme at the time. This process ensured that the scheme was always in touch with the needs of its members, and continued to evolve in line with the experiences of each cohort.

It should be noted that a number of particular factors enabled the scheme to flourish: Lancaster University's support, The South Cheshire ABI Service (with whom SW was working) giving me protected time to work on the project, and the enthusiasm of the original working party. Finally, I (SW) would emphasise the following factors as being core to the success of schemes such as this.

- The buy-in of as many stakeholders as possible.
- Shared ownership of the scheme.
- Having a self-sustaining structure.
- Being responsive to the needs of members.
- Using electronic surveys and emails as a form of communication.
- Ensuring there is "new blood" involved in all aspects of the scheme.
- Providing refreshments (helps to encourage a sense of nurturing).
- Holding sessions no more than monthly (thus reducing the time away from core work).
- Finding local clinicians/experts who will offer their time for free to facilitate workshop sessions.

The Qualification in Clinical Neuropsychology (QiCN)[1]

Since 2004, the Division of Neuropsychology within the British Psychological Society has administered a formal post-qualification process for clinical neuropsychological practitioners. Since 2010, the qualification has been known as the Qualification in Clinical Neuropsychology (QiCN). The QiCN is open to qualified clinical and educational psychologists. According to the *Candidate Handbook* (BPS, 2010), the QiCN

> is designed as an advanced professional qualification in the field of clinical neuropsychology. It confers eligibility for Full Membership of the Division of Neuropsychology and entry to the Division of Neuropsychology's Specialist Register of Clinical Neuropsychologists. It provides a standard of competence for practice as a Clinical

Neuropsychologist and is widely recognised as the professional qualification in this field. The objective of the qualification is to establish a standard of practice in clinical neuropsychology that will assure possession of the essential skills and underpinning knowledge for the expert and professional application of psychology in this field. It will enable competent practitioners to be identified and for the requirements for sound practice to be identified. (BPS, 2010, p. 5)

Candidates can undertake the QiCN in either Adult Clinical Neuropsychology or Paediatric Clinical Neuropsychology and must demonstrate competence in three domains: knowledge, research, and practice. Although candidates can choose to take examinations set by the Board of Assessors, most choose to take an accredited course in Clinical Neuropsychology at Glasgow, Nottingham, or Bristol universities, or the Institute for Child Health (paediatric course only) (at the time of writing). The accreditation process includes seeking evidence that the courses satisfy the broad curriculum set by the Board of Assessors of the QiCN. Details of the curriculum can be found in the *Candidate Handbook*, but it includes knowledge of neuroanatomy, acute onset and progressive disorders, psychometric assessment, and rehabilitation. The curriculum outline has been created and approved by experienced senior clinicians and represents a valid range of the knowledge one could reasonably expect of a credible junior neuropsychologist able to work in a range of UK-typical situations. Passing an accredited course confers an exemption from the knowledge dimension. Similarly, although a relevant research project can be completed, most UK applicants are given exemptions on the basis of completing their doctoral qualification in clinical psychology. Finally, the clinical practice competence domain is normally achieved by presenting a clinical practice portfolio for examination by *viva voce*. Again, details can be found in the *Candidate Handbook*, but the portfolio must show evidence via a logbook of at least eighty hours of supervised practice over two years (or pro-rata extensions of time should the candidate be working part time) and extended case studies.

Overall, the QiCN is a driver for ensuring that practitioners have received a thorough, rigorous, and governed training in the relevant domains of working in clinical neuropsychology. It is an important pump primer to CPD in early careers but can, through supervision provision and being able to attend course modules on an informal basis, also drive along CPD in more experienced clinical neuropsychologists

Conclusions

In this chapter, we hope we have confirmed that CPD is a vital component of professional governance, but also that it can be fun and can, with some imagination, range from the extremely small scale and personal to large scale full-blown courses of further study. In many senses, CPD is in the eye of the beholder; we hope that this chapter will help you to retain your sense of curiosity about your own development in the work that you do and begin to see CPD opportunities in every aspect of your work.

Note

1. GN was Chief Supervisor of the QiCN process from 2008–2011.

References

British Psychological Society (2009). *Continuing Professional Development Guidelines*. Leicester: BPS.
British Psychological Society (2010). *Qualification in Clinical Neurosychology Candidate Handbook*. Leicester: BPS.
British Psychological Society (2012). My CPD webpage: www.cpd.bps.org.uk/index.cfm?page=tabPlanAndRecord. Accessed 9 May 2012.
Department of Health (2012). Homepage: www.dh.gov.uk/. Accessed 6 June 2012.
Flynn, K., Weatherhead, S., & Daiches, S. (in press). Brain injury narratives: an undercurrent into the rest of your life. In: S. Weatherhead & D. Todd (Eds.), *Narrative Approaches to Brain Injury*. London: Karnac (in press).
Health and Care Professions Council (2012). *Our Standards for Continuing Professional Development*. Electronic version: www.hpc-uk.org/registrants/cpd/. Accessed 7 December 2012.

Maslow, A. H. (1987). *Motivation and Personality* (3rd edn). New York: Harper and Row.
Mental Capacity Act (2005). (c.9) London: The Stationery Office. Electronic version: www.legislation.gov.uk/ukpga/2005/9/contents. Accessed 23 May 2012.
Newby, G., & Coetzer, B. (2012). Facing down the elephant in the room: making your CPD log a successful part of your practice and development. *Clinical Psychology Forum, 236*: 46–49.
Newby, G., & Groom, C. (2010). Evaluating the usability of a single brain injury (ABI) rehabilitation service website: implications for research methodology and website design. *Neuropsychological Rehabilitation, 20*(2): 264–288.
Scaife, J. (2009). *Supervision in Clinical Practice: A Practitioner's Guide* (2nd edn). Abingdon: Routledge.
Skippon, R. H., Newby, G., & Simpson, J. (n.d.). The experience of being a parent with acquired brain injury. Manuscript awaiting acceptance.
Weatherhead, S., Newby, G., & Skirrow, P. (2012). Brain injury professionals' attitudes towards risk assessment. *Social Care & Neurodisability, 3*(2): 77–88.

PART IV

MAKING SENSE OF IT ALL: REFLECTIONS AND INSIGHTS

CHAPTER FIFTEEN

Epilogue: putting it into practice in the real world

Gavin Newby

By the time you get to this chapter, we hope you will have found the book to be readable, useful, and practical, and that you have already begun to test out some of its ideas in your own practice. In particular, we hope the book helps you to work with the type of real clients that we all see, but who rarely exist in textbooks: that is, the ones whose situations are messy, difficult, and challenging. But, as importantly, we would like to think that the ideas contained in this book will help you interpret the wood from the trees, and that you can start believing that you are working well with your clients..

As I sit here writing this, I am reflecting on a patient I have just seen—literally minutes ago. Bob is a twenty-five-year-old former professional sportsman who self-referred as he had just moved to our area. Leafing through copies of the medico–legal assessments in our notes that his solicitor was kind enough to send, I am reminded he was injured in a car accident over three years ago and suffered a severe-to-very-severe brain injury (Glasgow Coma Scale score of 3 and post trauma amnesia of over two weeks). CT scans suggested frontal contusions.

At the time of writing, I have seen Bob three times: once jointly with his partner, Lesley, and twice on his own. It was early days in our therapeutic relationship, but it was clear that there was a great deal of tension between the couple, frequent disagreements about the "true" state of their relationships, raised voices, and discord. Both highlighted Bob's temper and his low threshold for noise and frustration. Bob tended to talk over Lesley and ourselves, often talking quickly and misinterpreting or losing the thread of the conversation. He needed constant bringing back to the point of the conversation, but also reassurance that he was not being "rude". He thought he was "probably OK" and was a "good guy". With the cues from our semi-structured interview, he was able to acknowledge some problems with sleeping poorly, memory, and concentration. He said he could sometimes be "an idiot" when he had drunk whisky. It was hard to get a definitive account, but Bob and Lesley's brief accounts suggested he became garrulous, disinhibited, and shouted when drunk. Lesley said she "didn't want to be abused in another relationship". Bob said several times that he loved his ten-month-old son, Leo, and was scared he would lose him if anything happened to his relationship with Lesley.

Bob telephoned my manager two days ago to ask when his appointment was, despite having recorded it as a prompt on his mobile phone and having received a letter. Although he arrived for his appointment on the correct day, he was two hours early and in the wrong part of the hospital. A rather anxious, and slightly irate, receptionist telephoned to ask me to "come and pick up your patient". When I arrived at reception, Bob had been pacing up and down and looked highly agitated. While still in the reception area, he immediately began disclosing he had split up from his partner, had been living with his mother some distance away, and had left at 6.00 a.m. to see me. My attempts to stem the flow of his conversation in the corridor met with limited success, despite my worries about the loss of confidentiality.

In the next hour and a half (so much for a therapeutic hour!), Bob talked at speed about what had happened. Prior to Christmas, he had been cleaning the house he and his partner shared, he had overdone it, and "been a bit ratty". His partner asked him to slow down and he "just lost it". Although it was difficult to get precise details, it seems he began shouting and his partner reacted by asking him to leave. Recounting this story took Bob one hour and fifteen minutes. In the last fifteen minutes, we wrote down together some simple bullet points which included: get some advice on contact arrangements rights to his son via a Family Mediation Service, solicitor, or the Citizens Advice Bureau, see if his or Lesley's mother could look after their son while they chatted about their future, and rethink seriously about alternative accommodation (he was planning to spend the next few months in a hotel).

As you can see, this is an unfinished, unpolished, and red-hot active case. I need to be a man with a credible plan, and it needs to be formulated pretty sharpish.

Where to go next with Bob? Obviously, this is a work in progress; things might change, probably quite dramatically. However, I think it is reasonable and necessary to develop some sort of case conceptualisation to guide you through the chaos. These are my thoughts for the short, medium, and long term.

Short term: right here, right now fire-fighting

Whether or not you would conceptualise Bob's case psychodynamically, I think the transference generated creates the picture of a frightened, confused, and lonely "man-child". The man in Bob is trying to do the right thing, trying to protect his son and trying to be a good parent, trying desperately to be a good partner. The child in Bob needs protection himself, help and reassurance. Bob is putting a lot of faith in me and I have already become some sort of Father confessor character. He calls me "the boss". In among all of the chaos and uncertainty in his life, he needs a rock. Right here, right now, that rock is probably me.[1] He needs to be held therapeutically to feel these feelings of reverie that Bion and Kline talked about (e.g., see Waddell, 1988).

What might he need from this rock? He needs me to be present and to show interest. He will need me to be available, but boundaried. I am prepared to see him weekly, to answer his queries and questions by phone or text, but only during working hours. Who can be his "out-of-hours rock"? He needs me to be hands on, practical, and creative—I am guessing there is no space for fancy existential contemplation. With Bob, I have in my mind Maslow's (1954) hierarchy of need. I can imagine drawing out Maslow's famous triangle with Bob, helping him to see that some of his basic needs, such as safety, love, and belonging are under threat. This immediately sets out a very basic agenda. He might not have full insight and he might have memory difficulties that need assessing. However, potentially, he has nowhere to live, is in the middle of a relationship break-up, and is starting to worry about his access to his child.

So, let's start with: where is he going to live? It would probably be sensible to rent. I do not personally have the time and space, and it would probably cross some sort of boundary if I helped him to find a place. Maybe I could have a look at that genogram again—is there somebody within his family that might help? Could I encourage Bob to look through the newspapers? I wonder how much support he will need in choosing the right sort of place. I also think I need to encourage him to get some advice on his contact rights to his son. We could start with the Citizens Advice Bureau or family mediation service; I could download the web pages and maybe encourage him to speak to the solicitor that he has for his legal claim. Having some idea of his access rights that we can come back to in sessions might put some brake on him perseverating on this issue. However, a little alarm bell is going off in my head—what about his ability to look after this child without his partner present? (If I am wondering about this, surely others will, too, and he might face some roadblocks in the early stages of setting up arrangements to see his child. I will hold that thought as I consider the next move.) If I have understood Bob properly, I will probably need to be in the room with him when he telephones, perhaps helping him to draft some questions to ask, prompting him to clarify issues, and to write things down. We will probably need to debrief afterwards to check he has got the right end of the stick and to deepen his processing of what has happened. We will also need to find a way of noting down the information and keeping it in a safe place, maybe in his clinical notes for now?

In my next session, I also need to try to establish whether Bob's romantic relationship has irretrievably broken down, might do soon, or whether we are in for an "up and down ride" over the next few months. I need to ask Bob what help they as a couple might want or not want. Does he think the relationship is saveable?

Thinking about his solicitor also helps me remember he has an ongoing medico–legal case. It is three years in, but these cases rumble on. Many of the people I see find the whole medico–legal litigation process confusing and distressing. It can be confusing because you can lose who you are: you have '"your side" emphasising and magnifying your difficulties, and there is the "other side" minimising any problems and questioning your motivation. It is distressing because of the length of many of the medico–legal assessments, particularly the neuropsychological ones. Medico–legal assessments can also be quite confrontational. At this stage, and only a minor issue, I would also put into question whether I could and should test Bob's cognitive abilities. I would wonder what Bob's spare capacity is going to be for any testing. There could be both effort and practice effects to consider if he is going to be assessed medico–legally . . .

What is absolutely fundamentally and totally clear is that Bob is not a quick in and out case. For the service managers among you, a time-limited, session-limited approach just does not fit the bill.

Medium term: the next six months

There will be ups and downs, highs and lows, times of highly intensive effort and frequent phone calls. But, over time, as positions and feelings become clear, I could reasonably expect things to settle, at least a bit. There might be some space to start thinking about community rehabilitation in its widest sense. The best laid plans of mice and men . . . We have got to start somewhere.

Bob wants a job. He wants a job now, wants to race straight into it. However, using our eyes, ears, and experience, there is clearly a pretty potent mix for a rather unsuccessful return to work at this time. Bob is disorganised, has poor concentration, and poor memory. He has a short fuse—particularly when he drinks. We need time to get a good, decent picture; this might include testing, but all in good time. Perhaps the observations are enough to say "slow down Bob". It is perhaps time to work on increasing his mental stamina and fatigue strategies as well as increasing his weekly structure. He is a young and active man and wants to integrate with his new community. So far, I know that he likes the gym and would consider some sort of voluntary activity. Obviously, any voluntary activities need to fit in with his needs, wants, wishes, and aspirations. As we get to know him, perhaps my vocational rehabilitation occupational therapy colleague and I can help channel him into what is realistic. Alongside this, perhaps we can put him into our regular Fatigue Group. He would really benefit from a work preparation group to get back in touch with expectations around work, thinking about developing a *curriculum vitae*, etc., and maybe a trip to see the disability employment adviser (based in local Job Centres). But, above all, he could really benefit from immersing himself in his brain injury. He could hear about other people's experiences and learn about his own limitations; I can think of at least two or three other young men in a similar position—they would work well together. We could hold the group in that GP's surgery.

Longer term: acceptance, adjustment and the emergence of a new Bob

Over the next twelve to eighteen months,[2] I would hope he would continue to see me as a pathfinder who bears testament to his struggles, hears about his losses—that sporting career, all of his expectations of work and family life. Bob might well begin to experience his own grief. I would hope that our therapeutic relationship could be a safe space where he could begin to acknowledge and experience his doubts—will I be a good enough parent, can I cut it at work, am I a good enough partner? This adjusting and accepting process is hard to chart. It will have ups and downs, but I would hope that over the next eighteen months to two years he will begin to develop a more rounded view of himself. For example, as a parent he will hopefully recognise the downsides—his short fuse, reduced tolerance, and tendency to get overloaded. However, he might also begin to see how he has more time with his son than he would otherwise have had, that the whole experience has led him to really appreciate his time with his loved ones.

But hold on, before I get too carried away, I will probably need to think about his anxiety. Is he a worried well or is this a full-blown dual diagnosis? It will need to be a highly flexible and adapted approach. I wonder at this stage whether using cognitive analytic therapy might help him see the various roles he is starting to develop in his relationships; I will probably already have used some psychodynamic approaches to hold and contain him. There is no doubt that we will begin to look at some systemic patterns in previous, current, and future relationships. He is a texter. I wonder if I will be able to use this psychotherapeutically to help back up what we talk about, but, just at the moment, he is too concerned about whether his partner will see any texts. I wonder if we can get round this. I am also wondering if I will need any additional support. His partner experiences some extremes in his personality. She accuses him of being a "pretty boy" and "spending too much time in front of the mirror thinking only about himself". It is too early to say now, but I wonder if there are any narcissistic traits—could there be a personality issue or disorder here? Only yesterday, I met Mike Lloyd, who is an increasingly respected clinical psychologist working with people with diagnoses of a personality disorder within the same organisation that I work for (Cheshire & Wirral Partnership NHS Foundation Trust). He was interested in doing some training with our team; this could be an excellent opportunity for CPD and enhancing the skills of the team in screening/spotting personality disorders, as well as me working out how to manage any personality issues with Bob. I am going to read Mike's article in the *Health Service Journal* (Lloyd, 2011). Excitingly, he has some training DVDs—let's see where we can take the team.

Whether or not we end up doing any formal systemic family therapy work, I want to check in with the relationship on a regular basis, if they both want this. At least initially, I would imagine this would be a fairly simple regular meet up with myself and another therapist. Perhaps we will do a "divide and conquer", as Beth Fisher often calls it, with me spending time with Bob, and Beth spending time with Lesley before we come together to work out a shared understanding of the situation. Also, as Lesley has more than just hinted at previous relationship traumas and abuse of some sort, having dedicated individual time with Beth might draw out Lesley's own psychotherapeutic support history and current needs. Depending on how acute those current needs were, Beth might well signpost Lesley to such as the local IAPT[3] (Improving Access to Psychological Therapies) triage service. Perhaps there will be a willingness to do some work to look at the unhelpful repeating patterns and interactional difficulties. Perhaps they will let us do some in-room supervision to formulate and look at the mutual contributions to the difficulties. If there is a break-up, this will be an emotionally draining process on everyone and will restrict the space for working on difficulties. Maybe there will be a concern expressed by Lesley about Bob's ability to parent on his own. There will have to come a time when we, as a team, decide whether we are going to work with them or signpost them to the likes of Relate—an excellent UK-based relationship charity.

Now then, testing . . . I had almost forgotten about that. That is not because I have stopped valuing the contributions of neuropsychological assessments, it is just that I know they have their place and their time. It is horses for courses. Maybe early on, we could think about a Repeatable Battery for the Assessment of Neuropsychological Status (RBANS). It is good and indicative, but maybe rough and ready compared to a more comprehensive assessment based on such as a full Wechsler Adult Intelligence Scale (WAIS). At this stage, I have my doubts whether the full assessment kitchen sink will be needed—after all there is a medico–legal process where they might have at least two opposing lengthy assessments. However, the RBANS will tell me what the gross concerns are. Doing this reasonably early could be a good way of slowing Bob down in his race to get back to work. It could give me a good base to say, "Look, your memory, concentration, and speed aren't quite there yet". It might raise some concerns about driving—a hornet's nest, but somebody has to be brave. I wonder who might have to take the therapeutic relationship hit. It depends on how well Bob's relationship with the service and myself has continued. If we are still the main rocks in his life, it might need to be the GP whose relationship could be expendable in this circumstance. It could be the GP who bites the bullet and raises any concerns shown up by any testing.

There are lots of imponderables here, and there is bound to be something I have not thought about or could possibly have ever thought about. This is just one client . . . it is so complicated . . . and I thought I knew what I was doing. But I do have a road map!

Conclusion

I have at last come to the final section of this book. It has been an amazing journey for the other editors and myself. I hope that some of the insights and comments will stay with you and have some value in guiding you. I hope that Bob's case is a valuable nutshell in which to see the complexity of brain injury and that also, wherever you work, you can work well with complexity. It is possible to have a road map even although it might blow up in your face. Even if it does, dust yourself down, use that supervision, talk to your team, formulate, reformulate, and reformulate regularly, and so on. Hang on in there. For many of our clients with a brain injury, nobody else has ever hung on in there, so that makes you unique. I know I have left Bob hanging in mid-air. Maybe at some point in the future I will have the opportunity to tell you what actually did happen.

Notes

1. Of course, I do appreciate that not every reader would consider being a "rock" in this sense is either practicable or desirable, given its potential drain on therapeutic time and blurring of therapeutic roles.
2. I am well aware that for many clinicians, extended care episodes are not possible, with organisational restrictions on the number of follow-up visits. My employers are sympathetic to the long-term needs of clients with an ABI and I really appreciate having the time to work with Bob in the longer term. However, I hope that most readers could consider smaller possibilities within the larger plans I have outlined. Please be reassured that whatever you can provide, your time and informed consideration will inevitably add value to those clients with an ABI who are struggling and feel isolated.
3. IAPT is a UK-wide National Health Service delivery programme that provides talking therapy/counselling support (of predominantly cognitive–behavioural therapy orientation) for clients with anxiety and depression. Readers unfamiliar with this service could consult the IAPT website (IAPT, 2012) for more details.

Resources

Relate (2011). Home webpage. Accessed on 18 January 2012. www.relate.org.uk/home/index.html

References

Improving Access to Psychological Therapies (2012). About us webpage. www.iapt.nhs.uk/about-iapt/. Accessed 18 January 2012.

Lloyd, M. (2011). How investing in therapeutic services provides a clinical cost saving in the long term. *Health Service Journa*l (online):

www.hsj.co.uk/resource-centre/best-practice/care-pathway-resources/how-investing-in-therapeutic-services-provides-a-clinical-cost-saving-in-the-long-term/5033382.article. Accessed 29 May 2012.

Maslow, A. (1954). *Motivation and Personality*. New York: Harper.

Waddell, M. (1998). *Inside Lives: Psychoanalysis and the Growth of the Personality*. London: Duckworth.

INDEX

1MindTools, 325, 345

abuse, 144, 185, 366, 371
  alcohol, 126
  drug, 202
  substance, 53–56
  victim of, 93, 100
Access to Work, 235, 239, 341
Addenbrooke's Cognitive
  Examination (ACE), 40
Adler, L. E., 55, 62
aggression, 48, 75, 93, 120, 129–130,
  132, 144–145, 148 *see also*:
  behaviour(al)
Alderman, N., 42, 65, 206, 232, 243
Alderson, A. L., 213, 224
Alinder, J., 209, 212, 220, 223
Allgulander, C., 55, 62
Alzheimer's disease, 126
American Bar Association, 184, 193,
  206
American Brain Injury Association,
  133

American Psychiatric Association, 53,
  62
American Psychological Association,
  184, 193, 206
amnesia, 124, 145
  Korsakoff's, 17
  organic, 129
  retrograde, 123
  traumatic, 5, 45, 163–164, 214,
    365
Anderson, C., 185, 187, 207
Anderson, H., 110
Andrews, K., 166, 177
Andrykowski, M. A., 307, 319
aneurysm, 4, 22–23
  intracranial, 216
anger, 91, 93, 98, 108, 121, 134, 146,
  219, 247, 259, 279, 313
anosmia, 23
Ansell, B. J., 159, 176
Anselmi, V., 132, 147, 153–154, 156
Anton's Syndrome (cortical
  blindness), 20

375

anxiety, 8, 25, 30, 47, 52–53, 55, 68, 73, 77, 82, 84–85, 87, 89, 105, 125, 131, 134, 202, 220, 234, 249, 278, 309, 313, 315, 337, 366, 370, 373
  depressive, 6
  disorders, 52
  management, xxxi, 146
  provoking, 192, 285
  social, 275
Arango, J., 296, 318
Arango-Lasprilla, J. C., 211–212, 224, 272, 292
Arundine, A. L., 81, 111, 256, 268
Ashman, T., 56, 65
Ashwal, S., 172, 177
Atherton, H., 259, 268
attachment, 278
  enriched, 132
  relationships, 297–298, 312
  theory, 285
awareness, 8, 35, 43, 58, 68, 72, 74, 84, 95, 102, 120, 126, 134, 161–162, 166, 185, 220, 227, 284, 300
  see also: conscious, self
  body, 20
  immediate, 85
  impaired, 144
  insufficient, 276
  lack of, 88, 119, 144, 161, 174
  low, xx–xxi, xxiv, 5, 27, 29, 39, 44, 159–163, 165, 170, 173–174, 279
  marked, 160
  partial, 83
  poor, 150

Baguley, A. J., 56, 65
Bandura, A., 236, 240
Banos, J. H., 213, 224
Baptiste, S., 230–231, 233, 243
Barnes, C., 236, 240
basal ganglia, 6, 17, 22 see also: corpus striatum
Basford, J. S., 143, 155
Bashford, G. M., 210, 223
Bateman, A., 140, 156
Beardslee, W. R., 287, 292

Beattie, A., 54, 63, 132, 153
Beaumont, D., 227–228, 240
Beck Depression Inventory, 54
Becker, D. R., 234, 240
Beckner, V., 256, 268
behaviour(al) (*passim*)
  ability, 231
  activation, 82, 130
  aggressive, 75, 79, 129
  antisocial, 277
  approach, 124
  assessment, 142, 166–167, 174
  baseline, 168, 170
  challenging, xix, 48–50, 119
  changes, xx, 15, 21, 37, 68, 121, 145, 209
  cognitive, xix
  component, 82
  consequences, 40
  contingencies, 124
  coping, 128
  difficulties, xvii, 74, 131, 236
  effects, xvii
  emotional, 151
  experiments, 82
  function(ing), 13, 23, 24, 62, 92
  impairment, 234
  incentive, 129
  initiation, 117
  interpersonal, 144
  management programme, 132–133
  needs, xviii
  negative, 311
  neuroanatomy, xxiv, xxix
  observations, 28–29, 47, 170
  obsessional, 25
  offending, 56
  output, 24, 166
  patterning, 44
  perspective, 22, 34
  presentation, 38
  problems, 121, 131–133
  programme, 136, 140, 144–145, 151
  rehabilitation, 134, 150
  repertoire, 44, 167

research, 160
response, 37, 135, 174
reward programme, 129, 136
routine, 116
social, 8, 117, 129
spontaneous, 117
stability, 129
targets, 136, 140, 144–145
therapy, 68, 71–72
unhelpful, 8
unsafe, 212
unusual, 51
Behavioural Assessment of the Dysexecutive Syndrome (BADS), 42, 232
Belbin, 336–337, 339, 345
Bell, V., 215, 220, 223
Benn, K. M., 247, 252
Bennett, J. L., 273, 294
Bentall, R. P., 145, 154
Ben-Yishay, Y., 72, 111, 143, 153
Berberovic, N., 183, 207
Berman, P., 81, 112
Bernspang, B., 236–238, 242
Bertrando, P., 284, 291
Beutler, L. E., 71, 111
Bion, W. R., xxxii, 266, 367
Birkin, R., 232, 240
Bivona, U., 209, 222
Bjork, J. M., 56, 62
Black, F. W., 24, 26
Blackwell, H. C., 236, 242
Blankenship, J., 213, 224
Blitz, L., 228, 240
Bogdany, J., 54–55, 64
Bond, G. R., 234, 240
Bongar, B., 71, 111
Booth, J., xxxii, xxxv
Boscolo, L., 284, 291
Boss, P., 246, 253
Boudewyn, A. C., 307, 319
Bowen, A., 54, 62
Bowen, C., 245, 253, 271–274, 286, 288, 291
Bowen, M., 34, 62
Bradbury, C. L., 81, 111, 256, 268

brain (*passim*) *see also*: basal ganglia, brainstem, cortex, cranial nerves, frontal, limbic system, mater, occipital, parietal, temporal
cerebellum, 6, 18–19, 21
Circle of Willis, 21–22
falx cerebri, 19
foramen of Magendie, 18
foramina of Luscha, 18
sphenoid ridge, 15, 18
tentorium cerebelli, 19
thalamus, 6, 18
tumours, 4–5, 16, 18, 23
ventricles, 18
Brain Injury Rehabilitation Trust (BIRT), 42, 57, 62, 188, 201, 205, 287, 353
brainstem, 6, 18–19, 21, 161, 169
inferior colliculi, 18
medulla oblongata, 18
pons, 18, 21
reticular formation, 18
superior colliculi, 18
Brandau, S., 56, 65
Brands, I., 124, 156
Brenner, L. A., 55, 62
Brewin, J., 228, 230, 235–237, 240
British Geriatrics Society, 57, 63
British Medical Association (BMA), 186, 197, 205–206
British Psychological Society, 31, 63, 182, 203, 205–206, 212, 214, 219, 222, 349, 353, 359, 361
British Society of Rehabilitation Medicine (BSRM), xviii, xxii, 149–150, 153, 155, 226, 240, 326, 345
Broe, G. A., 296, 320
Brooks, D. J., 126, 155
Brooks, D. N., xviii, xxii
Brooks, N., 54, 63, 120, 132, 153, 211, 214, 222
Brouwer, W. H., 212, 222, 224, 259, 270
Brown, A. W., 164, 178
Brown, I. D., 211, 223

Brown, P., 57, 63
Brown, R. G., 81, 112
Browne, S., 164, 177
Buffington, A., 234, 237, 240
Burgess, C. N. W., 56, 65
Burgess, P. W., 42, 65, 206, 232, 243
Bushell, S., 260, 269
Bushnik, T., 211–212, 224
Busichio, K., 132, 153–154
Butera-Prinzi, F., 307, 319
Buttress, S., 30, 63, 210, 222
Byng, S., 290, 293

Calvert, M., 277, 292
Cameron, I. D., 56, 65, 164, 177
Campis, L. K., 249, 253
Campsie, L., 54, 63, 132, 153
Cantor, J., 56, 65
Car, J., 259, 268
Carlson, C. R., 307, 319
Carlson, N., 211–212, 224
Carlson, P., 273, 293
Carnevale, G. J., 132, 153–154
Carr, J., 258, 269
Carroll, E., 236, 240
Carter, B., 102, 111
case studies
    Bob, 365–373
    case example Chapter Two, 49, 51
    Dr P, 144–145
    Jack, 196
    James, 302–303
    Jeff, 218–219
    Joe, 129–130
    Keith, 201–202
    Lisa, 78–85, 87–95, 97–109
    Mary, 198–199
    Miss H, 39
    Mr A, 39
    Mr X, 38–39
    Mrs Z, 39
    Patient WG, 45
    Robert, 53–54
    Terry, 191–193
Cash, S., 286, 292
Caust, S. L., 210, 223

Cawthra, E., 55, 62
cerebro-spinal fluid, 18–19
Certified Brain Injury Specialist
    programme, 133
Chamberlain, M. A., 54, 62
Chanpong, G., 273, 294
Charles, N., 307, 319
Chaytor, N., 29, 63
Childs, N., 172, 177
Christensen, B. K., 81, 111, 256, 268
Christensen, J., 43, 10
Christie, N., 30, 63, 209–210, 212, 220, 222
Cifu, D., 211–212, 224
Clare, I., 194, 202, 205, 207
Clark, A., 248, 253
Clarke, J., 230–231, 233, 243
Classen, S., 212, 222
Coad, M., 273, 276, 294
Coelho, C., 257, 269
Coetzer, B. R., xxxiii, 33, 67–68, 72–74, 81, 111, 236–237, 240, 242, 245, 253, 262, 268, 350, 362
cognitive (*passim*)
    ability, 123–125, 136, 220, 231, 274, 369
    activity, 7
    aids, 140–141
    analytical therapy, xx, 78, 103, 370
    assessment, 24
    attributions, 144
    behavioural therapy (CBT), 68, 71–72, 78, 80–83, 134, 144, 146, 256, 373
    capabilities, 134
    changes, xx, 7, 44, 121
    competencies, 116
    complaints, 30
    consequences, 40
    dampening medication, 165
    deficits, 83, 109, 185, 202, 209, 211, 221, 235, 302
    demands, 127, 199
    difficulties, xvii, 15, 32, 44, 74, 81, 95, 108, 131, 146, 150, 212, 236, 258, 273

disabilities, 182, 202
dysfunction, xxix
effects, 56
examination, 51
failure, 85
flexibility, 103, 189
functioning, 13, 17, 20, 23–24, 31, 33, 36, 39–41, 47, 62, 92, 117, 122, 126, 139, 148, 187–190, 199, 210, 237, 280, 317
hypotheses, 124
impairment, 15, 18, 21, 30–31, 39, 41, 43, 68, 73, 76, 83, 89, 107–108, 117, 124, 131, 134, 138, 146–147, 149, 196, 220–221, 234, 259, 295, 313
interpretation, 145
issues, 51
limitation, 185
map, 118
needs, xviii
neuro-, 84
overload, 234
perspective, 22, 34
problems, 39, 44, 58, 98, 126, 133
processes, 117, 122, 193
profile, 108
reflection, 261
rehabilitation, xxxii, 67, 81, 89, 150, 153
resources, 127
response, 135
rigidity, 81–82
side-effects, 46
skills, 118, 187, 233
slip, 87
status, 40, 44
strengths, 24
test performance, 37
testing, 171, 181, 203
therapy, 71–72
underpinnings, 184, 193
weakness, 24
Cohen, Y., 183, 207
Cole, D., 230–231, 233, 243
Coleman Bryer, R., 213, 224

Collicut-McGrath, J., 34, 63, 280, 292
Collin, C., 307, 320
Collings, C., 246, 253
Coma Recovery Scale–Revised (CRS–R), 159, 169–170
Commission for Social Care Inspection, 298, 319
Community Head Injury Service, Aylesbury, xxxii
Conner, M., 54, 62
conscious(ness), 5, 18, 159–160, 162, 166, 176, 340 *see also*: unconscious(ness)
  awareness, 86
  incompetence, 347
  loss of, 164
  minimal, 161–162, 172
  state, 44, 162–163
continuing professional development (CPD), xxi, xxiv, xxix, 34, 323, 347–354, 357–358, 360–361, 371
Cooper, B., 229, 243
Cooper, E., 281, 288, 293
Cope, J., 122, 154
Cordan, G., 56, 65
Cordova, M. J., 307, 319
corpus striatum, 17
  caudate nucleus, 17, 46
  globus pallidus, 17
  putamen, 17
Corrigan, J. D., 55, 63
cortex, 6, 17, 19
  auditory, 6
  primary somatosensory, 20
Costandi, M., 4, 10
Cotter, I., 260, 269
Coughlan, A. K., 42, 63, 205, 296, 320
Coughlan, T., 296, 320
Cox, W. M., 55, 64
Cranford, R., 172, 177
cranial nerves, 6, 18, 22–23
  abducens, 22
  accessory, 22
  auditory, 22
  facial, 22
  glossopharyngeal, 22

hypoglossal, 22
oculomotor, 22
olfactory, 22–23, 170
optic, 6, 21–22
trigeminal, 22
trochlear, 22
vagus, 22
Crawford, J. R., 42, 63, 205, 296, 320
Crittenden, P. M., 297, 319
Crossman, A. R., 13, 26
Cruse, D., 162, 177
Culbert, J. P., 295, 320
Cully, C., 259, 269
Cunningham, L. L., 307, 319
Curtiss, G., 290, 294

Daiches, S., 351, 361
Daisley, A., 259, 269, 272–273, 287, 292, 294–295, 311, 319–320
Dallos, R., 96, 98, 110–111, 297, 319
Davis, M., 229, 234, 236, 240
Dean, A., 260–261, 269
Dean, D., 33, 64
De Bono Group, 345
Dedda, K., 183, 207
Degeneffe, C. E., 288, 292
Delhomme, P., 211, 222
Delis, D. C., 42, 63, 205
Delis-Kaplan Executive Function System (DKEFS), 42, 189, 198
Delmonico, R., 9–10, 140, 154
DeLuca, J., 147, 156, 209, 224
dementia, 4–5, 37, 51, 53, 126, 160
Demm, S. R., 245, 253
Dental Plus, 258, 269
Department for Constitutional Affairs, 179, 206
Department of Health, xviii, xx, xxii, 150, 154, 226, 237, 241, 295, 319, 345, 355, 361
    Knowledge and Skills Framework (KSF), 348
    Social Services Inspectorate, 6, 10
Department of Transport, 213, 222
Department of Work and Pensions, 226–227, 241

depression, 24–25, 49, 53, 55, 68, 73, 125, 134, 202, 234, 236, 249, 275, 287, 306, 315, 373
    severe, 52
Deutschle, J. J., 55, 63
development(al), 83, 116, 122, 128, 247, 296, 300, 302–303, 309, 347, 350 *see also*: self
    child, 116, 314
    disorder, 247
    early, 14
    emotional, 312
    experience, 33
    neuropsychological, 119
    normal, 285
    professional, xxi, xxiv, xxix, 34, 185, 323, 327, 347
Dezfulian, T., 296, 318
Diamond, J. B., 329, 346
Dick, L. P., 307, 319
Diehl, N. N., 164, 178
Dikmen, S., 29, 63
Diller, L., 72, 111
D'Ippolito, M., 209, 222
Disability Rights Commission, 227, 241
Disler, P., 228, 239, 241
Dobson, L., 256, 269
Dodd, K., 205
Drake, R. E., 227, 234, 240–241
Draper, R., 96, 110–111
Driver and Vehicle Licensing Agency (DVLA), 210, 213–223, 341
    Medical Branch, 215–220
Drummond, A. E. R., 81, 112
Dryden, W., 71, 111
Duchnick, G. C., 290, 294
Dudley, M., 281, 288, 293
Duncan, J., 87, 111
Dunn, G., xviii, xxii
Dunn, M., 103, 111
Du Toit, P., 236–237, 240
dysexecutive
    difficulties, 87, 211
    functioning, 121
    problems, 87

Syndrome, 42, 232
dysfunction(s), 123, 128
   cognitive, xxix
   executive, 15, 118–119, 124, 153
   organic, 52
   sexual, 261

Edwards, A., 274, 292, 304, 319
Eisenberg, H. M., 164, 178
Ekin-Wood, A., 307, 320
Ellison, B., 209, 212, 220, 222
Elman, R. J., 290, 292
Elsass, L., 273, 292
Elton, R. A., 59, 64
Emerson, E., 48, 63
Emslie, H., 42, 65, 87, 111, 206, 232, 243, 259, 270
Enderby, P., 205
epilepsy, 7, 15, 27, 37, 125, 150, 213, 218, 246, 341
Epston, D., 90, 113, 284, 294
Equality and Human Rights Commission, 227, 241
Eriksson, G., 286, 292
Evans, J. J., 42, 55, 64–65, 88, 113, 140, 146, 156, 206, 232, 243, 259, 269–270

Family Head Injury Semantic Differential Scale, 249
Family Mediation Service, 367–368
Feeney, T., 283, 294
Fenske, C. L., 56, 65
Fischer, J. S., 28, 43, 64
Fisher, A. G., 232, 241
Fitzgerald, J., 164, 177
Flaada, J. T., 164, 178
Flanagan, S., 119, 155
Fleming, J. M., 229, 241
Fleminger, S., 55, 64, 81, 113, 126–127, 154
Flynn, K., 351, 361
Focht-Bikerts, L., 287, 292
Foley, C. C., 273, 294
Formisano, R., 209, 222
Foulkes, M. A., 164, 178

Fox, G. K., 210, 223
Fraas, M. R., 277, 292
Frank, A., 227, 230, 234, 239, 241
Freer, C., 87, 111
French, J., 176–177
Frenchay Aphasia Screening Test (FAST), 188–189
frontal
   bone, 14
   contusions, 144, 365
   craniotomy, 46
   lobe, 14–15, 19–20, 23, 46, 211
   system, 119
Froud, B., 183, 207
Fugl-Meyer, A. R., 286, 292

Gautille, T., 164, 178
General Medical Council (GMC), 214, 223
genogram, 34, 98–101, 104, 185, 279, 281, 368
Gentleman, S. M., 126, 155
Gergen, K., 110–111
Gerson, R., 34, 64
Ghadiali, E., 125, 154
Giacino, J. T., 159, 172–174, 177
Gills, D. J., 288, 292
Gill-Thwaites, G., 166, 177
Gill-Thwaites, H., 29, 45, 64, 159, 169–170, 172, 177
Gioia, G. A., 125, 155
Giustini, M., 209, 222
Gladman, J. R. F., 81, 112
Glasgow Coma Scale (GCS), 5, 45, 163–164, 365
Glass, C., 125, 154
Godfrey, H., 291–292
Godwin, E. E., 272, 292
Gontkovsky, S. T., 245, 253
Goodkin, D. E., 307, 319
Goolishian, H., 110
Gordon, W. A., 56, 65
Gorske, T. T., 30, 58, 64, 285, 292
Government Equalities Office, 227, 242

Gracey, F., 69, 81, 87–90, 103, 111, 113–114, 122, 140, 154, 156, 274, 292
Grant, S. J., 56, 62
Grayson, G., 209, 212, 220, 222
Green, R. E., 81, 111, 256, 268
Greenwood, R. J., xviii, xxii, 234, 237–238, 242
grief, 72, 85–86, 125, 175, 246, 370
Groeger, J. A., 211, 223
Gronseth, G., 176, 177
Groome, C., 217, 223, 258, 261, 269, 290, 293, 351, 362
Grote, M., 211–212, 224
Gudjonsson, G. H., 202, 206
  Suggestibility Scales (GSS), 202
Gurd, J., 3, 6, 10, 28, 64
Gurr, B., 81, 111

Hackman, J. R., 335, 345
Hadfield, C., 232, 243
Haffey, W. J., 175, 178
Haig, J., 227–230, 233–236, 238, 242
Hall, T., 245, 253
Hallet, J. D., 286, 292
Hamill, M., 87, 89–90, 113
Hamilton, J., 183, 207
Hanks, R., 213, 224
Hannay, H. J., 28, 43, 64
Hardy, G. E., 262, 269
Harris, A., 4, 11, 128, 156
Harris, J., 291–292
Hart, K. A., 140, 154
Hartman, A., 281, 293
Harwood, J. E., 55, 62
Hague, G., xxxii, 7, 153, 228
Hawken, P., 325, 346
Hawley, C. A., 211, 214, 222
Hayden, M., 228, 231, 236–237, 242
Hayes, N., 236–237, 240
Hayes, S. C., 72, 112
Hazell, A., 228, 230, 235–237, 240
Head Injured People in Cheshire, 250, 253, 334, 341
Headway, xviii, xxxiv, 103, 289, 334, 341

Health and Care Professions Council, 348, 350, 361
Health and Social Care Information Centre, 4, 10
Henwood, K., 88, 113
Herisenau, R., 56, 65
Herman, S., 7, 10
Heslin, J., 234, 237–238, 242
Hibbard M. R., 54–56, 64–65, 273, 276, 294
High, W. M., 140, 154
Hinshelwood, R. D., 86, 112
hippocampus, 17
Hirsch, J., 174, 177
Hobday, A., 282, 293
Hoc, J., 213, 223
Hogan, B., 96, 112
Holland, A., 194, 202, 205, 207
Homaifar, B. Y., 55, 62
Hopewell, C. A., 125, 154
Horn, S., 29, 44, 65
Hospital Anxiety and Depression Scale (HADS), 54, 198, 249
House of Commons Health Committee, 4–5, 10
Howard, C. A., 273, 294
Howard, I., 256, 268
Howard, K. I., 70–72, 77, 112, 256, 262, 268–270
Howard, M., 227, 242
Howard, P., 232, 243
Howieson, D. B., 211, 223
Hsu, N., 132, 154, 296, 319
Huckvale, C., 259, 268
Humle, K., 284, 294
Humphrey, M., xviii, xxii, 274, 294
Husbands, S., 81, 112
hydrocephalus, 18
hypopituitarism, 165–166
hypoxia, 46, 165

Improving Access to Psychological Therapies, 371, 373
Innes, E., 230, 233, 242
intervention, xxi, xxxii–xxxiii, 49, 58, 83, 88–89, 93–97, 102, 119–121,

125, 130, 134–135, 146–150, 152, 173, 203, 221, 228, 233, 236, 238
educational, 98
group-based, 245
neuropsychological, xxi, 130
perspective, 232
psychotherapy, 68
rehabilitation, 52, 67, 129, 140
surgical, 78
systemic, 102, 146
technique, 98
therapeutic, 47, 71
iPlato organisation, 258, 269
Isquith, P. K., 125, 155

Jackson, H. F., xxxii, 7, 121, 125–126, 128, 133, 145, 153–155, 228
Jackson, R., 119, 154
Jacobs, K., 229, 231, 242
Jaffe, M., 273, 276, 294
Jahoda, M., 229, 236, 242
James, M., 42, 65
Japp, J., 237, 242
Jenkins, D., 296, 320
Jenkins, R., 4, 11, 128, 156
Jennett, B., 5, 10–11, 160, 163, 172, 177–178, 263, 270
Jerome, J. S., 245, 253
Jha, A., 296, 318
Job Centre Plus, 226, 242
Johansson, U., 229, 236–238, 242
Johns, L. C., 30, 64
Johnson, R., 87, 111
Johnston, J., 273, 293
Johnston, M. V., 132, 147, 154, 156
Jones, K., 205
Joyce, T., 204, 206
Judd, D., 68–69, 112
Jurjevic, L., 164, 178

Kabat-Zinn, J., 72, 113
Kahn-Bourne, N., 81, 112
Kalmar, K., 159, 174, 177
Kaplan, E., 42, 63, 205
Kaplan, R. S., 345–346
Kaplan-Solms, K., 72, 83, 112

Kapp, M. B., 187, 206
Katz, D. I., 172–174, 177
Katzenbach, J. R., 326, 346
Kayes, N., 73, 114
Keenan, J. E., 159, 176
Kelly, J., 172, 177
Kennedy, M. R. T., 257, 269
Kennedy, P., 307, 320
Kepler, K., 54–55, 64
Kerr, I. B., 103–104, 108–109, 113
Ketchum, J., 296, 318
Kidd, G., 59, 64
Kielhofner, G., 229, 231–232, 234, 242
King, C., 164, 177
King, N. S., 52, 64, 249, 253, 272, 294, 311, 320
Kinsella, G., 183, 207, 273, 292
Kischka, U., 3, 6, 10, 28, 64
Klauber, M. R., 164, 178
Klein, M., xxxii–xxxiii, 86–87
Klonoff, P. S., 72–73, 112
Klüver-Bucy syndrome, 17
Knight, P., 291–292
Knowledge@Whorton, 336, 346
Kolakowsky-Hayner, S. A., 245, 253
Kosch, Y., 164, 177
Koshy, E., 258, 269
Kowalske, K., 228, 231, 236–237, 242
Kramer, J. H., 42, 63, 205
Kreutzer, J. S., 9–10, 132, 140, 154, 174, 178, 245, 253, 272, 292, 296, 318–319
Kritzinger, R., 81, 111
Kurtyka, J., 147, 156

Labbe, D., 211–212, 224
Lanford, D., 212, 222
Langlois, J. A., 239, 242
Lau, M. A., 81, 111, 256, 268
Laureys, S., 160, 166, 177–178
Law, M., 229, 243
Law Society, 186, 197, 205–206
Leach, J. P., 4, 10
Leach, K., 183, 207
Leadbeater, M., 258, 269
Lebowitz, M., 256, 270

Ledder, H., xviii, xxii
Lehan, T., 272, 292
Leibson, C. L., 164, 178
Letts, L., 229, 243
Levy, C., 212, 222
Lezak, M. D., 28, 43, 64, 117–120, 154, 211, 223
life (*passim*)
  adult, 85
  changing, xxviii, 317
  child's, 314
  cycle, 102, 185
  day-to-day, 6, 166
  emotional, 124
  events, 32, 52, 127–128, 146
  everyday, 29, 59, 85, 125, 131, 144
  expectancy, 203
  experience, 104
  family, 34, 296, 306, 370
  interpersonal, 84
  meaningful, 153, 279
  mental, 88
  preserving, 18
  priorities, 237
  quality of, 239
  real, 31, 144, 231
  roles, xviii
  satisfaction, 211, 236
  school, 314
  span, 203
  style, 116, 142, 144, 183, 236
  threatening, 9
  trigger, 87
Likosky, W., 307, 319
limbic system, 17–18, 23, 25
  amygdala, 17, 25
  cingulate gyrus, 17
  formix, 17
  hippocampal formation, 17
  hypothalamus, 17–18, 22
  septum, 17
Lincoln, N. B., 81, 112, 191, 207
Linn, R., 273, 276, 294
Livesey, A., 205
Llewelyn, S., 262, 269
Lloyd, M., 371, 373

Lloyd-Williams, K., 282, 293
Lobato, D. J., 288, 293
Logie, R., 59, 64
Longo, E., 209, 222
Loring, D. W., 28, 43, 64, 211, 223
Lovestone, S., 127, 154
Luerssen, T. G., 164, 178
Luis, C. A., 290, 294
Lulham, J. M., 296, 320
Lundqvist, A., 209, 212, 220, 223
Lundwall, R., 307, 319
Luria, A. R., 118, 152, 154
Lusby, B., 228, 231, 236–237, 242
Lyman, R. D., 249, 253

Machamer, J., 29, 63
Mackenzie, J. A., 191, 207
Main, L., 227–230, 233–236, 238, 242
Mair, J. M. M., 275, 291, 293
Maitz, E. A., 286, 293
Majeed, A., 258, 269
Majerus, S., 166, 177
Malan, D., 84, 89, 112
Malec, J. F., 143, 155, 164, 178, 234, 237, 240
Malone, R., 174, 177
Manchester, D., 81, 112, 121, 125, 133, 154–155
Mandrekar, J. N., 164, 178
Mann, W. C., 212, 222
Marcos, C., 230–231, 233, 243
Margison, S., 248, 253
Markus, H., 122, 155
Marlow, L., 205
Marmarou, A., 164, 178
Marshall, J. C., 3, 6, 10, 28, 64
Marshall, L. F., 164, 178
Marson, D. C., 189, 193–194, 207
Marwitz, J. H., 132, 154, 296, 319
Maslow, A., 347, 362, 367, 374
Mason, B., 187, 207
Mateer, C. A., 125, 155
mater
  arachnoid, 19
  dura, 19
  pia, 19

Mathe, J., 213, 223
Matheis, R. J., 209, 224
Matsuzawa, Y., 256, 270
Matthews, S., 150, 156
McCaffrey, R. J., 273, 293
McCall, M. A., 273, 293
McCarthy, D., 212, 222
McCarthy, P., 287, 293
McColl, M. A., 247, 252
McDonald, S., 119, 155
McGaugh, J. L., 173, 178
McGaw, S., 298, 319
McGoldrick, M., 34, 64, 102, 111
McGrath, J. C., 69, 88, 90, 103, 114, 239, 242
McKenna, K., 143, 155
McKenna, P., 42, 64, 211, 215, 220, 223
McKinlay, W., 54, 63, 132, 153
McKinstry, B., 59, 64
McLellan, L., 29, 44, 65
McMillan, R., 5, 10
McMillan, T. M., xviii, xxii
McPherson, K., 73, 114
Meade, M. A., 245, 253
Mechanic, D., 228, 240
Meehan, M., 232, 240
Megginson, L. C., 127, 155
Melia, Y., 150, 156
memory, xxvii–xxviii, 7, 13, 17–20, 23–24, 37, 40, 45, 51, 59, 79, 81, 85, 91–95, 104, 106, 127, 129, 146, 173, 192, 196, 233, 274, 313, 366, 372
  aids, 74, 79
  auditory, 333
  autobiographical, 32, 188
  deficits, 80, 120
  delayed, 46
  difficulty, 251, 267, 273, 368
  external, 142
  function, 17, 173
  impairment, 15, 17, 22, 25, 129, 146, 196
  lapse, 76
  loss, 79
  poor, 76, 369
  problems, 7, 68, 73, 76, 79, 107, 131, 138, 146, 296
  procedural, 103
  prospective, 87
  research, 173
  short-term, 46
  strategies, 109, 312
  verbal, 42, 188
  visual, 42
  working, 42, 188, 202
Mental Capacity Act, 179, 204, 207, 355–356, 362
Mental Health Act, 182, 355
Mercer, G., 236, 240
Merry, P., 132, 155
Mewse, A. J., 56, 65
Meyer, B., 59, 64
Michon, J. A., 220, 223
Miller, L., 131, 155
Milleville-Pennel, I., 213, 223
Mills, S. R., 132, 153
MindTools, 325, 340, 345–346
Minnes, P., 273, 293
Moffat, N., 119, 154
Mohamed, S., 87, 89–90, 113, 122, 154
Mohr, D. C., 256, 268, 307, 319
Monti, M. M., 160, 178
Morris, J. R., xviii, xxii, 298, 300, 304, 320
Morton, M. V., 273, 293
Moss, B., 290, 292–293
Mossman, D., 187, 206
mother, xx, xxxiii, 53, 79–80, 84, 86–87, 89–91, 93–94, 100–101, 106–107, 198–199, 246–250, 366–367
  –infant interactions, 309
motivation, 17, 30, 47, 58, 86, 98, 118, 126, 129, 134, 137, 143–144, 201, 275, 285, 335, 369
Moye, J., 189, 193–194, 207
Mudaliar, Y., 56, 65
Muir, C. A., 175, 178
Mullaly, E., 183, 207
Multi-Society Task Force on PVS, 161, 172, 178

Munday, R., 29, 45, 64, 159, 170, 172, 177
Murphy, L. D., xviii, xxii
Murray, G., 263, 270
Myles, S., 90, 112

Nampiaparampil, D. E., 55, 64
Nangle, N., 260, 269
National Health Service (NHS), xxiii, xxxi, 57, 89, 227, 238, 258, 295, 325, 327–328, 330, 332–333, 340–341, 343–344, 348, 356, 371, 373
National Leadership Council (NLC), 325, 328, 346
Nayyar, V., 56, 65
Nead, R., 209, 224
Neary, D., 13, 26
Neath, J., 183, 207
Neumann, V., 54, 62
neuroanatomy, xix, 13–14, 21, 23, 26, 360
  behavioural, xxiv
  functional, 6, 13, 171
Newberry, A. M., 184–185, 207
Newby, G. J., 30, 63, 91, 113, 185, 187, 191, 207, 209–212, 214, 217, 220, 222–224, 245–246, 253, 258, 260–261, 269, 290, 293, 300, 302, 307, 320, 343, 346, 350–351, 362
Newman, T., 298, 319
NHS Institute for Innovation and Improvement, 327, 346
Niemczura, J., 234, 237, 243
Nimmo-Smith, I., 205, 232, 243
Nochi, M., 90, 112
Nosek, M. A., 273, 294
Nouri, F., 217, 224
Novack, T. A., 211–213, 224

object, 121, 246
  decision, 42
  foreign, 4
  internal, 85–86
  localisation, 170
  neglecting, 86
  paternal, 86
  recognition, 170
  relations theory, 86
  usage, 161
objective, 82, 163, 327, 336, 360
  assistance, 186
  identification, 83
  observation, 25
  psychometric indication, 202
  scoring, 58
  service, 326
occipital
  bone, 14
  lobe, 14, 20–21
Oddy, M., 42, 63, 150, 156, 205, 296, 320
O'Dell, J., 87, 89–90, 113, 122, 154
Odhuba, R. A., 30, 64
O'Driscoll, K., 4, 10
Ogden, J., 281, 288, 293
Oldham, G. R., 335, 345
Oldham, P., 81, 111
Oliver, D. L., 55, 64, 127, 154
Ollier, K., 282, 293
Olney, M. F., 288, 292
Olsen, J., 43, 10
O'Neil-Pirozzi, H. F., 296, 318
Onsworth, T., 143, 155
Orlinksy, D. E., 70–72, 77, 112, 256, 262, 268–270
Orsillo, S. M., 273, 293
Owen, A. M., 160, 162, 177–178
Ownsworth T., 274, 292

Pachet, A. K., 184–185, 207
Pallant, J., 228, 239, 241
Palmer, S., 122, 154, 271–274, 286, 288, 291
Panting, A., 132, 155
Pappadopulus, E., 273, 276, 294
Parenting Locus of Control (PLOC), 249
parietal
  bone, 14
  lobe, 6, 14, 20
Parr, S., 290, 292–293

Parry-Jones, B. L., 55, 64
Partridge, F., 291–292
Pedersen, M. G., 43, 10
Pellett, E., 73, 114
Perez, K., 56, 65
Perkins, P. K., 164, 178
Perlesz, A., 307, 319
Pessar, L., 273, 276, 294
Peterson, C. B., 7, 10
Petheram, B., 290, 293
Pettigrew, L. E., 263, 270
Pfaff, A., 164, 178, 296, 320
Piasetsky, E., 143, 153
Pijnenborg, G. H. M., 259, 270
Pinn, J., 307, 319
Pinnock, H., 59, 64
Pitsiavas, V., 56, 65
Plenger, P., 228, 231, 236–237, 242
Plum, F., 160, 177
Pollard, C., 307, 320
post traumatic
   amnesia, 5
   brain injury, 54
   seizures, 15
   stress disorder (PTSD), 53, 55, 57
Pothier, J., 213, 223
Powell, J. M., 211–212, 224, 234, 237–238, 242
Powell, T., 3, 6, 10, 307, 320
Praamstra, A. J., 81, 113
Prangnell, S. J., 33, 64
Pratt, J., 229, 231, 242
Prentice-Dunn, S., 249, 253
President's Commission for the Study of Ethical Problems in Medicine and Biomedical and Behavioral Research, 160, 178
Priestly, N., 121, 125, 155
Prigatano, G. P., 69, 113, 118–119, 155
Primrose, W., 183, 207
Psaila, K., 87, 89–90, 113, 122, 154

Quirk, K., 259, 270

Rapport, L., 213, 224
Rasquin, S. M., 81, 113

Rattok, J., 143, 153
Reardon, R., 230–231, 233, 243
Rice-Varian, C., 105, 113
Richardson, J. C., 126, 155
Ridby, P., 229, 243
Riddick, A., 132, 154, 296, 319
Ridgeway, V., 205, 232, 243
Rinaldi, M., 229, 234, 236, 240
Rintala, D. H., 273, 294
Ripley, D., 211–212, 224
Roberts, C., 236, 242
Robertson, I. H., 205, 232, 243
Robillard, D., 273, 276, 294
Rodriguez-Moreno, D., 174, 177
Ronnberg, J., 209, 212, 223
Roosen, E., 147, 156
Rosenberg, J., 172, 177
Rosenthal, M., 9–10, 140, 154, 234, 237, 243
Rossi, C. D., 273, 294
Roth, R. M., 125, 155
Rothengatter, J. A., 212, 224
Round, A., 4, 11, 128, 156
Rous, B., 122, 154
Rous, S., 81, 113
Royal College of Physicians, xviii, xxii, 149, 155, 226, 233, 240, 243
   Working Group, 172, 178
Ruddle, J., 236, 240
Russo, D., 307, 319
Rutland-Brown, W., 239, 242
Ruttan, L. A., 81, 111, 256, 268
Ryle, A., 103–104, 108–109, 113

Sachs, P. P., 286, 293
Sacks, A. L., 56, 65
Salisbury, D., 213, 224
Sander, A. M., 9–10, 140, 154
Sastre, M., 126, 155
Savill, T., 30, 63, 209–210, 212, 220, 222
Scaife, J., 351, 362
Schiff, N., 173–174, 177
Schmidt, W. H., 329, 346
Schnakers, C., 174, 177
Schneider, J. J., 213, 224

Schönberger, M., 284, 294
Schultheis, M. T., 209, 224
Schwartz, T., 147, 156
Sebough, J., 287, 293
Seel, R. T., 211–212, 224
Segal, Z., 72, 113
self, 85, 87–88, 90–91, 122–123, 161, 247–248, 274, 282–283
 -ability, 274
 -appraisal, 119
 -assessment, 328, 331
 -awareness, 25, 31, 70–72, 74–77, 81–82, 120, 122, 149, 161, 262, 264, 328
 -belief, 236
 -belonging, 256
 -blame, 315
 -care, 129, 144–145, 310
 -concept, 81–82, 95, 245
 -confidence, 226, 229, 236, 274, 336
 -constructs, 123
 -control, 117, 126
 -correction, 119–120
 -critical, 120, 275
 -determined, 136, 152
 -development, 323
 -direction, 118
 -discipline, 336
 -disclosure, 221
 -doubt, 52
 -efficacy, 226, 230
 -esteem, 31, 126, 137, 141–142, 144, 152, 236, 312
 -evaluation, 81–82, 134, 144–145, 274
 -evident, 150
 -experience, 84
 -focused, 279
 -fulfilment, 73
 -generated, 96
 -harm, 48
 -identity, 122–123, 142–143
 -important, 175
 -instruction, 124
 -interest, 194
 -knowledge, 74, 122
 -management, 143, 327
 -medicate, 230
 -monitoring, 32, 79, 82, 94, 141, 143–145, 313
 -motivated, 252
 -perception, 230, 238
 -prompting, 116
 -protection, 185
 -reflection, 146
 -regulate, 119–120, 139
 -reinforcing, 106
 -relatedness, 71, 262, 264
 -rewarding, 140, 145
 -schema, 122
 sense of, 123, 274
 -serving, 132
 -stimulation, 48
 -structure, 131, 134–135, 139, 142, 144
 -sustaining, 252, 358–359
 -worth, 211, 272
Semantic Differential, xxix, 249
Sensory Modality Assessment and Rehabilitation Technique (SMART), 159
Sensory Stimulation Assessment Measure (SSAM), 29
Shaikh, U., 258, 270
Shannon, H., 230–231, 233, 243
Shaw, K., 122, 154
Sheikh, A., 59, 64
Shellenberger, S., 34, 64
Sherer, M., 211–212, 224
Sherman, E. M. S., 28, 65
Shiel, A., 29, 44, 65
Sidenius, P., 43, 10
Silver, J., 54–55, 64
Silver, S., 143, 153
Simpson, J., 302, 307, 320, 351, 362
Sinclair, S., 230–231, 233, 243
Skippon, R. H., 302, 307, 320, 351, 362
Skirrow, P., 351, 362
Slewa-Younan, S., 56, 65
Smith, D. K., 326, 316

Smith, S. R., 30, 58, 64, 285, 292
Snaith, R. P., 206, 249, 253
Snoek, J. W., 212, 224
Social Exclusion Task Force, 298, 320
Social-Moral Awareness Test (SMAT), 189, 205
Sohlberg, M. M., 125, 155
Solms, M., 72, 83, 112
Soo, C., 147, 155
Sopena, S., 81, 113
South Cheshire Acquired Brain Injury Service, 258, 270
Specialist Driving Assessment Centres, 214
Speileman, L. A., 56, 65
Spillane, J. P., 329, 346
Spreen, O., 28, 65
Stapert, S., 124, 156
Stedman, J., 98, 111, 248, 253
Steffen, V., 246, 253
Stewart, D., 229, 243
Strauss, E., 28, 65
Strettles, B., 296, 320
Strong, J., 229, 241
Strong, S., 229–231, 233, 243
Strosahl, K. D., 72, 112
Strub, R. C., 24, 26
Struchen, M. A., 140, 154
Stuckey, R., 229, 243
Summers, F., 183, 207
Suto, I., 194, 202, 205, 207
Sutton, L., 87, 89–90, 113
Swift, T. L., 92, 113
Symington, C., 54, 63, 132, 153

Taggi, F., 209, 222
Tajfel, H., 122, 156
Tannenbaum, R., 329, 346
Tate, R. L., 147, 155, 164, 178, 296, 320
Taylor, D., 174, 178
Teasdale, G. M., 5, 11, 163, 178, 263, 270
Teasdale, J., 72, 113
Teasdale, T. W., 284, 294

Temkin, N., 29, 63
temporal
  bone, 14–15
  contusions, xxxiii
  dementia, 51
  lobe, 6, 14–15, 20–21, 23
  seizure, 17
Tennant, A., 54, 62
Tham, K., 229, 237, 242, 286, 292
therapy (*passim*) *see also*: behaviour, cognitive
  commitment, 72
  couples, 89, 271, 286
  family, 73, 271, 371
  group, 245
  narrative, xx, xxix, 78, 90, 246, 248, 284, 354
  occupational, xxxiv, 31, 133, 191, 203, 369
  opportunistic, xvi
  personal construct, 291, 354
  psychological, 70–71, 73, 81, 83, 109–110, 275
  speech and language, 133, 203
  systemic, xx, 78, 96
  talking, 373
  vocational, 354
Therapy Today, 256, 269–270
Thomas, J. R., 258, 270
Thomas, M., 236, 243
Thompson, J., 57, 63
Thurgood, J., 227, 230, 234, 239, 241
Tiersky, L. A., 147, 156
Timmerman, M. E., 259, 270
Todd, D., 185, 187, 207
Tonks, J., 56, 65
Transitional Rehabilitation Unit (TRU), 129, 144, 148, 151, 153
Trescoli, C., 81, 112
Tsaousides, T., 256, 270
Turner-Stokes, L., 238, 243
Tyerman, A. D., xviii, xxii, xxix, xxxii, xxxv, 30, 63, 150, 156, 209–210, 212, 214, 220, 222, 224, 232, 238, 243, 249, 253, 272, 274, 294, 296, 320

unconscious(ness), 5, 53, 85, 340
    see also: conscious(ness)
    permanent, 160
Urbach, J. R., 295, 320
US General Accounting Office, 149, 156
Uysal, S., 54–55, 64, 273, 276, 294

van den Bosch, R. J., 259, 270
van den Broek, M. D., 30, 64
Vanderploeg, R. D., 37, 65, 290, 294
Van de Sande, P., 81, 113
Van Heugten, C. M., 81, 113, 124, 156
Van Zomeren, A. H., 212, 224
Vaslamatzis, G., 266, 270
Vaughan, F. L., 55, 64
Vella, L., 256, 268
Vestergaard, M., 43, 10
Vickery, C. D., 245, 253
Vignally, P., 209, 222
Visual Object and Space Perception Battery (VOSP), 42
vocational rehabilitation (VR), xx, xxiv, 9, 143, 150–151, 225–232, 234–239, 276, 289, 369
Vogenthaler, D., 119, 156

Waddell, M., xxxii, xxxv, 367, 374
Wade, D., 205
Waid-Ebbs, J. K., 212, 222
Wald, M. M., 239, 242
Waldman, J., 55, 62
Wall, J., 234, 237, 243
Wallace, J. J., 245, 253
Walsh, B., 245, 253
Walsh, F., 276, 294
Walsh, V., 132, 154
Warburg, R., 125, 154
Ward, T., 205, 232, 243
Warrington, E. K., 42, 64–65
Wates, M., 300, 304, 320
Watson, M., 29, 44, 65
Watson, N., 290, 293
Watson, P., 59, 64
Weatherhead, S. J., 91, 113, 245–246,
    253, 300, 320, 343, 346, 351, 361–362
Webster, G., 272–273, 287, 292, 294–295, 311, 319–320
Wechsler, D., 42, 65, 206
    Abbreviated Scale of Intelligence (WASI-II), 189, 201
    Adult Intelligence Scale Version Four (WAIS-IV), 42, 188, 372
    Memory Scale (WMS-IV), 188
Weed, W., 213, 224
Wehman, P., 273, 293
Wells, D. L., 288, 292
Wessex Head Injury Matrix (WHIM), 29, 44
Western Neuro Sensory Stimulation Profile (WNSSP), 159, 169–170, 172
Wetters, K., 288, 294
White, M., 90, 95, 113, 284, 294
Whyte, J., 159, 172, 177
Whyte, M., 183, 207
Willer, B., 273, 276, 294
Williams, K., 132, 154, 296, 319
Williams, M., 72, 113
Williams, P., 87, 111
Williams, W. H., 4, 11, 55–56, 64–65, 81, 113, 128, 146, 156
Wilson, B. A., 29, 42, 44, 65, 81, 113, 140, 156, 206, 232, 243, 259, 270
Wilson, J. T., 263, 270
Wilson, K. G., 72, 112
Wilson, M., 183, 207
Wilson, S. L., 68–69, 92, 112–113
Winek, J. L., 97, 113
Winnicott, D. W., 51, 65, 309, 320
Withaar, F. K., 212, 222, 259, 270
Wittgenstein, L., 176, 178
Wolters, G., 124, 156
Wood, R. L., 81, 112, 132, 156, 296, 320
Wood, V., 205
Woodford, L., 273, 293
Woods, B., 290, 293
world, 76, 95, 104, 122–123, 130, 141, 153